Treating the Tough Adolescent

THE GUILFORD FAMILY THERAPY SERIES
Michael P. Nichols, *Series Editor*

TREATING THE TOUGH ADOLESCENT
A Family-Based, Step-by-Step Guide

Scott P. Sells

Forewords by Jay Haley and Neil Schiff

THE GUILFORD PRESS
New York   London

Library of Congress Cataloging-in-Publication Data

Sells, Scott P.
    Treating the tough adolescent: a family-based, step-by-step guide/ Scott P. Sells; forewords by Jay Haley and Neil Schiff.
        p.   cm. — (The Guilford family therapy series)
    Includes bibliographical references and index.
    ISBN 1-57230-422-7
    1. Problem youth—Counseling of.   2. Family psychotherapy.
    3. Problem youth—Family relationships.   I. Title.   II. Series.
    RJ506.P63S45   1998
    616.89′00835—dc21
                                       98-39683
                                               CIP

To my family, who taught me to never give up.

*And to Dr. Thomas Smith, who believed
in me when others did not and stuck
by me through good times and bad.*

About the Author

Scott P. Sells, PhD, is Associate Professor of Social Work at Savannah State University and Clinical Director of Savannah Family Institute, Savannah, Georgia. Dr. Sells has personally treated over 300 difficult children and adolescents, is a consultant for the Department of Juvenile Justice, and has been invited to speak on the topic of tough adolescents by such national professional organizations as the American Association for Marriage and Family Therapy, the National Association of Social Workers, and the American Academy of Child and Adolescent Psychiatry. He has developed a 5-week parent training education program, "Taking Charge: Regaining Authority and Nurturance," for parents of difficult children and teenagers, which was adopted as a standard model in Las Vegas, Nevada, and Savannah, Georgia, by those states' juvenile probation agencies, and has been working with an inner-city neighborhood in Savannah to establish a community center and clinic that will treat at-risk children and adolescents using the principles presented in *Treating the Tough Adolescent*. In addition to *Treating the Tough Adolescent*, Dr. Sells is the author of over 10 major publications in refereed journals and a book chapter.

Acknowledgments

I want to thank the many people who supported me through the years to help this book become a reality. God, who has continued to protect and watch over me all these years. My grandfather, who was never educated formally but had wisdom and kindness beyond his years; his memory and long talks on the porch in Eagle River and Florida continue to inspire me. My grandmother, who is so full of life and who never allowed me to get down on myself; she taught me never to give up. My father, who spent hours with me as child teaching me compassion and how to become a man. My mother, whose courage, love, and belief in me guided me through dark times and allowed me to emerge a stronger and better person. Sally, whose love, patience, and encouragement gave me the strength to finish this book. My sister Nancy, my niece Ashley, and Chris, who have always stuck by me.

Special thanks to Dr. Tom Smith, my mentor, and Kitty Moore, my editor at The Guilford Press. Both of them believed in me and gave me a chance when others did not. This is also true of Dr. Neil Schiff, Jay Haley, and Dr. Neil Newfield. Without their vision and kindness, this book would not have been possible. I also wish to thank Dr. Charles Fishman and his family. When I was a young graduate student in the summer of 1991, he allowed me to live with his family. I sat in Charles's basement for hours, editing tapes and talking to him about process research and difficult adolescents. These early experiences blazed the path for this book and some of the ideas contained within.

I am grateful to the social work faculty at Savannah State University, Dr. Carlton Brown, Dr. Joseph Silver, the residents of the Midtown community, and the many students whom I have taught over the years. Their kindness and faith in me has helped heal old wounds and bring me to the next level.

Finally, I wish to thank the parents and teenagers whose stories, trials, and courage are the reason this book was written. Each family touched me in a profound way and taught me that they are the teachers, if we only listen to the tremors beneath the surface. I only hope that we as counselors will listen and provide what you want. . . . A detailed road map to follow and AAA service along the way only if needed.

Forewords

FOREWORD BY JAY HALEY

Treating the Tough Adolescent offers a sensible and strategic approach to resolving the family problems of difficult adolescents. Essentially the work is concerned with changing the hierarchy of families in trouble when the problem adolescent is in charge of the family and the parents are not. What is unique, and should be common in the field, is the way the therapy is supported by research data.

Having been a participant in Scott Sells's research endeavors, I have learned to admire the systematic way he presents his ideas. He writes clearly and concisely and focuses on his subject while being comprehensive in his presentation. Neil Schiff and I were asked to contribute a case for the research and so experienced Dr. Sells's approach firsthand. The case was an extremely difficult one, which took 28 interviews to resolve. Dr. Schiff was the therapist and I was the colleague behind the mirror. The interviews were transcribed for systematic study, and we were asked to comment step by step through the videotaped drama of a family where a problem son's behavior was finally corrected by parents who took charge. Actually, we were nagged to comment, as Dr. Sells pursued us until he had gathered the data he wanted. This book reflects the tenacity required to create a research contribution, and which is reflected in the therapy approach.

I recall the period in the field of family therapy when therapists typically joined adolescents against their parents. The sympathy went with the adolescents, whose parents struggled with each other and did not appreciate youth. The therapist was not thinking hierarchically and so did not notice that he or she was giving power to the adolescents by joining them against the parents. The trend in the field today is to help parents organize the family so *they* are in charge. This book outlines dozens of ways this can be done and expresses the new concern with authority in the family. Years ago, we also did not have the idea that an adolescent could harm himself or herself

ix

as a way of helping and stabilizing parents in trouble. This theory of motivation makes it possible to appreciate the problem adolescent while also being concerned about the parents. The art of therapy with families with problem adolescents is to side with the young person and also with the parents while they are in conflict with each other.

This is a valuable book that wedges research-supported ideas into practical guidance for therapists struggling with exasperating adolescents and their families.

FOREWORD BY NEIL SCHIFF

Treating the Tough Adolescent is a book about changing the behavior of problem young people who engage in a range of often extreme behavior that is destructive to themselves and to those who love them and cannot stop them. It is a family-based approach that is informed by important ideas that have been in circulation in the field for some time but heretofore have not been adequately organized, explicated, codified, tested, and systematically described in sufficient detail such that they could be easily replicated by members of the practitioner community. Here, in straightforward language and exhaustive detail, Scott Sells methodically describes in successive steps the empirically tested family interventions, both large and small, that are required to succeed in resolving the frequently grave problems presented by adolescents in the context of their families. Dr. Sells's approach, which is theoretically derived, extensively researched, and carefully refined, is logical, considerate, eminently practical, and easy to follow. His explanations of what to do, why to do it, and how to do it should be accessible and useful to all.

This is also, perhaps preeminently, a book about how to do research on psychotherapy and the ways in which good research should illuminate and inform effective therapy. For the conceptually inclined, it may be worthwhile to begin the book by reading the last chapter first. Dr. Sells took the field literally. He went to the library, identified the major models in the field, developed a model that operationalized the major ideas in each approach, tested these ideas by carefully analyzing a complete case in great depth, revised his model, tested his revised model by application, and then further refined his approach. The careful and protracted work involved, the integration of clinical and research findings, and the constant testing of ideas on paper, by reference to longtime practitioners, and by repetitive application are exemplary and should set a standard for all of us.

On a personal level, I enjoyed participating in Dr. Sells's endeavor, although until I first read the manuscript, I had no idea about how extensive and laborious his undertaking was. I admire his energy, enthusiasm, idealism, and diligence. More simply, his interest in psychotherapy and curiosity about every aspect of the process was a profound pleasure to me. Though the work was quite painstaking, certainly more on his part than on my own, the opportunity to parse interactions (all recorded on videotape), session by session, in a difficult and complex case I had worked on with Jay Haley was extremely satisfying. In fact, it was gratifying just to talk about the strategy and mechanics of fomenting change—essentially the art of psychotherapy— in great detail with someone who was so obviously interested in it during a time when psychotherapy sometimes appears as though it may become a disappearing art.

This is a good book that presents a useful, easily understood clinical model. It is an example of the use and benefits of good research, and sets a standard for the integration of the two.

Contents

PART ONE

A FAMILY-BASED MODEL FOR TOUGH ADOLESCENTS

CHAPTER 1

Introduction

Severe behavioral problems in adolescents currently account for one-third to one-half of all adolescent clinic referrals (Webster-Stratton & Dahl, 1995). Moreover, the prevalence of these behavioral problems is increasing dramatically, creating a need for services that currently exceeds the availability (Alexander, Pugh, & Newell, 1995; Chamberlain & Rosicky, 1995). Without effective interventions, these difficult adolescents are at high risk for developing antisocial personality disorder as adults (Loeber & Schmalling, 1985). They are often recipients of emotional or physical abuse, and are involved in drug use and violent crimes (Chamberlain & Rosicky, 1995). The economic impact on society is also great, with the average cost of incarceration per juvenile exceeding $60,000 per year (Webster-Stratton & Dahl, 1995). Finally, recent studies suggest that when these adolescents become parents, they pass along antisocial behaviors to their children, thus initiating a multigenerational chain of problematic behaviors (Patterson & Chamberlain, 1994).

A comprehensive review of treatment research with adolescent behavioral problems reveals that outpatient therapy with this population presents extraordinary challenges and fails with alarming frequency (Gould, Shaffer, & Kaplan, 1985; Kazdin, 1993; Prinz & Miller, 1994). One reason for this failure is that the majority of counselors have not been trained to work with defiant adolescents and have difficulty in obtaining improved outcomes (Kazdin, 1994; Liddle, 1995). Accordingly, there has been a call for treatment manuals that outline specific procedures to treat specialized populations such as difficult adolescents (see Crits-Christoph & Mintz, 1991; Lambert & Bergin, 1994).

WHY A FAMILY-BASED MODEL?

To address these issues, I have developed a 15-step family-based model from a 4-year process–outcome research study (the study is described in detail in

3

Chapter 12). The model is family-based because it is believed that changes in the family environment during adolescence have a tremendous impact on a teenager. These changes include those within individual family members (e.g., depression, substance misuse) and those in the family as a whole and its life cycle (e.g., divorce, parental job loss, children's leaving home). The adolescent is extremely vulnerable to these changes and will often react with behavior problems. From both developmental and systems theory perspectives, this interconnectedness indicates that the family itself, not just the adolescent, must be transformed.

Developmental Issues

Developmentally, adolescents are in the process of formulating identities separate from their families. Teenagers are still dependent on their parents in many ways, and yet seek complete independence. If individual family members' problems remain unresolved, or family difficulties persist, adolescents risk developing identities that are associated with problem behaviors. For example, when parents have severe marital problems, depression, or drug or alcohol problems, their children are likely to demonstrate these same problems when they reach adulthood (Kazdin, Siegel, & Bass, 1992; Scherer, Brondino, Henggeler, & Melton, 1994). Furthermore, they are extremely vulnerable to changes in their social surroundings as they struggle with their identity formation.

Systems Theory

From a systems theory perspective, adolescents often develop behavioral problems because of difficulties within either the immediate family or the broader social environment (Goldenberg & Goldenberg, 1991). The problem moves from psychopathology within the individual to a social context that is faulty or oppositional. For example, an adolescent who has failing grades or skips school is probably being enabled by others to continue this behavior. This "help" may take the form of a teacher's failing to notify the parents of poor grades, or of parents' refusing to collaborate with school personnel because they falsely assume that the teacher blames them for the problem. As long as the school and the parents fail to work together, the adolescent is inadvertently allowed to maintain both failing grades and truancy.

In this example, the adolescent's dysfunctional behavior can be viewed as a product of flawed transactional patterns between the family and the school system, rather than simply as an internal problem (e.g., a learning disability or chemical imbalance). Change is possible when a school counselor can act as a mediator and bring the two parties together to rectify faulty assumptions and enhance communication. If this mediation is successful, the teacher will contact the parents by phone whenever the teenager is truant or does not complete an assignment. In turn, the parents can now implement consequences that will stop these behaviors. With this improved communication, the problem behavior ends. These changes also tend to be maintained because the family and the broader environment are being transformed, not just the individual teenager.

In sum, it is easier to change a behavioral problem by addressing all the outside forces that are maintaining it. This point is often illustrated when adolescents are placed in residential facilities. After an initial "honeymoon" period of relative calm upon returning home, the adolescent frequently returns to his or her old ways of functioning. This is because the conditions within the family and external environment have a greater influence on the difficult teenager than any other factor.*

WHO ARE OUR TOUGH ADOLESCENTS?

It is important to understand just what the designation "tough adolescent" means. An adolescent is labeled "tough" or "difficult" when his or her behavior includes hostility, threats of violence, theft, destruction of property, vandalism, lying, fire setting, truancy, threats of suicide, or running away. Engaging in these activities impairs the adolescent's ability to function at home, school, or work. Parents and society regard these adolescents as unmanageable. These problems eventually drive many parents to seek professional help, and they can challenge even the most skilled counselors. Often the behaviors are so extreme that counselors have difficulty coming up with effective strategies to stop them. As a result, the counselors either give up, refer the families elsewhere, or recommend institutionalization for the adolescents.

Adolescents labeled "tough" will generally be diagnosed as suffering from oppositional defiant disorder or conduct disorder; these labels have been most recently defined in the *Diagnostic and Statistical Manual of Mental Disorders,* fourth edition (DSM-IV; American Psychiatric Association, 1994). Oppositional defiant disorder often begins in childhood and results in an open defiance of adult rules, accompanied by a negative, hostile attitude (Quay, 1986). Conduct disorder encompasses oppositional behavior but also produces more serious deviations from societal norms, such as violence or

*Recent meta-analytic studies support the contention that a family systems approach is the most effective treatment modality for severe behavioral problems in both adolescents (Chamberlain & Rosicky, 1995; Shadish, Montgomery, Wilson, Wilson, & Okwumabua, 1993) and children (Estrada & Pinsof, 1995).

aggression to people or animals, destruction of property, theft, running away, setting fires, and truancy (Kazdin, 1987). Therefore, for the purposes of this book, "tough adolescents" include young people between the ages of 12 and 18 who meet the DSM-IV diagnostic criteria for either oppositional defiant disorder or conduct disorder, exhibit significant impairment in functioning at home or school, and are regarded as unmanageable by their parents or teachers.

BASIC PRINCIPLES OF TREATMENT

The theoretical orientations of both structural therapy (Minuchin, 1974) and strategic therapy (Haley, 1976; Madanes, 1991) form the foundation of the treatment model presented in this book. The book integrates key concepts and principles from both theories.

Integrating Structural and Strategic Approaches

Extreme behavior problems in adolescents often emerge when the family hierarchy has become reversed: The teenager runs the household, and parents are unable to enforce rules and consequences effectively. The adolescent assumes control, determines the mood of the household, and neutralizes the parents' ability to regain control. This structure establishes the way family members interact. A basic premise of this model is that in order to eliminate behavioral problems, the counselor must establish a hierarchy in which the parents are in a position of authority.

One way to establish this hierarchy is through the use of strategic approaches that employ specific and directive tasks. If an adolescent runs away, for example, the counselor helps the parents design a creative consequence that would make the teenager give up that behavior rather than suffer the punishment. For example, the counselor can suggest that the parents put up posters with their teenager's photo at school, with a reward for any information regarding his or her whereabouts. Many teenagers would rather give up the extreme behavior of running away than suffer the embarrassing consequence of having their pictures posted all over school. Once the threat of running away is removed, the probability that rules will be followed increases dramatically.

This blend of structural and strategic approaches gives a counselor both a road map and a set of techniques for negotiating the twists and turns of the family maze. Structural theory provides such concepts as "hierarchy" and "boundaries" to show counselors the need to return parents to a position of authority. Strategic methods show counselors how to make these structural

changes possible through specific techniques and directives (rules and consequences, troubleshooting, paradox, etc.). Thus a combination of the two approaches can be used to restructure the family hierarchy and eliminate adolescent behavior problems.

Major Assumptions

One assumption of this model is that once family and environmental problems have been addressed, behavioral problems will diminish. The central focus is the alleviation of the presenting problem through the parents' return to
a position of authority, which changes the structure that is maintaining the
behavioral problem. A counselor needs to be highly directive in giving a family and adolescent precise instructions and in troubleshooting all the things
that could go wrong.

A second assumption is that an adolescent's problem must be defined as
one that can be solved by the parents. A behavior problem that is diagnosed
as a chemical imbalance (e.g., attention-deficit/hyperactivity disorder) or
mental illness (e.g., schizophrenia) becomes more difficult to solve than the
behavior of a rebellious adolescent who is stuck in a rut, stubborn, or in need
of parental guidance. Even though a problem may involve both medical and
behavioral causes, it is often more productive to define treatment from a behavioral perspective (although of course the medical aspects must be adequately addressed). Otherwise, the risk is great that parents will believe that
their teenager is not responsible for the problem. If this happens, parents will
resist the notion that they must take charge, and instead will look for external
solutions such as medication or hospitalization.

Another assumption is that clearly defined rules and consequences are
crucial to treatment success. Rules and consequences may look good on paper, but they are often ineffective unless counselors show parents how their
buttons are pushed during confrontations. Adolescents are typically more
skillful than their parents in the art of confrontation. In order to change the
timing and direction of confrontations, parents must learn the tools they
need to play the game better than their teenagers.

A final assumption is that hierarchy is maintained by both a "hard" and
a "soft" side. The hard side of a hierarchy is sustained by the parents' ability to
determine the rules and consequences for, as well as the process and timing
of, confrontations. However, hierarchy is also maintained by a soft, nurturing
side. Parents are responsible for soothing the pain of their children and helping them feel loved and needed. Parents are also responsible for providing
special outings or times during the week that promote positive parent–child
interactions. One aspect of hierarchy without the other will only lead to temporary changes in a teenager's problem behavior.

PLAN OF THE BOOK

This book is designed to accomplish three objectives. First, I present the treatment model, which includes 15 specific procedural steps for treating difficult adolescents and their families. Part I of this book offers six basic assumptions about the causes of severe behavioral problems, and then presents the treatment model, with the guidelines necessary to address each of these six causes. Actual case examples are used to highlight and clarify major points within each step of the model.

Second, I hope to teach counselors how to engage an uncooperative adolescent, empower parents to change parent–adolescent communication, stop the adolescent's most severe behavioral problems, and restore nurturance and tenderness between parents and teenager. Part II of this book presents five key principles within the 15-step model that are essential for change: (1) setting clear rules and consequences; (2) troubleshooting; (3) changing the timing and process of confrontations; (4) neutralizing the adolescent's "five aces" (running away, truancy/poor school performance, suicidal threats or behaviors, threats or acts of violence, and disrespect); and (5) restoring nurturance and tenderness. Part III outlines specific strategies addressing special treatment issues, such as working with outside systems (peers, school, etc.); single-parent families; divorce and stepfamily problems; and alcohol and drug use.

Finally, in Part IV (Chapter 12), I describe how process–outcome research was used to refine key theoretical concepts within this model. The integration of theory and research into clinical practice is designed to enhance counselors' understanding and utilization of the treatment model.

CHAPTER 2

Point of Entry
Why Difficult Teenagers
Have Problems

A point of entry into this area of treatment is to unravel the mysteries of why difficult teenagers have behavior problems. The family-based model suggests six basic assumptions about the causes of severe behavioral problems in adolescents. First, an incongruous hierarchy exists in which the adolescent is in charge and more powerful than the parents. Whenever the parents try to restore their authority, the difficult adolescent will use extreme behaviors (e.g., running away, becoming truant, or threatening suicide) to intimidate the parents into giving their authority back to the teenager. Second, the parents often turn to outside forces (judges, police, counselors, medication, hospitalization) to stop their teenager's problem behavior, but in the process they inadvertently undermine their own authority and effectiveness. Third, an adolescent's problems are often a conscious or unconscious attempt to shift the family's focus away from more threatening problems, such as marital conflict, depression, or alcohol/drug misuse. As long as parents or other family members remain focused on the adolescent's problems, the other issues may be ignored. Fourth, the adolescent operates on the basis of the pleasure principle, or whatever feels good at the moment. The teenager would rather suffer the consequences of his or her behavior than give up the immediate gratification it brings. Fifth, difficult adolescents often possess the ability to think two steps ahead: They foresee the number and type of sequential steps necessary to unravel any rule or consequence. Finally, adolescents are more skillful than their parents during confrontations. They know how to push their parents' buttons through words or actions so that the parents will become angry and lose control. By determining the general mood or direction of the argument, the adolescents are able to maintain their status quo position of authority.

AN INCONGRUOUS HIERARCHY

Adolescents with severe behavioral problems are hierarchically more power-ful than their parents. When parents ask a difficult adolescent to comply with basic rules, the teenager may counter with verbal threats or even violent be-havior to maintain his or her authority. Jerome Price (1996) has termed this ability "parent abuse"; he describes it as the adolescent's ability to use de-structive behaviors to demoralize, intimidate, or subjugate the parents into doing whatever the adolescent wants. This kind of power can mirror the ef-fects of an addictive drug. Initially, being in charge feels very good. However, to keep and maintain this power, the teenager must use increasingly destruc-tive behaviors.

When this "upside-down" hierarchy occurs, it also inadvertently places the adolescent in a double bind. If the teenager behaves without causing prob-lems, he or she will lose power and control. However, to maintain power and control, the teenager must continue to intensify the self-destructive behaviors. Hence, the adolescent cannot behave without problems and be in charge at the same time. The adolescent is then caught between a rock and a hard place.

CLINICAL EXAMPLE

The parents of 14-year-old Mary reported that they were unable to get her to clean her room or perform other chores. The parents said that each time they asked Mary to do something, she would swear and yell until they backed down. During counseling, the parents were able to stop backing down and make Mary complete the chores. However, Mary did not like losing her power, so to regain it she went from swearing to threatening to kill the mother and father with a knife while they were sleeping. In turn, this created a double bind: Mary could not give up her power and be in control at the same time.

Such a situation makes conventional treatment extremely difficult. The adolescent perceives that giving up any authority is an unacceptable loss, and will use whatever methods are necessary to stay in charge.

MISUSE OF OUTSIDE FORCES

When a teenager's self-destructive behavior persists or intensifies, parents of-ten seek help outside the family to restore their authority and help the teenager. These outside forces can include the police, the court system, a mental hospital, medication, and/or a psychiatrist or other counselor.

Unfortunately, there are several problems with this approach. The main one is that using outside forces disempowers the parents to an even greater degree. Initially, the threat of resorting to these forces may have some effect, but this can quickly diminish. When this happens, the adolescent views the parents as powerless.

CLINCAL EXAMPLE

Every time 13-year-old Michael threatened to throw a brick through the window, his single-parent mother would call the police to the house. Each time, the police would leave after telling Michael to stop threatening his mother. The first few occurrences of this had the desired effect, and Michael's threats stopped temporarily. However, over time the effect of the police's coming to the house lessened, and Michael resumed his threats of violence the next day. In addition, the police department grew annoyed with the mother's constant calls and stopped coming to the house. The mother was disempowered when Michael saw that these outside forces could not stop his behavior.

When seeking outside assistance involves hospitalization, residential treatment, or incarceration, two things can happen. The adolescent's behavioral problems may lessen or stop with these environments, but it does so because of counselors or because of the structured setting itself. The parents are not the ones who have brought about this change. After an initial "honeymoon" period, the parent abuse may recur because the adolescent is still in charge. In addition, the parents may now view these outside systems as the only option to stop their teenager's behavior. The result is a vicious cycle in which the adolescent is constantly in and out of institutions.

Finally, if hospitalization or medication is used, the definition of the problem shifts from a misbehaving or stubborn teenager in need of parental guidance to someone who is not responsible for his or her own behavior (Madanes, 1991). Medication or hospitalization can be a useful aspect of treatment in some cases. Hospitalization or residential care is sometimes needed if there is a potential for suicide or if the parents are initially unwilling or unable to provide the necessary structure. The risk is that parents may come to believe that their teenager is a mental patient who cannot function without these external forces. If this happens, there is little incentive to treat the teenager as a normal adolescent who is in need of parental guidance to get out of a temporary rut.

CLINCAL EXAMPLE

When 16-year-old Rick put his fist through a window, his parents immediately hospitalized him. The next day, the counselor asked the parents why they had called the hospital rather than calling the police to press charges. In essence, the counselor was telling the parents that the son was normal and responsible for his actions, rather than mentally ill and not responsible.

THE PROTECTIVE FUNCTION OF BEHAVIOR PROBLEMS

In some cases, the adolescent's problem is a conscious or unconscious attempt to shift the focus away from more threatening issues in the family, such as marital conflict, depression, or substance use problems. If the parents or other family members get stuck on the adolescent's problem, other issues are not addressed. This theory can easily be tested if the presenting behavioral problems are solved but other problems begin to emerge soon after.

CLINCAL EXAMPLE

Thirteen-year-old Nicole had severe behavioral problems of chronic truancy, running away, and threats of suicide. Immediately after these problems began to decrease, the mother began to complain of symptoms of depression, and the father complained of severe back pain. Nicole told the counselor privately that she was extremely concerned and worried about her parents. The next week, Nicole relapsed by running away. Afterward, the mother no longer seemed depressed and the father reported that his back was fine. This cycle of the parents' problems surfacing and the daughter's relapsing continued several more times, until finally the parents were able to "fire" their daughter from worrying about their problems.

This connection between adolescent problems and parental problems is defined as "triangulation" (Haley, 1980). Sometimes the adolescent exhibits extreme psychotic symptoms or self-destructive behaviors that prevent him or her from leaving home to pursue the next developmental level (i.e., going to college, establishing a career, or becoming self-supporting). Every time the adolescent begins to function normally and without problems, the family becomes unstable and other problems surface. The adolescent must again function incompetently to shift the focus away from these other problems, so that the family can restabilize itself. Jay Haley (1980) hypothesizes that this connection often goes unnoticed, because many counselors have not been trained to solve problems long enough to see other family issues emerge. In addition, a counselor helping to medicate or institutionalize an adolescent may believe that he or she is an agent of change, when in reality the counselor is being used to stabilize the family so that change does not occur. Therefore, unless the counselor can effectively solve other family problems, there is no reason why the adolescent will not have another relapse.

Cloé Madanes (1991), however, cautions that this connection is not always the rule. Many times, what starts off as a protective function leads to a permanent reversal in the hierarchy and a shift in power, independent of what set it off. For example, an adolescent who consistently exhibits self-destructive behavior whether or not another family problem surfaces has lost this connection.

It is important not to point out this connection to the family. On a deeper level, each family member may already be aware of it, but verbalizing it may prove too threatening and may scare the family away. Instead, the counselor can ask the following question: "If your teenager were concerned about someone in the family, even though he [she] might not be aware of it, who would it be and why?" This question is a respectful way to get to the heart of this connection without scaring off family members.

THE PLEASURE PRINCIPLE

Adolescents' behavior is based on the pleasure principle, or whatever feels good at the moment. This process is comparable to smoking or eating fatty foods: Even though these habits are destructive and can lead to death in the long term, people still engage in these behaviors because they receive immediate gratification from them. In the same way, the difficult adolescent gets immediate pleasure from skipping school to be with friends, or attention and power from self-destructive acts.

CLINCAL EXAMPLE

The parents of 15-year-old Adam were extremely angry and frustrated. They had promised that if Adam stayed in school and maintained a C average, they would buy him a car at the end of the school year. It was not logical to Adam's parents that he would give up this positive reward to ditch school. Yet Adam continued to skip school and was grounded every weekend. Adam told the counselor privately that he did not think about his future. He skipped school because it was fun at the moment and because he could go to the mall and drink. In addition, he was grounded on the weekends and did not want to wait to be with his friends (who were also truants) for the 2 weeks necessary to get off grounding. Adam would thus rather suffer the consequences than give up any immediate gratification; he could not see past tomorrow, and therefore a long-term reward such as a car seemed a lifetime away.

Such scenarios are common with difficult adolescents who are impulsive. This makes conventional consequences like grounding ineffective. Consequences must therefore be immediate and extreme enough to make the adolescent want to give up any immediate pleasure. A menu of such consequences is presented in Chapter 6.

THINKING TWO STEPS AHEAD

Tough adolescents seem to possess an uncanny ability to think two steps ahead and unravel even the best-laid plans. Jim Keim (1996) describes this behavior as "enhanced social perception," or the ability to imagine the number and type of sequential steps necessary to achieve a desired end result.

CLINCAL EXAMPLE

During a parent–teen conference, the school counselor asked 15-year-old Roger how he was able to get himself suspended so frequently. Roger smiled mischievously and stated:

> "It's easy. First you kick someone under the desk. Once you do this, that person will yell and point to me. Then the teacher will get mad and tell me to stop. Then if I mimic the teacher with her voice and facial expressions, the other kids will laugh, causing the teacher to get embarrassed. Finally, once the teacher gets embarrassed, she will have to do something to save face and act like she is in charge by suspending me."

This seven-step sequence for achieving suspension was easily constructed by Roger. He played out in his mind as many different scenarios as needed until he found one that worked.

With this skill, teenagers like Roger can find a loophole in any rule or consequence. As a result, parents must learn how to develop their own set of social perception abilities to think two steps ahead of their teenagers.

BUTTON-PUSHING SKILLS

Adolescents are often more interested in determining the mood or direction of an argument than the actual issue being argued. If they can determine the mood, teenagers can get their parents to lose control of their emotions. Once a parent has lost control, rules and consequences are ineffective. This also allows adolescents to maintain their position of authority.

CLINICAL EXAMPLE

Jim's parents were willing to extend his curfew by 1 hour. However, Jim wanted the curfew to remain at 9:30 P.M. The parents argued that this was an increase in time. The son stated that he was aware of this fact, but that he would determine when his curfew would be raised, not his parents. In this case, the parents were outcome-oriented (a 1-hour curfew extension), while Jim was more process-oriented (deciding when his curfew would be extended).

Tough adolescents will deliberately seek confrontations in which they can push the buttons of authority figures to gain control over a given situation. These buttons commonly consist of phrases such as "You're not my mother, so don't tell me what to do," "You don't love me," "I hate you," or "You never let me do anything." These comments are designed to paralyze, frustrate, or anger the parents into doing whatever an adolescent wants. The more time the parents spend trying to give an explanation for a particular decision, the more debilitated they can become. For instance, after one long, heated argument, a mother said to her counselor:

> "At the beginning of the argument I was 45 years old, but after 10 minutes of constant bickering I felt that I was 25. As we continued, I was suddenly at my daughter's age [16 years old], and it felt like two kids battling for power and control."

During these confrontations, stubborn adolescents are unwilling to back down and take responsibility for their behavior. They are vociferous in demanding equal treatment and authority over adults. This is the reason why many parent training programs, such as those described in the books *Back in Control* (Bodenhamer, 1988) and *Tough Love* (Neff, 1996), are ineffective: The principles and techniques are often sound, but they fail when the parents are confronted with an extremely skillful teenager who is unwilling to back down. The parents often lose control of their emotions and are unable to be consistent or to enforce rules or consequences. This can lead to what is called a "symmetrical communication feedback loop," which neither the teenager nor the parents take a one-down position or are willing to back down (Becvar & Becvar, 1988). If this happens, the adolescent's and/or parents' behavior will escalate to threats and possibly acts of violence.

CHAPTER 3

A Model for Change

Figure 3.1 depicts the 15-step family-based treatment model for treating adolescents with severe behavioral disorders. Many of these steps can also be modified to treat behavior problems in younger children. The steps are not intended to be rigid procedures, but rather guidelines that are systemic yet flexible enough to adapt to novel situations. The sequence of the steps in this model was discovered within my process–outcome research study (see Chapter 12).

STEP 1: ENGAGEMENT

"Engagement" is defined as the counselor's ability to enlist both the parents' and the adolescent's cooperation by developing rapport, reducing blame, and developing meaningful goals for both parties (Liddle, 1995). Recent studies reveal that engaging both parents and teenagers is paramount to successful treatment, and that a negative alliance is difficult to reverse (Henggeler, Melton, & Smith, 1992; Horvath & Greenberg, 1994; Liddle, 1994). Therefore, a core component of this model is successful engagement with the parents and adolescent throughout the counseling process. Depending on the particular case, engagement may also include enlisting the cooperation of extrafamilial systems (e.g., school personnel, other mental health professionals, probation officers, the juvenile justice system, or peer groups).

Since few people want therapy, especially when they think it means exploring past problems, it is important for the counselor to begin the engagement process by asking the parents to "help solve the teenager's problems," rather than to "have therapy" (Haley, 1980). If a family member is reluctant to participate, the counselor asks that person to attend a session simply to help the counselor do a better job by providing needed information. This request should be made directly instead of being communicated through other

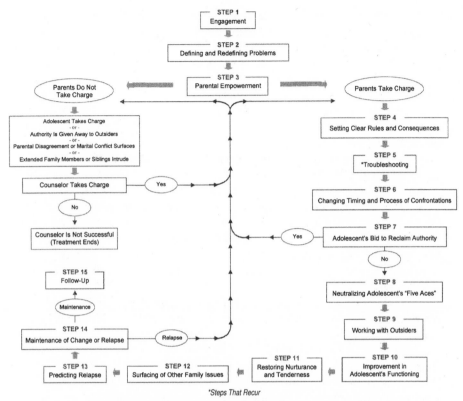

FIGURE 3.1. The 15-step family-based treatment model.

family members. Once the reluctant family member is at the session, it is easier to obtain a commitment from him or her to continue attending. This is done by respecting and acknowledging this person's point of view and helping the person see that he or she has something to gain from improvement in the adolescent's behavior. If the family member still refuses to come, the counselor works with those who are cooperative to build trust and rapport. Successful engagement with them will often lead to the participation of the reluctant family member, whether voluntarily or though persuasion from the other family members.

To strengthen the engagement process further, the parents' despair and hopelessness must be addressed directly. Parents need to voice how angry they have been with their son or daughter, and how they feel they are losing the struggle. When this occurs, the counselor should not counter too quickly with concrete solutions. Rather, the counselor should listen in a nonjudgmental fashion and should stress the normality of the parents' feelings of resentment, anger, and disappointment. The adolescent should not be present at this venting process, so that parents can express themselves freely and without the worry of how their statements will affect their son or daughter. By the same token, the adolescent should also have the opportunity to vent his or her feelings and frustrations when speaking with the counselor privately.

After the parents have vented, the counselor must be concrete and specific in his or her discussions. This is especially critical when the counselor and parents define the desired outcomes of treatment. For example, instead of "improved behavior," the counselor and parents should specify "no drug use," "no running away," or "completion of chores." Many goals will probably exist, but the family may feel overwhelmed and unable to undertake the multiple actions necessary to complete each goal successfully (Hepworth & Larsen, 1995). It is therefore important to limit goals to three behaviors at a time, in order to increase the chances for success, build momentum, and instill hope. By focusing on the problems in a more concrete and manageable manner, the counselor is able to strengthen the engagement with the parents, and everyone is better equipped to begin working with the adolescent to solve behavior problems.

Another way the counselor can strongly engage the family is to address issues and goals that are important to the parents and the adolescent individually. Studies show that "working both sides of the fence" by generating meaningful goals for both parties is a difficult but necessary process in effective treatment (Liddle, 1995; Selekman, 1993; Selekman & Todd, 1991). When meeting with the adolescent alone, the counselor attempts to find out whether there is any way he or she can act as the adolescent's advocate with the parents. The counselor does this by asking, "How can I be helpful to you?" or "Is there something you would like me to go to bat for with your parents?" Most adolescents are shocked at these questions, because their parents' desires have usually taken precedence in the past. Moreover, resistant adolescents tend to cooperate with counselors who pay attention to their goals and incorporate them into the treatment process (Selekman, 1993).

Another way to involve adolescents and to secure engagement with them is to designate them as expert consultants in solving their own problems. Adolescents almost always want their parents or other adults to "get off their backs" and leave them alone. If this is an adolescent's goal, the counselor can ask the following questions: "Starting tomorrow, if your parents were off your back, what would you be doing or saying differently so that they would no longer be on your case?" and "What would your parents be saying or doing differently with you that would make it easier for you to get them off your back?" With questions like these, the counselor fosters a cooperative working relationship by defining the adolescent as an expert who can solve his or her own behavioral problems in specific and concrete ways.

STEP 2: DEFINING AND REDEFINING PROBLEMS

When parents view their difficult teenager as frail, incapable, or mentally ill, they will typically hand over their authority to outside agents—probation officers, judges, police, medication, or institutionalization (Madanes, 1991). To determine how individual family members see the problem, the counselor asks, "What is your understanding or theory of the reasons why your teenager has these problems?" If one or both parents indicate that their son or daughter has medical or psychiatric problems, the counselor must carefully reframe the problem so that it is viewed instead as a controllable and changeable behavior.

CLINICAL EXAMPLE

Ben, a 13-year-old boy, was referred to counseling because he frequently lost his temper and hit other children in the classroom. The mother was convinced that Ben's problem was a chemical imbalance that prevented him from controlling his temper. Her only solution was to try different medications. The problem had worsened over the years, and Ben had seen eight different psychiatrists without success.

When the counselor asked Ben's mother whether there was ever a time her son could control his temper, she paused and said that Ben's temper tantrums seemed to stop when he really wanted something. The counselor replied that he had never heard of a chemical imbalance in which the resulting behavior could be controlled in one setting and not in another. The counselor was tactfully and skillfully redefining the problem as one that the son and mother had control over, rather than as a chemical imbalance that was out of their control.

Parents who do not want to take charge will protest these kinds of reframes and explain that other experts have recommended years of counseling, institutionalization, or the need to accommodate to their son or daughter. If this hesitation persists, current treatment efforts will inevitably be thwarted. As stated earlier, even though some problems can be helped with medication (e.g., depression), it is important to reframe a majority of the problem behaviors as solvable through parental intervention. In the case of the adolescent with temper tantrums, the problem was redefined from being the result of a chemical imbalance to one of an explosive yet controllable temper that could be stopped through severe consequences. Once the problem is successfully reframed, the counselor is ready to proceed to Step 3 and empower the parents to take charge.

STEP 3: PARENTAL EMPOWERMENT

The counselor begins Step 3 by emphasizing to the parents that their teenager's problem is one that they can handle if they outline clear rules and enforce effective consequences. The counselor must be able to convince the parents that once they are in charge, their son or daughter will behave normally. If this is not the first time the parents have sought professional help, the counselor can assert that since these other "experts" were unable to change the teenager's behavior permanently, it must be up to the parents rather than outsiders to solve the problems. The counselor's role is simply to teach the parents how to gain the skills and maintain the authority necessary to do this. If the parents choose to give their authority to other counselors or to outside systems such as institutions or hospitals, then the probability is great that their son or daughter's problem behaviors will endure.

If the parents are still reluctant, the counselor can ask this question: "Is what you are doing now effective in solving or improving the problems?" If the parents answer "No," the counselor can state that a new approach must be tried and that more of the same treatment will not work. Armed with these facts, the counselor asks the parents to try an experiment: Would they be willing to follow the treatment plan for only 1 or 2 weeks if it would result in even one small improvement? If the plan does not work after 1 or 2 weeks, the parents can always return to their previous methods. The counselor knows that from a systems theory perspective, one small change can increase the likelihood that more difficult problems will be solved. The counselor tells the parents that outsiders do not know their child better than they do themselves. As a result, they possess the necessary power to get their teenager back on track. If the parents are still reluctant, the counselor can point to the fact that outside experts have failed to achieve permanent change. In this context, most parents are willing to tolerate 1 or 2 weeks of experimentation before giving up or handing their authority to outside forces.

CLINICAL EXAMPLE

The single mother of 13-year-old Amy worked long hours, and her schedule prevented her from being home to enforce rules or consequences. As a result, Amy ran away from home on a regular basis. At first the mother was unwilling to modify her work schedule. However, when the counselor asked the mother to experiment by changing her schedule for only 2 weeks, she agreed. The mother even had time to take Amy on a special outing once a week. Just 1 hour a week of time together restored tenderness in the mother–daughter relationship. This decreased Amy's anger and bitterness, as well as her desire to run away. Empowered by the success of this experiment, the mother voluntarily decided to modify her work hours and devote the time necessary to tackle these difficult issues.

At this stage in treatment, the parents and counselor reach a proverbial fork in the road: The parents can either decide to take charge and proceed directly to establishing clear rules and consequences, or refuse to take charge. If the parents refuse to take charge, the counselor must take charge by persuading the parents to rethink their position or by blocking outside forces from undermining the counselor's credibility. If the counselor is unsuccessful with either of these goals, treatment will probably end prematurely.

The Parents Refuse to Take Charge

If one or both parents refuse to take charge, one of four things will happen: (1) The adolescent takes charge and makes decisions instead of the parents; (2) the parents formally or informally transfer their authority to outside sources and rely on those sources' decisions; (3) the parents quarrel and disagree, thus ensuring that neither one will take charge or exert joint authority: or (4) other extended family members or siblings will interfere and prevent the parents from exerting their authority. If one or more of these events takes place, the counselor must convince the parents of his or her expertise and ability to treat the case. If the counselor is successful, the parents will take charge and proceed to Step 4. If not, treatment is likely to end prematurely.

The Counselor Takes Charge

Ironically, once the counselor is in charge, he or she must begin to insist that the parents take charge before going further in treatment. The counselor does this by patiently and repetitiously clarifying the parents' responsibility for solving their adolescent's problem. The counselor states that the best hope for the adolescent is the involvement of the parents rather than outside experts, and he or she blocks outside influences (e.g., grandparents, other practitioners, siblings) from undermining the parents' authority. The counselor also insists that the parents stop fighting, take charge, and present a united front until their teenager is functioning without behavioral problems.

CLINICAL EXAMPLE

Marcus, a 16-year-old boy, presented problems of frequent truancy, poor grades, running away, lying, and refusing to obey his parents. Throughout the first meeting, the parents argued bitterly and could not agree on any rule or consequence. The counselor discovered that when the parents argued at home, the mother would immediately call her mother-in-law to complain that her son was a bad husband and father. The mother-in-law would then call her son and berate him; he would then get more upset with his wife. All the while, Marcus continued to defy his parents. In addition, whenever the counselor proposed that the parents take charge, they would say they had been told by other doctors that Marcus would need long-term residential care. They came to counseling in the hope that the counselor would get this process started.

The counselor's response was to take charge by the following methods. First, by using concrete examples of how experts' interventions had only made matters worse, he convinced the parents that they were the best hope for their son. The counselor argued successfully that the parents knew their son best, and that a majority of locked facilities such as prisons had failed to rehabilitate teenagers. Second, he used concrete examples to demonstrate how involving the mother-in-law had prevented the parents from working through their problems and uniting as a team. Finally, the counselor asked the parents to consider all the ways their disagreements helped their son remain in charge and continue his problematic behavior.

Counselor Is Not Successful and Treatment Ends

If the counselor is unsuccessful in convincing the parents to take charge, treatment will undoubtedly end: The parents will either terminate treatment permanently or seek out other counselors. The counselor should encourage the parent to return if other treatment approaches fail. In fact, the counselor can offer to call the parents in 2 months to check on current events. This proactive call is a safety valve; it is assumed that most families will not call on their own or that they will wait until it becomes too late for the counselor to intervene. Two months is enough time to allow other treatment methods to fail, yet still permit the counselor to salvage the troubled family. If the other treatment approach is successful, the counselor should congratulate the parents on their good fortune.

CLINICAL EXAMPLE

In the case of 16-year-old Julie, her parents were caught in the middle between a psychiatrist who wanted to use medication and hospitalization to control Julie's chronic truancy, and a counselor who wanted to use the present treatment model to place the parents in charge. When the counselor used this model to stop the truancy, Julie reacted with the more extreme behavior of running away to get the parents to weaken their position and give their authority back to Julie.

At this point, the psychiatrist intervened and advocated for hospitalization. The counselor called to discuss the matter, but the psychiatrist refused to change his mind. The parents reported to the counselor that they felt caught between the two different treatment philosophies. The parents finally decided to go with the psychiatrist's recommendation because they were tired and "burned out." Instead of getting angry or defensive, the counselor empathized with their dilemma and stated that if things did not improve, his door was always open. The only conditions would be that they would have to agree to having only one helping professional involved in the case, and that they would have to commit themselves to taking charge. When the daughter returned home from the hospital, her problem behavior resumed as the counselor had predicted. The parents then returned to the counselor and the 15-step treatment model.

The Parents Take Charge

Once the parents agree to take charge, treatment can proceed to Step 4. Realistically, however, not all cases will progress in such an orderly and systematic fashion. At any point in the treatment process, one or both parents may insist that they are unable or unwilling to take charge because of their teenager's extreme behavior and/or series of relapses. When confronted with tired or worn-out parents, the counselor must be ready to take charge and convince the parents to go through the storm.

STEP 4: SETTING CLEAR RULES AND CONSEQUENCES

Setting clear rules and consequences is the basic work of this therapy model and is arguably the most important step in the overall treatment process. This step provides the foundation for all subsequent steps and must be carried out successfully if the parents are to have any chance of retaining and maintaining a position of authority. This is because difficult teenagers suffer from what could be called "literal disease." Every rule and consequence must be literally spelled out and concretely defined, or the teenager will find a loophole and fight both the parents and the counselor.

CLINICAL EXAMPLE

Thirteen-year-old Billy had a problem of running away every time he did not want to comply with a rule or request. During counseling, the mother developed a contract that included the consequence of being grounded if Billy ran away in the future. However, this contract failed to specify what constituted running away or how long Billy would be grounded for each offense. A few days later, Billy went to a friend's house without permission, because he did not consider this act running away. The mother than grounded Billy for a week. He became extremely bitter and resentful, since there was nothing in the contract about going to a friend's house or being grounded for an entire week. Billy's sense of fairness had been violated, so he retaliated with behavior that was even more extreme: He destroyed the paint job on his mother's car with a key.

Every rule and consequence in the contract must include details about how and when compliance with the rule will be monitored and enforced. The first step for the counselor is to help the parents state precisely what it is they expect their son or daughter to be doing. For example, if parents say they want their son to show respect, the counselor asks what their son would be doing or saying to demonstrate respect. Words like "respect" and "better behavior" are abstract terms that mean different things to different people. Furthermore, "respect" is not a solvable problem, whereas swearing at one's parents is. It is also imperative that rules be limited to what the parents see as the teenager's three worse behaviors. As noted earlier, trying to address more than three rules at a time may overwhelm the parents or adolescent, thereby preventing any meaningful progress. Once the top three are targeted and successfully solved, other problems can be addressed.

When determining consequences for not obeying rules, the counselor should consider the following four guidelines:

1. Consequences should be operationally defined and written down in a contract format. For example, a consequence such as "no phone use" or "grounding" is too general and lacks specification. "No phone use" should include when the consequence is enforced, for how long, and who is responsible for monitoring and/or enforcing this consequence.

2. The counselor should solicit and use the parents' ideas for consequences whenever possible, to reinforce the contention that they are the experts. Research shows that success increases when clients' ideas are incorporated directly into the treatment process (Luborsky, Crits-Christoph, Mintz, & Auerbach, 1988).

3. The adolescent's expertise should also be incorporated whenever possible. Ironically, adolescents are often knowledgeable about what consequences work best with them, if they are only asked the right questions. (See Chapter 4 for additional guidelines on this topic.)

4. The counselor should listen patiently to any skepticism voiced by the parents, prior to offering reassurance that the current treatment process will succeed.

Each rule and consequence should be written down in a contract. This format directly incorporates the principles of Reid and Epstein's (1972) task-centered model; details on formulating contracts are outlined with illustrations in Chapter 4. Securing each relevant person's signature is desirable as a symbol of commitment. If the adolescent refuses to sign, the parents are told to avoid a power struggle by simply telling the adolescent that he or she is still bound by the contract. Parents are then asked to read the contract each day, so that the rules and consequences become second nature.

STEP 5: TROUBLESHOOTING

Before implementing a particular consequence, the counselor must first troubleshoot with the family everything that could go wrong beforehand. After the intervention is outlined, the counselor asks the parents and/or adolescent what things could go wrong with the plan. If the family cannot come up with anything, the counselor should suggest some possibilities to begin discussion. Interventions are then outlined for each possible contingency. Troubleshooting is critical because teenagers with behavioral problems have enhanced social perception abilities, as noted in Chapter 2. Unless troubleshooting takes place, an adolescent will be able to foresee the sequential steps necessary to unravel any plan.

Parents must be taught that their son or daughter will often triangulate or enlist the help of outsiders to regain any lost authority. This possibility must be anticipated beforehand, and the parents must decide what their response will be if it should happen.

CLINICAL EXAMPLE

The counselor told the parents of 15-year-old Sue that if they prevented her from leaving the house, she might enlist the help of outside authorities by claiming child abuse. The counselor and the parents then engaged in troubleshooting to determine how the parents would handle such an occurrence. The next day Sue intentionally threw herself against the bathroom wall to create bruises on her arms and shoulders. When Sue reported the bruises to child protective services, the parents were prepared. As planned, the parents called the counselor to intervene with the protective services worker. In this way, the rapport and trust between parent and counselor were strengthened, and the parents were not disempowered by child protective services. The father reported later that if he had not been prepared, he would have been so angry with his daughter that he would have left home, never to return again.

Troubleshooting is critical to treatment success, but is often the most overlooked part of the entire intervention process. Both counselors and parents often assume that the enforcement of a rule or consequence will run smoothly if outlined in concrete terms. Unfortunately, this is not always the case. The counselor must go through as many "what if" scenarios as are necessary to enable the parents to think two steps ahead of the adolescent and increase the chances of success. This is the case with any intervention initiated. Troubleshooting is used as a separate step after rules and consequences are outlined, but also as a necessary procedure following any intervention. The rationale is that the difficult teenager has enhanced social perception abilities. Consequently, the parent must use troubleshooting whenever a new intervention is introduced. Because of this fact, troubleshooting is listed as a re-curring step throughout the treatment process. Chapter 4 provides examples of such scenarios.

STEP 6: CHANGING THE TIMING
AND PROCESS OF CONFRONTATIONS

In order for consequences to work, changes in the timing and process of con-frontations must be made. Parents must recognize through concrete exam-ples what buttons they allow to be pushed during an argument. "Buttons" in this sense are words or actions that adolescents use to get parents to lose con-trol of their emotions by becoming angry, frustrated, or defensive. The par-ents are then easily thrown off track and unable to administer consequences effectively.

If this button pushing continues, an adolescent will be able to determine the content, direction, and general mood of any argument (Keim, 1996). When this happens, the adolescent is in charge because the parents are unable to remain calm and enforce rules.

CLINICAL EXAMPLE

Whenever the parents of 13-year-old Jill enforced a rule, she would go through a predictable series of button-pushing statements to throw her parents off track. Jill would begin with statements such as "You don't love me any more," and "I hate you," to induce guilt or get her parents to lose control through personal character attacks. If this did not work, Jill would move to the next level and say that she was going to kill herself. This threat was used to intimidate her parents and get them so scared that they would back down. At each level, the goal was the same: to manipulate her parents' emotional states so that Jill could retain her po-sition of authority.

A key element of this approach is educating the parents about the me-chanics of the process, especially how the adolescent locates the parents' points of vulnerability. Parents must understand that this is a key reason why previous consequences have been ineffective. The adolescent is not bad or mean-spirited, and the parents should not feel weak or blame themselves. The adolescent simply perceives confrontation in a different way and up until now has been able to derail the parents skillfully. The counselor can show parents how they have also inadvertently pushed their teenager's buttons through preaching, lectures, or guilt trips. For example, one 15-year-old boy complained that each time his grades improved, his father preached that he could do better; over time, the boy stopped trying because nothing he did was good enough. Educating all parties helps take the sole blame off any one party and creates a situation in which both the parents and the adolescent must change their confrontational style of communication. Once this is done, the counselor can give the parents specific strategies—for instance, exiting and waiting, staying short and to the point, and using deflectors to respond to their teenager in a nonreactive but firm manner. These and other strategies are explained further in Chapter 5.

STEP 7: THE ADOLESCENT'S BID TO RECLAIM AUTHORITY

After the parents take charge, the adolescent will often make a powerful bid to reclaim his or her lost authority. The primary method of doing this is an increase in the frequency or intensity of the most extreme or destructive behavior (e.g., suicidal threats, violence, running away), in order to demoralize, intimidate, or weaken the parents into returning things to the status quo. If this defiant behavior continues, the parents will either relinquish their authority or proceed directly to the next step of neutralizing the adolescent's "five aces." If the parents choose to relinquish their authority, the counselor must again take charge and try again to keep the parents in a position of authority. The counselor has to convince the parents that their teenager is doing whatever possible to regain control over the parents, and that this signals that the parents are on the brink of victory if only they can endure a little longer. If they relinquish their authority now, the teenager will walk away with the clear message that he or she can always win against the parents by using these tactics.

STEP 8: NEUTRALIZING THE ADOLESCENT'S "FIVE ACES"

The best poker players often seem to have an ace hidden up a sleeve to defeat their opponents at the precise moment the opponents appear to be winning. By the same token, a difficult adolescent seems to have the uncanny ability to defeat his or her parents by using the "five aces" of running away, truancy/poor school performance, disrespect, suicidal threats or behaviors, and threats or acts of violence. These "aces" must be neutralized; that is, the consequences for extreme behavior must be severe enough that the teenager will give up the extreme behavior rather than suffer the consequences (Haley, 1984). The difficulty with this theory has been finding consequences that are effective in stopping these types of extreme behaviors without being abusive. This is one of the key reasons why counseling with this population often fails. When traditional consequences fail, the most common interventions used are hospitalization, residential treatment, medication, or incarceration. However, the adolescent often returns to the same behavior when he or she finally returns home, since the family structure has remained largely unaltered. Specific methods to counter each of these "five aces" are detailed in Chapter 6.

STEP 9: WORKING WITH OUTSIDERS

While the counselor works with the parents to solve the teenager's problems, he or she must simultaneously consider the influence of the larger environmental system. Difficult adolescents are often involved with the juvenile justice system, local police departments, school personnel, and other mental health care providers. As a result, the counselor must act as a mediator between the adolescent and family on the one hand, and these other systems on the other, to increase cooperation and collaboration.

The influence of these outside systems cannot be underestimated. When a counselor sets changes to parental authority in motion, the outside environment will also react to these changes. Sometimes the reaction is positive and supportive: School personnel may begin calling the parents when the teenager is truant, or extended family members may rally in support of a single parent. At other times the reaction is negative and unsupportive: A psychiatrist may advise parents that the therapist is wrong and recommend residential care, or a child protective services worker may believe a teenager's claims of child abuse. The teenager may also enlist the support of peers in establishing a network of "safe houses" so that he or she can successfully run away.

It is critical for a counselor to understand how these outside forces affect the family and the difficult adolescent. The counselor must understand how to mediate a better fit with outsiders (e.g., getting church members and a single parent to collaborate) while simultaneously neutralizing any outside influences that might impede parental effectiveness (e.g., negative peer influences, unsupportive probation officers). To accomplish this goal, counselors must be willing either to leave the comfort of their offices and go into the outside environment or to bring these outsiders into their offices. Specific methods of work with outsiders are detailed in Chapter 8.

STEP 10: IMPROVEMENT IN THE ADOLESCENT'S FUNCTIONING

When the adolescent's "aces" are neutralized and there is a collaboration with larger systems, the adolescent's behavioral problems begin to recede on a more permanent basis. A period of calm often ensues, as the communication no longer centers exclusively around negative parent–teenager interactions. At this point, many families declare treatment a success and want to end therapy. The less chronic a problem was before treatment, the more likely it is that treatment can actually be ended at this point, with only periodic sessions for maintenance purposes. If the counselor has the opportunity to treat problems when they first appear, the chances are smaller that negative interaction patterns have become entrenched. In addition, treatment can probably be terminated at this stage if the adolescent's problem is not a conscious or unconscious attempt to shift the focus off more threatening problems such as marital conflict, depression, or alcohol or drug misuse.

However, if the problem is chronic or there is a dearth of tenderness between parent and child, treatment must proceed to Step 11. Otherwise, the behavioral problems are likely to return in the future. If a problem is chronic, old patterns will return when stressful events return. In addition, without nurturance, negative communication patterns will lead to bitter confrontations and a return to behavior problems. Even if these issues are not addressed, parents may indicate that they want to terminate or take a break. If this happens, it is wise to schedule a follow-up appointment for several weeks or a month away. This communicates to the family members that they have worked hard and have earned a respite, in addition to giving them an opportunity to try out new skills. It also indicates to the family members that they can contact the counselor if there is a problem in the future.

STEP 11: RESTORING NURTURANCE AND TENDERNESS

To maintain changes in a difficult adolescent's behavior, the soft, nurturing side of the hierarchy must be addressed, in addition to the hard, disciplinary side. Nurturance is often maintained by the parents' ability to provide special outings on a regular basis, healthy physical touch, and soothing communication patterns that include encouragement and praise. Addressing one side of the hierarchy and excluding the other can result in behavioral problems that resurface again and again. For example, if there is nurturance without rules, teenagers may have little respect for authority and may be unable to tolerate constraints on their behavior. They may need instant gratification and grow up extremely self-centered. On the other hand, if there are only rules and no nurturance, teenagers can grow up extremely bitter, angry, and unable to trust. They may not have the ability to show empathy with or nurturance for other people, and may often retaliate with extreme and destructive behavior.

Given years of stress and negative communication, parents who enter a counselor's office may love their teenager but no longer like him or her. The counselor must understand this fact and move cautiously. In some cases, the counselor will be able to address the hard and soft sides of the hierarchy simultaneously. For example, while the parents are establishing a contract of rules and consequences, they can also set up specific times and dates for special outings. However, in most cases, the soft side cannot be addressed until a teenager's functioning has improved. Years of conflict and bitterness have usually taken a toll on the parent–child relationship: The parents feel out of control, helpless, and disempowered. Wounds cannot heal until the bleeding has stopped. Only after the adolescent's extreme behaviors have been neutralized will the parents have the peace of mind, time, and energy necessary to inject tenderness back into the relationship.

CLINICAL EXAMPLE

Fifteen-year-old Tony was referred to counseling by the probation department for stealing, chronic truancy, and assault on his mother. The mother, a single parent, was so angry at her son that all she wanted was for him to be locked up and out of her life forever. When the counselor made a home visit, the mother took the counselor on a tour of the home and relayed a story for each hole in the wall and every piece of broken glass. She even pulled out a knife from under the bed and told the counselor that Tony had threatened to use this knife on her while she was sleeping.

The counselor then made the mistake of suggesting that maybe Tony was crying out for attention and only needed special outings and quality one-on-one time with the mother. The mother reacted by stating that other counselors had told her that again and again. This only made her feel blamed as a parent. In addition, each time she tried following their suggestions and let her guard down, Tony would take advantage of her kindness.

The counselor regrouped and focused on neutralizing Tony's "aces," beginning with his threats and acts of violence. He accomplished this by mobilizing neighbors and church leaders. If Tony threatened violence, one or more of these people were available at a moment's notice to come to the house and support the mother. With this strong show of support, the mother was able to regain her authority and stop Tony's problem behavior. Armed with this success, the counselor again approached the issue of nurturance and tenderness. The mother stated that she now felt ready to address this issue and organize special outings. She stated that the counselor was the only one who had been successful in helping her son change. As a result, she trusted his judgment and was willing to take the risk of getting hurt again by trying to instill nurturance.

In this case, the counselor first had to restore order and give the mother some peace of mind before attempting to inject nurturance back into the family household. By putting the parent back in charge and neutralizing the teenager's "aces," the counselor gained rapport and trust with the parent. In turn, the parent was more willing to face the difficult and challenging task of being vulnerable and soft. Specific methods to address this issue are detailed in Chapter 7.

STEP 12: SURFACING OF OTHER FAMILY ISSUES

If the adolescent's functioning begins to improve, the focus may now shift to more threatening problems in the family, such as marital conflict, depression, or alcohol and drug misuse. Previously, the parents or other family members could focus their attention on the adolescent's problems. When these problems are resolved, other issues have the opportunity to surface. Consequently, the counselor must be skilled at using various treatment modalities (i.e., family, group, marital, and individual) to treat a variety of specialized treatment issues (e.g., depression, substance use problems, domestic violence, marital conflict). Otherwise, the adolescent may have a relapse in response to these unresolved issues. Even if the teenager's problems do not serve a protective function, the tension and stress these other issues bring can trigger a relapse of the problem behavior.

CLINICAL EXAMPLE

Sixteen-year-old Margie repeatedly failed in school and had bouts of severe depression. When asked whether she was concerned about someone in the family, Margie reported that she was worried that her mother was lonely and depressed. Further exploration revealed that the mother and daughter were extremely close, while the father remained emotionally unavailable.

The mother became even more depressed and lonely immediately after Margie began to function better. Marital conflict surfaced as the husband wanted more of the wife's time, now that she was not exclusively involved in the daughter's problems. As these issues began to arise, Margie became anxious and worried about her mother's problems and soon relapsed. This cycle continued until the counselor helped the parents resolve their marital conflict and the mother's loneliness while treating the daughter's behavioral problems. Once these problems were addressed, the connection was broken, and the daughter was free of the emotional burden of the mother's problems.

At this point, the counselor should offer a new treatment contract to address other family issues that may have surfaced. If the family resists further treatment, the counselor might warn family members about the risks associated with not treating these other issues. Parents can be told that unresolved tension in specific areas can lead to a stressful environment for the entire family; this can eventually increase the risk of a relapse by the adolescent. If family members still decline this offer, the counselor can conduct "tune-up" sessions as needed while leaving the option of future therapy open. Often the parents need time to see how unresolved family issues can lead to relapse. Finally, the counselor can proceed to Step 13, predict a relapse, and ask the family to reconsider the new treatment contract if the prediction proves to be true.

STEP 13: PREDICTING RELAPSE

When other family problems emerge or when things are going too well, the risk of relapse increases. The new change in family structure and in methods of interaction produces normal anxiety and tension. Even though family members rationally accept that this new way is better, emotionally they are still used to the old way of interacting, no matter how chaotic it seemed. The old patterns were at least familiar and predictable. A conscious and unconscious pull to return to old ways of functioning thus remains until the changes become better established over time.

To decrease this risk of relapse, the counselor tells the adolescent and parents that things are going too well and that a relapse may happen within the next couple of weeks. Parents should prepare themselves by outlining a specific plan if a relapse occurs. This intervention is paradoxical; it is designed to provoke the parents and adolescent into *not* relapsing by rebelling against the counselor's message. In essence, by predicting a relapse, the counselor hopes that the adolescent will want to prove the counselor wrong by not relapsing. However, if a relapse does occur, the parents and adolescent have a contingency plan in place and will be prepared.

CLINICAL EXAMPLE

Fifteen-year-old Chip relapsed by continuing to run away soon after things were going well. The stunned parents were immediately ready to terminate treatment, because they felt that all their time and effort had been wasted. This changed when the counselor realized his mistake and normalized relapses as common when change first happens. He told the parents the goal was to extend the time between relapses until they disappeared completely, while at the same time preparing for their occurrence.

Chip's parents were now ready for relapses as a normal part of the overall therapeutic process. Chip, however, did not like anyone telling him that he was going to relapse. He rebelled and wanted to prove everyone wrong by stubbornly refusing to have another relapse. Chip eventually did relapse months later, but his parents did not get upset and instead initiated the agreed-upon steps to get things back on track as quickly as possible.

This skillful use of a paradoxical message encourages the adolescent or family to rebel against the counselor by not relapsing. Even if a relapse should occur, the parents are not caught off guard and have the tools necessary to take charge of the situation.

STEP 14: MAINTENANCE OF CHANGE OR RELAPSE

After the relapse is predicted, the adolescent will either maintain the changes in behavior or relapse as predicted. If the adolescent does not relapse, the counselor proceeds directly to Step 15 for follow-up. However, if the adolescent does relapse, the parents must again take charge of the problem and retrace some or all of the previous steps from 4 through 15. This usually involves simple "tune-up" procedures with several of the steps, rather than a major overhaul or a new beginning. However, if one or both parents refuse to accept a position of authority, the counselor must again take charge and convince the parents to make one final push to help change their teenager's behavior permanently.

STEP 15: FOLLOW-UP

Follow-up is critical to the overall treatment process. Without good follow-up, adolescents and their families may attain first-order but not second-order changes. This means that the adolescent and/or parents may solve the presenting problem (first-order change) but may fail to change the structure or social environment that "helped" the problem continue to survive and thrive (second-order change) (Becvar & Becvar, 1988). This failure to achieve second-order change is evident when adolescents' problem behaviors are "cured" while they are in therapy but resurface soon after the completion of treatment. This happens when a fundamental aspect of the family environment (e.g., marital discords) is unaltered and the counselor is no longer available to mediate and force the parents to exert their joint authority.

Ideally, second-order change occurs when the hierarchy is reversed and the parents are able to maintain their authority over time. However, this second-order change is new and often tenuous at best. If the family or adolescent experiences stress in the form of unresolved family issues, an unexpected crisis, or developmental changes, the adolescent may again experience problems.

CLINICAL EXAMPLE

In the case of 15-year-old Tom, the father lost his job and the family went bankrupt soon after treatment was completed. The stress of this unexpected financial crisis resulted in marital problems and in the father's becoming clinically depressed. Earlier changes were reversed as the father again became distant from the family and could not support his wife in providing discipline or nurturance. The son then began to exhibit earlier behavioral problems. Without subsequent follow-up sessions, Tom would have relapsed.

To maintain or initiate second-order change, the parents and adolescent are taught preventive anticipatory guidance strategies. With the counselor's help, the family openly discusses possible future crises or problems. The counselor shows the family members how they can use strategies and tools acquired during treatment to avoid becoming overwhelmed in the future.

Treatment sessions are spaced out gradually over weeks and then months, to convey the message that the family can solve its own problems and to give parents time to implement new techniques. The counselor also makes himself or herself available for "callbacks" (phone calls from the parents throughout the week, to enable them to touch base and seek guidance before a minor conflict becomes a major problem). The counselor is still supportive if needed, but becomes less involved as the family maintains second-order changes. This slow but steady weaning process is extremely effective in helping achieve this goal.

After the weaning process is completed, the counselor reassures the family members that the door is always open if they should need help in the future. The counselor will proactively contact the parents in 2 months to check on their progress. If further sessions are needed, they should be viewed as "tune-ups" rather than "therapy." The goal of these meetings is to help maintain changes or get the family back on track as quickly as possible. In this way, family members are not given the message that therapy is always needed, but are shown that it is normal to have maintenance sessions as needed to maintain existing changes. Within this framework, the family is likely to contact the counselor in the future if a crisis emerges that members cannot solve.

PART TWO

SPECIFIC PRINCIPLES
AND GUIDELINES

CHAPTER 4

Setting Clear Rules and Consequences
The Basic Work of Therapy

Setting clear rules and consequences—Step 4 of the 15-step family-based model—is the foundation on which parents can regain their authority and successfully realign the family hierarchy. If specific consequences are not established, parents are anxious and unsure of what to do when their teenager breaks a particular rule. This can lead to arguments, violence, and a worsening of the teenager's behavior. However, once rules and consequences have been predetermined, the parents' need to nag, remind, or lecture is greatly reduced. They now have the ability to enforce planned consequences and will not be forced to make "off-the-cuff" decisions.

CLINICAL EXAMPLE

A constant power struggle ensued between 15-year-old Brian and his mother over chores. Every night the mother would remind Brian, and every night Brian would either drag his heels or not do the chores at all. After counseling, the mother wrote each chore on a contract with the stipulation that they had to be completed by 6:00 P.M. If all the chores were not completed by that time, the money for doing the chores would be given to Brian's younger brother, and Brian's phone privileges would be taken away the next day. With planned actions rather than impromptu reactions, the mother no longer had to nag or justify her behavior. The need for power struggles and confrontations was eliminated.

The bulk of this chapter is devoted to a detailed discussion of strategies for constructing effective rules and consequences. A brief discussion of troubleshooting (Step 5 of the 15-step model) is also included, since troubleshooting is inextricably bound up with the setting of rules and consequences and is vital to its success.

STUMBLING BLOCKS FOR PARENTS

To become successful in establishing clear rules and consequences, counselors must first understand the stumbling blocks that parents often face. There are six primary reasons why parents have difficulty in setting clear rules of consequences.

1. Rules and consequences are not clearly operationalized before a rule has been broken.
2. Rules are optional rather than mandatory.
3. There are too many rules to master at any one time.
4. Consequences are not effective enough.
5. Parents do not follow through on a consistent basis, or they change rules or consequences in midstream.
6. Rules and consequences are not written down in a contract format.

These potential stumbling blocks are described in a handout for parents (Figure 4.1).

Rules and consequences not clearly operationalized	Rules optional, not mandatory	Too many rules at one time	Consequences not effective	No consistency	Rules not written in contract format
Teenagers are extremely literal and will continue to get into arguments about the interpretation of rules or consequences. Therefore, rules and consequences must be clearly operationalized before a rule has been broken.	A mandatory rule is one that the teenager must obey. However, if the rule is not clearly stated, it becomes optional and ineffective.	Rather than focusing their time and energy on the most important issues, parents often want to correct every negative thing the teenager does at one time.	Consequences are often not severe enough. Therefore, the teenager has no reason to give up the extreme behavior.	Parents do not follow through on a consistent basis, or they change the rules or consequences as they go along.	Rules and consequences are not written down in a contract format. As a result, both parents and adolescent get confused as to what was said and how the rule was to be enforced.

FIGURE 4.1. Parent handout: Potential stumbling blocks in establishing clear rules and consequences. From *Treating the Tough Adolescent* by Scott P. Sells. Copyright 1998 by The Guilford Press. Permission to photocopy this handout is granted to purchasers of *Treating the Tough Adolescent* for personal use only (see copyright page for details).

STRATEGIES FOR CONSTRUCTING EFFECTIVE RULES AND CONSEQUENCES

The six potential stumbling blocks can be countered with the following seven strategies: (1) getting the parents to agree upon the top three behaviors that they want to improve; (2) getting parents to convert unacceptable behaviors into clearly operationalized rules; (3) constructing effective consequences to reduce or eliminate extreme behavioral problems; (4) showing parents how to put together a written contract; (5) incorporating the adolescent's expertise in setting his or her own consequences; (6) getting parents to follow through on a consistent basis; and (7) consideration of family dynamics.

It is important to note that with the exception of Strategy 5, each of these strategies should initially be undertaken without the adolescent present. This is done for two reasons. First, at this stage in the overall treatment process, the adolescent is still in charge. One way of maintaining this authority is to know everything that is going on and then to use this information to eliminate any perceived threats. Therefore, it is important that parents not reveal their strategies until these are defined and operationalized. Keeping the adolescent "in the dark" limits his or her ability to sabotage the parents' plan of action. It also creates a boundary between parents and teenager, because the adolescent is no longer involved in every executive decision. Second, if the adolescent is in the room, he or she may disrupt the process of constructing clear rules and consequences.

Strategy 1: Reaching Consensus on the Top Three Behaviors to Change

Before the counselor helps the parents establish clear rules and consequences, they all must reach a consensus on the exact behaviors the parents feel are most important to change. Parents can list as many as they like on their individual lists (see below), but should rank the three most important from most to least critical. With more than three, the risk of "burnout" increases. From a systems theory perspective, one small change can have a ripple effect on other subsystems or problems. For example, when parents can collaborate and reach agreement about rules and consequences, this can have a positive effect on such marital issues as poor communication. In addition, a positive change in one behavior can also create hope, momentum, and renewed strength for addressing more difficult problems in the future.

Rationale for Limiting the Focus to Three Behaviors

Getting the parents to limit their focus to three key behaviors can be a challenging task even for the most seasoned counselor. When parents try to win every little battle, they lose the energy necessary to deal with the major issues, such as running away, truancy, or violence. To address this stumbling block, the counselor can use a simple metaphor of telling the parents that they begin each day with one tank of gas. If the parents use up half their tank dealing with small issues, they won't have the gas necessary to address the big ones. In addition, when the parents choose to fight every battle, the probability that the teenager will misbehave increases. This is because the parents are reinforcing every minor misbehavior by the teenager with attention and power, but are not able to expend the energy necessary to resolve each misbehavior. Their focus may be divided among a dozen small problems instead of three larger ones, so none of them gets the attention needed. Parents can usually relate to this rationale and often change their perspective on the need to win every battle.

CLINICAL EXAMPLE

Sixteen-year-old Wendy would often run away and be gone for up to 3 weeks at a time. Many times, teenagers will run away when there is something toxic within the family environment. In this case, the mother would constantly nag Wendy about everything—from how she brushed her hair to how she walked and talked. This created a very poisonous relationship between mother and daughter. Arguments usually led one of them to slap the other. This cycle would repeat itself until the daughter ran away. When the mother reacted to every issue, she had no energy left over to deal with the bigger ones, such as Wendy's running away or staying in school. Trying to win every battle only ended in a power struggle and in the mother becoming more agitated.

Procedures for Reaching a Consensus

Once the counselor convinces the parents to focus only on crucial behaviors, he or she must show the parents how to reach a consensus. These procedures are adapted from Stanley Turecki's (1989) work with difficult young children and have been modified for parents with difficult adolescents. To help facilitate this process, parents are given a handout (Figure 4.2) that provides an example of how to list and rank relevant behaviors.

Construction of Two Relevant Behavior Lists. The counselor asks the teenager to leave the room and each parent to construct a list of relevant behaviors. These are defined as behaviors that parents feel they must take a stand on. They will share their lists later, but for the moment each parent completes one privately. Parents are instructed to write down each behavior and ask themselves the following four questions: (1) "Is this behavior really important?" (2) "Could I let this behavior go for now?" (3) "What would happen if I just waited?" and (4) "Could I lose by doing nothing?" When each be-

Mother's list	Father's list
Son will not go to school. (1)	Son sulks, always in a bad mood. (4)
Son is disrespectful through swearing and not doing what I ask him to do the first time. (3)	Will not listen to me. (2)
	Does not appreciate us as parents. (3)
Son will not come home on time for curfew. (2)	Lying. (1)
Son fights with brother. (4)	

Combined relevant behavior list (rank order of priority)

1. Son will not go to school.
2. Son will not come home on time for curfew.
3. Son is disrespectful through the following behaviors: Swearing, lying, not following directions.

FIGURE 4.2. Parent handout: Example of how to list and rank relevant behaviors. From *Treating the Tough Adolescent* by Scott P. Sells. Copyright 1998 by The Guilford Press. Permission to photocopy this handout is granted to purchasers of *Treating the Tough Adolescent* for personal use only (see copyright page for details).

havior has passed this four-question test, the parents rank them from most important to least important.

Exchange of Lists and Production of One Combined List. After completing their lists separately, the parents exchange lists and note which behaviors they agreed upon and which they did not. If the lists are different, the counselor asks the parents to reach a consensus and put aside any differences for the sake of solving their teenager's problem. Compromise is especially difficult when the parents have conflicting parenting styles or marital problems. When this is the case, the counselor must give concrete examples of how different parenting styles have allowed the teenager to divide and conquer. The greater the number of concrete examples, the more likely it is that the parents will agree upon one list of relevant behaviors.

If the parents are still unable to reach an agreement, the counselor suggests a rationale for choosing the behavior that he or she feels should be addressed first. However, it should first be a collaborative process between the parents and counselor until the parents get "stuck" and cannot move forward. When this happens, the counselor must take charge to solve the problem.

CLINICAL EXAMPLE

Thirteen-year-old Jerry set fires because it was the best way he knew to communicate his anger at his father for always working and ignoring his needs. For the first half-hour of the session, the parents argued and disagreed on what behaviors they should address and their order of priority. The father thought that the first relevant behavior should be the fire setting and said that all Jerry needed was "a good whipping." The mother stated that the father was never home and wondered how he could know what to do.

The mother also noted two other problems: Jerry never listened, and he regularly picked on his baby sister. The parents then began to argue, with the mother maintaining that the father was too harsh, and the father accusing the mother of being too soft. At this time, the counselor took charge by using concrete examples to show clearly how the parents' disagreements were limiting their effectiveness. The counselor pointed out that as long as they could not agree and failed to exert joint authority, Jerry would continue to have problems. He also reminded the parents that setting fires was very serious and dangerous: if no action was taken, their house could burn down.

Until the parents could agree on which behaviors were relevant, the counselor asked for permission to proceed as the unbiased mediator and suggest the top three behaviors to work on. When phrased in this manner, both parents agreed. The counselor chose fire setting, the father's absence from the family, and the son's disrespectful behavior.

If the counselor works with a single parent, the exchange of lists is of course skipped, and the parent immediately proceeds to outlining rules and consequences for each identified relevant behavior. The counselor may still have to make suggestions if the single parent has failed to identify certain relevant behaviors. For example, one such parent failed to address a teenager's suicidal behavior as relevant. For reasons of safety, the counselor must be ready to take charge actively and convince a parent that certain issues must be addressed immediately. After the top three relevant behaviors have been identified and ranked, the counselor proceeds directly to Strategy 2.

Strategy 2: Converting Unacceptable Behaviors into Clearly Operationalized Rules

Rationale for Predetermining Rules and Consequences

Before proceeding with Strategy 2, the counselor must provide the parents with clear reasoning on the importance of predetermining both rules and consequences. Without predetermined rules and consequences, the adolescent is given the opportunity to bargain, demand an explanation, plead his or her case, or point out inconsistencies in the parents' behavior. This allows the adolescent to control the mood and direction of the conversation. Predetermined rules and consequences can reverse this trend. The adolescent knows ahead of time what will happen if he or she crosses a particular line or breaks a particular rule. This predetermination is referred to as "tagging" of the inappropriate behaviors; it is preferable to spontaneous reactions to such behaviors. The parents are now able to enforce a rule without the need to explain and without the teenager's pleading his or her case.

Specifying Each Rule in Concrete Terms

After providing rationale, the counselor asks the parents to take each relevant behavior on their combined list and specify in concrete terms what their teenager would be saying or doing if he or she were performing each behavior. For example, "disrespect" can mean different things to different people. The parents must write down all the things the teenager says or does that clearly indicate that the teenager is being disrespectful. In one family disrespectful behavior may consist of swearing or lying, while in another family not following directions may be considered disrespectful.

Questions include what the rule is (e.g., son must come home on time for curfew), when is it to be done (e.g., curfew time will be 5:00 P.M. on school nights and 9:00 P.M. on weekends), how often it is to be done (e.g., every day), how long the rule is in effect (e.g., until the parents decide otherwise), and how the rule will be monitored (e.g., one or both parents will be there to see whether the son is home on time). It is important to note that monitoring a rule is a critical but often overlooked piece of the overall process. For example, parents may tell their teenager that a rule is for the teenager to attend every class each day. However, the rule will fail without monitoring. The adolescent will quickly realize that the parents are unable to create a set of rules that can be effectively monitored and enforced.

Parents are told to inform their teenager ahead of time that each rule is subject to change at the parents' discretion, *not* the teenager's. However, the parents must notify the teenager before a new or modified rule goes into effect. This caveat gives parents the flexibility to modify or create rules in the future. The only stipulation should be that possible modifications should be brought to the counselor's attention ahead of time. If the counselor is not involved, parents may make sudden changes that could be ineffective and that do not give the existing rules enough time to work.

CLINICAL EXAMPLE

The rule was that 15-year-old Angela could not spend the night at a friend's house until she came home on time for 2 full weeks. Unfortunately, after only 1 week, Angela nagged the father until he rescinded the earlier rule and gave Angela permission to sleep over. Neither the mother nor the counselor was consulted beforehand. This caused the mother's and counselor's authority to be undermined. Since the rule was modified too quickly, the daughter did not come for curfew, and the father took this action as a personal "slap in the face." As a result, he took an overly harsh stance and grounded Angela for a month, which only caused her to rebel more and make his wife more angry and frustrated. The mother later told the father that this could have been avoided if they had consulted with each other and the counselor ahead of time.

Figure 4.3 is a parent handout that illustrates how rules can be operationally defined and stated in behavioral terms. Please note that each rule is very literal and defined as if it came out of a dictionary. Each rule is also designed to custom-fit what behaviors occur within the particular family. For example, the behavior of truancy is defined very explicitly. Instead of simply saying that John has to attend school every day, the rule explicitly states that school attendance includes being present at every class period with no tardies. In addition, it outlines the exception of a medical emergency in anticipation of John's finding a loophole. The rule also clarifies how the parents will monitor John's school behavior. This type of clarity decreases chaos, clarifies roles, and leaves nothing to chance.

Rule 1 (Son will not go to school) Beginning Monday, John will ride the bus at 8 A.M. and attend school every day. This includes every class period with no tardies, unless there is a medical emergency that requires John to be taken to the doctor's office. The parents will determine this and will contact the attendance officer each morning to monitor John's attendance.

Rule 2 (Son will not come home on time for curfew) John's curfew time will be 5 P.M. on school nights (Sunday through Thursday) and 9 P.M. on weekends (Friday and Saturday). If John returns even 1 minute past the curfew hour, he will be considered late. These times will not be changed or altered until the parents decide otherwise. Therefore, John's trying to change them on his own also breaks this rule.

Rule 3 (Son is disrespectful through the following behaviors: Swearing, lying, not following directions) John's behavior will be considered disrespectful if he does one or more of the following:

   (a) Swears or uses obscene gestures such as giving the finger.
   (b) Tells a lie (and it is proven that he told a lie as determined by a parent).
   (c) Refuses to complete a task (homework, chores, etc.) even after one warning is given.

Please note: We as parents reserve the right to change both rules and consequences within this contract, and we will give prior notice if and when this occurs.

FIGURE 4.3. Parent handout: Example of how to specify rules in concrete terms. From *Treating the Tough Adolescent* by Scott P. Sells. Copyright 1998 by The Guilford Press. Permission to photocopy this handout is granted to purchasers of *Treating the Tough Adolescent* for personal use only (see copyright page for details).

Strategy 3: Formulating Effective Consequences

Underneath each rule in the contract, consequences for breaking that rule are outlined. Like rules, consequences must also be explicitly stated. Parents must address what each consequence will be, how it will be monitored, who will deliver it, when it will be enforced, and how long the consequence will last.

Using Both Positive and Negative Consequences

Whenever possible, consequences should be both negative *and* positive—negative if a particular rule is broken, and positive if that same rule is consistently followed. This formula mirrors the real world and gives the adolescent a choice: to be positively rewarded, or to have some restriction placed on him or her until the rule is followed. This also avoids a strictly negative stance and can promote a more cooperative and positive relationship between parents and teenager. An example of how both negative and positive consequences can be provided is given below for the rule of obeying curfew (Rule 2 in Figure 4.3).

> John's curfew time will be 5 P.M. on school nights (Sunday through Thursday) and 9 P.M. on weekends (Friday and Saturday). If John returns home even 1 minute past the curfew hour, he will be considered late. These times will not be changed or altered until we as parents decide otherwise. Therefore, John's trying to change them on his own also breaks this rule.

Consequence A (negative)	*or*	Consequence B (positive)
For every night John is late, he will be grounded for the next day plus the next weekend night. If he is late again that same week, the same thing happens. If he runs out of weekend nights, then the grounding will be carried over to the next weekend.		If John comes home on time, he will receive 1 hour added to his curfew time the next night. If the next night is a school night, the curfew will be 6:00 P.M. and if it is a weekend night, it will be 10:00 P.M.

In this example, John has a choice: following the rule of curfew and receiving the reward or positive consequence (an extra hour of curfew), or choosing not to follow the rule and receiving a negative consequence (being grounded the next day plus one weekend night).

Whenever possible, each consequence should be related to the particular rule. For example, giving an adolescent $5 every time he or she comes home on time is a positive consequence, but it does not relate to the rule of curfew. However, receiving an extra hour of curfew for being on time is related. Without this direct relationship, both positive and negative consequences are often ineffective.

Having both positive and negative consequences can place the burden of responsibility on the adolescent instead of the parents. Parents only have to "tag" the inappropriate behavior and enforce the predetermined consequence, rather than assume responsibility for the choices an adolescent makes. In addition, parents with difficult adolescents tend to focus only on the negative and therefore to give only punitive consequences. By administering both types, they model the real world and create a situation in which the adolescent can choose to be either positively rewarded or penalized with a predetermined negative consequence.

Exceptions to the inclusion of a positive consequence are made when the behavior is extreme (running away) or the adolescent is in crisis (threatening suicide). In these situations, the adolescent does not care about positive rewards. Instead, either the teenager is hoping to regain or maintain a position of authority, or he or she is in the middle of a crisis. Consequently, the counselor must take charge and design a consequence with the parents that is severe enough to stop the extreme behavior or stabilize the current crisis. These strategies are discussed in detail in Chapter 6.

The Art of Creating Effective Consequences

Parents must also be taught the art of constructing creative and effective consequences. The counselor must tell the parents that the number and range of consequences that make a difference to teenagers decrease dramatically as they enter adolescence. A 9-year-old child responds to numerous consequences, but by 12 years of age the range of effective consequences becomes smaller and smaller. As a result, the counselor must brainstorm with the parents all the possible consequences that matter to their particular teenager. These custom-fit consequences are then written down and ranked from most to least effective. Parents are told that the top eight consequences for most teenagers concern the following: (1) money; (2) cars, driving privileges, and parental transportation; (3) telephone privileges; (4) clothing; (5) freedom; (6) loosening of restrictions; (7) going out; and (8) being treated like an adult. The counselor then gives each parent a handout (Figure 4.4) listing nine rules of thumb for constructing effective consequences.

Rule 1: Make a List of Both Positive and Negative Consequences. Parents are asked to take each rule on their list and write both a positive consequence (what happens if the rule is consistently followed) and a negative consequence (what happens if the rule is broken). For example, if the rule is that household chores must be completed by 6 P.M., then consequences involving telephone use can be both a negative (phone privileges are taken away the next day if chores are not completed) and positive (the adolescent gets an extra half-hour of phone time if all the chores are completed by 6 P.M.). If

1. Make a list of both positive and negative consequences.
2. Give a reward immediately after the desired behavior occurs.
3. Do not allow the teenager to take rewards for granted.
4. Keep consequences straightforward and manageable.
5. Make consequences helpful.
6. "Highball" or "lowball" the adolescent.
7. Establish a hierarchy of consequences.
8. Look for positive behaviors and traits.
9. Be patient and endure.

FIGURE 4.4. Parent handout: Nine rules of thumb for constructing effective consequences. From *Treating the Tough Adolescent* by Scott P. Sells. Copyright 1998 by The Guilford Press. Permission to photocopy this handout is granted to purchasers of *Treating the Tough Adolescent* for personal use only (see copyright page for details).

phone use is set for a reasonable period of time to begin with, increasing that time by a half-hour is not inconvenient for the parents and can motivate the adolescent to complete the chores in a timely fashion. This same formula can be used for other consequences as well. If the consequences involve car use, this can be increased or limited, depending on the rule and the severity of any infractions. The counselor can teach the parents how to vary the type and degree of consequences according to their teenager's behavior.

Rule 2: Give a Reward Immediately after the Desired Behavior Occurs. The counselor must inform the parents that a reward's effectiveness is based on how closely it follows the desired behavior. As stated in Chapter 2, adolescents are impulsive and are governed by the pleasure principle, or whatever seems or feels good at the moment. Consequently, they cannot see beyond the next day, let alone the next week. For example, if the problem is chronic truancy, the teenager will have a difficult time maintaining a week of perfect attendance. However, the parents can tell their teenager that for every day of school attendance, he or she will receive an immediate 1-day reduction off each week of grounding. If the reward is immediately attainable, the probability of success in following the rule is increased. Negative consequences do not have to be immediately enforced after a rule is violated.

Rule 3: Do Not Allow the Teenager to Take Rewards for Granted. The counselor should tell the parents that if their teenager takes a reward for granted by never being satisfied or expecting more, they can remove the rewards for a particular rule until the adolescent can consistently follow that rule. The parents can specify a time limit for this to happen, or can decide for themselves when the time is right and inform their teenager at that time. The negative consequences will remain intact, but instead of material rewards, the adolescent will be praised for coming close to following the rule on a consistent basis. Something nice and unexpected may be done to celebrate that the rule has been followed (dinner, a movie, etc.). Parents are cautioned that they do not have to reward the following of every rule; they can experiment with different combinations until they hit upon the right formula for their particular teenager.

Rule 4: Keep Consequences Straightforward and Manageable. For consequences to be effective, they must not be elaborate or harder for the parents to enforce than for the teenager to obey. For example, one parent had five different consequences for one rule, and another parent grounded his teenager for 2 months at a time. In both cases, not only were the consequences unmanageable and unrealistic, but they were also very difficult to monitor and administer. In the second case, if the father had to be home every weekend for 2 months, the consequence would have been harder on him than on the adolescent. In turn, such consequences breed resentment and bitterness between parents and teenager. To counter this problem, the counselor should advise parents to implement only one or two consequences for each rule and to enforce them when it is convenient for them.

CLINICAL EXAMPLE

A single parent grounded her 13-year-old son, Darryl, during the week for missing school. However, she was unable to monitor him because she had to work at the time he came home from school. As a result, Darryl would leave home immediately after school, and the mother had stomach problems all day worrying about whether Darryl was leaving home without permission. Therefore, the consequence was changed to grounding on 1 weekend day and evening for each missed school day. If more school days were missed during that same week, the consequence was postponed until the following weekend.

In this way, the mother could enforce this consequence at a time when it was convenient for her, while at the same time making a bigger impact on Darryl. In addition, the mother needed Sunday as a day of rest and rejuvenation, so a consequence was not given on this day.

In this example, the consequence was enforced when it was convenient for the parent. In addition, the mother kept the consequence simple and manageable: Darryl was grounded on a 1:1 ratio—1 day of grounding on a Saturday for each day of school missed. Simplicity and convenience are keys to the success of consequences.

Rule 5: Make Consequences Helpful. Typically, when a teenager breaks a rule, the consequence is negative and does not benefit either the parent or the teenager. It is simply a punishment designed to increase the probability that the same rule will not be broken again. However, if the consequence is written so that it helps another person and/or the teenager, it can build the teenager's character and value system while simultaneously decreasing the likelihood that the rule will be broken in the future. For example, a teenager who damages property or steals from another person has inflicted trauma or pain on that person. However, it is often more beneficial for both the teenager and the injured party if the adolescent makes reparation instead of going to jail. Reparation can take the form of getting a job or earning extra money at home to pay the victim back for damages or emotional pain. Even though reparation is mostly symbolic. It is important that the adolescent do something beneficial for the victim that involves long-term sacrifice. This will help ensure that the adolescent will not forget what happened and will not commit the same offense again. In addition, it will help the adolescent to heal, because good deeds can help one forgive oneself.

Similarly, this method can be used for other infractions. While an adolescent is grounded for missing school or breaking curfew, he or she can be required to do volunteer work at a homeless shelter or a retirement home. The consequence will help others while helping the teenager grow and mature.

Rule 6: "Highball" or "Lowball" the Adolescent. The sixth rule of thumb allows the adolescent to feel that he or she has won, when in actuality it is the parents who come out on top. When a customer goes to buy a new car, the salesperson usually quotes a high price, and the customer negotiates to bring the price down. The customer walks away feeling that he or she has gotten a great deal and bested the salesperson. However, little does the customer know that the price he or she has paid is still higher than what the car is worth or what the salesperson may have been willing to sell the car for. The salesperson just started the bidding at an inflated or "highball" rate. Dropping the price is merely a psychological ploy to make the customer think that he or she is getting a better deal. Parents can similarly "lowball" consequences with their teenager—beginning the negotiation by restricting all privileges, and ending by offering some as a sign of good faith. The teenager walks away thinking that he or she has gotten the best of the parents, when in actuality they may have been willing to concede much more.

CLINICAL EXAMPLE

The parents of 14-year-old Rob were coached to "lowball" him by stating that curfew would be 8 P.M. on weekends. After much debate, Rob countered with 11 P.M. and the parents in turn offered 9 P.M. Rob then settled for 9:30 P.M. and felt that he got the better of his parents, even though they were originally prepared to go up to 10 P.M.

This same procedure can work for other consequences (chores, grounding, loss of car, etc.). The parents can either "highball" or "lowball" the teenager and allow the teen to believe that he or she has won; this increases the chances of compliance.

Rule 7: Establish a Hierarchy of Consequences. A hierarchy of consequences is a particularly effective approach if the adolescent engages in the same misbehavior many times during the day or throughout the week. Consequences can get more severe if the teenager is disrespectful and refuses to cooperate several times on a single day, or breaks curfew or misses school several times during the same week.

For example, a teenager who refuses to follow directions can first be given a verbal warning. If the behavior continues, the teen is placed in the bathroom for 15 minutes of time out. If the teen keeps refusing to follow directions, time out is increased to 30 minutes, 45 minutes, and so on. Similarly, if a teenager misses school, the first offense may be grounding the next day plus one weekend day and evening. However, if it happens again the same week, one or both parents will attend school and sit next to the teenager. The teenager may also be fined $5 for every hour the parents have to take off work to sit with their son in class. In this way, the consequence starts out small, but gets more and more severe until the problem behavior stops.

Rule 8: Look for Positive Behaviors and Traits. While consequences are being initiated and implemented, it is critical that the counselor explain the importance of looking for positive behaviors or personality traits in the adolescent. Before coming to counseling, parents and adolescents often no longer like each other and focus only on the negative. However, by doing this, the parents unknowingly reinforce the very behaviors or traits they want stopped. Parents are therefore asked to keep an imaginary giant magnifying glass in their back pocket at all times, and to take it out regularly during the week between each counseling session to find positive things about what their teenager is saying or doing.

If the negative trend is not reversed, consequences will only have a temporary impact. After counseling is completed, a family has a tendency in times of stress to revert to previous communication patterns. The counselor must therefore educate parents about this likelihood by pretending to be the teenager while the parents practice looking for and focusing on anything positive about a behavior or personality trait. (This is done without the teenager present in the room.) Through these role plays, the counselor can locate potential problems and correct them before the teenager is subjected to more negative criticism. A more detailed discussion of this topic is provided in Chapter 7.

CLINICAL EXAMPLE

Sixteen-year-old Janet was a chronic runaway. One of the primary reasons for this behavior was the fact that her mother was extremely harsh, punitive, and critical. The mother maintained that she could be positive any time she wanted. However, during the role play, every attempted compliment was coupled with a "but" statement that contained a negative criticism. This criticism completely negated the previous compliment. The counselor was able to identify this problem and help the mother correct it. This subtle but important change greatly improved the mother–daughter relationship and contributed to stopping the runaway behavior.

Rule 9: Be Patient and Endure. Counselors must forewarn parents that many consequences will have to be implemented on a trial-and-error basis until the right combination is found. If the consequence appears to be ineffective, the rule of thumb is to wait at least 1 or 2 weeks before switching. This is because the adolescent may "play possum" by intentionally trying to make the parents believe that the consequence is not effective. Parents must also be warned that things will usually get worse before they get better. As soon as the parents start using consequences that work, it will seem like trying to saddle a wild stallion. The adolescent will fight, resist, and do everything possible to get the parents to give up. Parents have to be told that they must endure this until the adolescent, like the wild stallion, gets used to being controlled and calms down. Once this happens, there will be green pastures ahead: The adolescent will begin to feel secure and even at peace, once there is clarity about family roles and the parents maintain their position of authority. However, for this to happen, the parents must not let go of the reins until the worst is over.

Parents will need much support and guidance through these trying times. Therefore, the counselor must be willing to go the distance with such a family and be on call 24 hours a day, 7 days a week until the crisis has passed and the consequences are effective. This includes home visits and meeting on weekends. Hence, the counselor's commitment and availability become the fulcrum of the therapeutic process. If the family members do not have the counselor's 24-hour-a-day support, they are likely to feel lost and alone. The tide will often turn simply because both the parents and the counselor are more stubborn than the adolescent and refuse to give up and be defeated.

Strategy 4: Putting the Written Contract Together

Once these nine rules of thumb are explained, the counselor asks the parents to list the consequences under each rule to create their first written contract. They are told that this first contract is a working document and can be refined if there are unanticipated glitches. However, this contract should remain the primary document from which to develop future agreements. The counselor works in close collaboration with the parents to develop this contract before the teenager is brought into the process.

It is extremely important for the parents, *not* the counselor, to come up with both rules and consequences. Otherwise, if the rules or consequences are ineffective, then the parents can easily blame the counselor instead of themselves or their teenager. On the other hand, if the interventions are effective, parents can become dependent on the counselor instead of relying on their own abilities. The counselor should ideally serve as a sounding board by offering possible suggestions and providing a template to follow while the parents fill in the fine details.

CLINICAL EXAMPLE

A single mother was trying to come up with rules and consequences to eliminate 12-year-old Vinnie's disrespectful behavior. However, the counselor made the mistake of telling the mother what behaviors he thought were disrespectful, rather than asking the mother how she would define "disrespect" in her particular household.

COUNSELOR: So what does Vinnie do that's disrespectful?

MOTHER: I'm not sure.

COUNSELOR: Well, here are some things I see. He swears at you, doesn't do as he is told, and yells at your boyfriend.

MOTHER: I guess you're right.

Instead of giving the mother a chance to figure out what disrespectful behavior meant to her, the counselor took charge much too soon and defined the behavior for her. This undermined the mother's "expert status" and threatened her ability to take charge. If the counselor had gone on doing this, the mother might have felt relieved that the counselor was doing all the work for her, but in the long term she might have deferred to the counselor as the expert instead of struggling with the difficult process of defining rules and consequences.

The counselor in this case made another mistake by outlining for the mother what the consequences would be for disrespectful behavior in the future. He explained the time-out procedures and had the mother write them in a contract format. Again, the problem was that the counselor was deciding the best course of action for treating Vinnie without the mother's input. This could have been a lose–lose situation: If the procedure worked, the mother would have become dependent on the counselor; if it failed, the mother would have left counseling or felt more hopeless. However, after supervision, the counselor was able to come back to the mother before the session ended and do some damage control. The counselor redefined his role as that of a coach and the mother's as that of the expert. After the counselor provided the opportunity, the mother was able to communicate her expertise and personal knowledge of what consequences would mean the most to her child.

COUNSELOR: I want to apologize for jumping the gun a bit. I came up with the consequence of time out before I even asked what you thought would work best for Vinnie.

MOTHER: Thanks for saying that. I was feeling a little overwhelmed. Yeah, I was thinking that before we go to time out, maybe I could try taking his candy away for a day when he is disrespectful. I know it may sound strange, but Vinnie really loves candy and would just die if I took it away.

COUNSELOR: Sounds like a winner. I was just wondering if you could take me step by step through how you would take away his candy. Would you give him a warning first and then take it away? Would it be all of his candy, or just some of it? What if he refuses to give it up? What is Plan B if that happens?

Note how the counselor provided a directional outline that allowed the mother the means to construct a clear, concrete plan of action that would custom-fit her family's needs rather than the counselor's.

In sum, the counselor's goal is to provide direction and help the parent formulate clear rules and consequences for up to three behaviors at a time. The counselor is active in defining rules and consequences only if the teenager exhibits extreme behaviors such as chronic running away, chronic truancy, suicidal threats, or violence. Under these circumstances, there is no time for exploration. The counselor must give the parents specific consequences to stop the behavior so that they can maintain their authority long enough to bring about lasting change. However, whenever possible, the counselor still incorporates ideas from the parents into the treatment plan and remains knowledgeable about their strengths and limitations.

Working within this framework, the counselor provides the parents with a handout (Figure 4.5) that is a template for designing a contract, and refers to this handout with the parents as the contract is put together. Please note how each consequence relates directly to the rule broken. It is also important to note that not all consequences must contain positive and negative aspects; this depends on the particular rule and what the parents feel will work best with their particular teenager.

Strategy 5: Incorporating the Adolescent's Expertise

After the initial contract is written, the counselor should invite the adolescent back into the room to incorporate the adolescent's expertise into the determination of effective consequences. Both counselors and parents are

Rule 1	(Son will not go to school) Beginning Monday, John will ride the bus at 8 A.M. and attend school every day. This includes every class period with no tardies, unless there is a medical emergency that requires John to be taken to the doctor's office. The parents will determine this and will contact the attendance officer each morning to monitor John's attendance.
Consequence A	If it is discovered that John did not attend school, was tardy, or missed even one class, the following consequences will occur: *First offense*: John will be grounded the next day plus 1 weekend day and evening. This means no phone calls, no TV, and no friends over. *Second offense*: Mother or father will attend school and sit next to John in as many classes as possible the first available day either parent can get time off from work. John will be fined $5 for every hour a parent has to take off work to sit with him in class.
Consequence B	Each day that it is determined from the attendance officer that John has abided by Rule 1, he can have 1 extra hour of phone time.
Rule 2	(Son will not come home on time for curfew) John's curfew time will be 5 P.M. on school nights (Sunday through Thursday) and 9 P.M. on weekends (Friday and Saturday). If John returns even 1 minute past curfew, he will be considered late. These times will not be changed or altered until the parents decide otherwise. Therefore, John's trying to change them on his own also breaks this rule.
Consequence A	For every night John is late, he will be grounded the next day plus the next weekend night. If he is late again that same week, the same thing happens. If he runs out of weekend nights, then the grounding will be postponed to the next weekend. If John happens to be grounded for breaking curfew on the same day he is grounded for missing school, one of the days will be postponed until the next available date.
Consequence B	If John comes home on time, he will receive 1 hour added to his curfew time the next night. If the next night is a school night, the temporary curfew will be 6 P.M., and if it is a weekend night, it will be 10 P.M..
Rule 3	(Son is disrespectful through the following behaviors: Swearing, lying, not following directions) John's behavior will be considered disrespectful if he does one or more of the following: (a) Swears or uses obscene gestures such as giving the finger. (b) Tells a lie (and it is proven that he told a lie as determined by a parent). (c) Refuses to complete a task (homework, chores, etc.) even after one warning is given.
Consequence A	If John is disrespectful, he will be given a verbal count of 3 to stop swearing, tell the truth, or complete the task. If he refuses, he will be escorted to the bathroom for a time out. For the first offense, he must stay in time out 15 minutes. Each additional offense on the same day will result in a 15-minute addition to the penalty. John will begin each day back at 15 minutes. The timer does not start until he is quiet. His total time is cut in half if he goes to the time-out area on his own and quietly completes his time.

Please note: We as parents reserve the right to change both rules and consequences within this contract, and we will give prior notice if and when this occurs.

FIGURE 4.5. Parent handout: Example of a written contract. From *Treating the Tough Adolescent* by Scott P. Sells. Copyright 1998 by The Guilford Press. Permission to photocopy this handout is granted to purchasers of *Treating the Tough Adolescent* for personal use only (see copyright page for details).

often surprised to realize that many adolescents can clearly define what consequences work best for them. They only have to be asked the right questions.

CLINICAL EXAMPLE

Thirteen-year-old Matt had diabetes but would constantly eat too much sugar, putting himself at risk of a diabetic coma. The father tried all kinds of negative consequences for this behavior, but was unsuccessful in stopping the problem. The father then asked Matt to think of the worst punishment he could imagine. Matt responded by stating that for the first offense, he should be required to pick up stones in the backyard for 1 hour in the hot sun. Each additional offense would add another hour to his time picking up stones. This would continue until Matt stopped eating too much sugar. The father agreed to try this, and the behavior quickly ended.

Rarely are adolescents asked for their opinions in the course of treatment; instead, they are told what they can and cannot do. Developmentally, adolescents have an emotional need to feel important and validated as they struggle to form their own identities and to separate from their families. By incorporating the adolescent's expertise, parents are addressing this developmental need while at the same time encouraging cooperation. When adolescents have shared ownership in a plan of action, they have a greater investment in adhering to the plan.

Techniques for Eliciting the Adolescent's Views on Consequences

Parents are told that they are still in charge and therefore have final approval of the contract. The parents inform their teenager of this fact before they begin discussing the contract, so that the teenager is not surprised or resentful if some of his or her own consequences are not incorporated. After this stipulation is presented, the parents try to elicit possible consequences from the adolescent. The counselor can give the parents this sample script to follow:

> "[Teenager's name], before we finalize a contract of consequences for the rules we are putting down, we want to ask you a couple of questions for your expert opinion about what might work best for you. However, while we want your opinion and will try to include your ideas, we as parents will decide what ultimately gets put into the final draft."

The parents then ask these questions:

1. "If you could stop this problem [name the specific problem] tomorrow, what positive consequences or rewards do you think would help end the problem or decrease it?"
2. "If you could stop this problem [name the specific problem] tomorrow, what negative consequences or punishments do you think would be in place to end the problem or decrease it?"
3. "What would you say is the single worst punishment that would stop you in your tracks or slow you down if you broke this rule [name the specific rule]?"

If the adolescent says "I don't know" in response to each question, the parents or counselor can ask the adolescent to "guess." Most adolescents will be able to come up with something. If the adolescent is unwilling to guess, the parents can throw out possible answers that will require the adolescent either to refute or to agree with their statements. This gets the adolescent talking and the momentum started. The following session excerpt will help clarify this process.

CLINICAL EXAMPLE

PARENT: Michael, to make you stop missing school beginning tomorrow, what punishment would be in place to end this problem or even slow it down? [The parent used a hypothetical solution-focused question to help Michael formulate an idea of what punishment would best fit him.]

MICHAEL: I don't know.

PARENT: Let's say you did know. What would you say might work? [The parent was asking the son to guess, in such a way that it would be hard for him not to try at least.]

MICHAEL: Mmmm . . . still have no clue.

PARENT: Let me guess. . . . How about having your stereo taken away for 6 months? [The parent purposely went overboard or "highballed" the consequence to entice the son to disagree vehemently with something so harsh, and thus force him to come up with a better solution.]

MICHAEL: Are you kidding me?! Maybe a week, but that's it. You know how I love my music. [Michael took the bait and unknowingly produced a custom-fit consequence that would work for him.]

PARENT: I don't know. Maybe 2 weeks? [The parent had been coached by the counselor to resist and continue with the "highball" strategy. This would allow the teenager to feel that he had ultimately achieved a real victory.]

MICHAEL: Hey, come on. Give me a break. One week is plenty. [The teenager became even more invested in the process.]

PARENT: OK. I will write it in the contract and we'll try it. Let me read this back to you, then. For every day the attendance officer reports that you miss school from this point on, including tardies, skipping a class, and so forth, you will lose your stereo privileges for 1 week. [The parents showed Michael that they were incorporating his idea into the contract, while summarizing in very specific terms how the rule would be enforced. Again, this allowed Michael to feel that he had achieved a victory over the parents, and it promoted the spirit of collaboration.]

MICHAEL: Sounds fair to me. [Adolescents value fairness, so if they think that a rule and consequence are fair, the likelihood that the rule will be followed increases dramatically.]

It is important to note that the parents had already prepared a set of written consequences before beginning these collaborative discussions. The adolescent was in the other room and had no idea what was initially contained within the contract. As a result, the parents, with the counselor's coaching, could take the conversation in a direction that allowed Michael to feel that he not only created his own consequences (both positive and negative), but won the battle with his parents.

Parents can role-play this technique before the adolescent enters the room, with the counselor playing the part of the adolescent, so that the parents can practice and fine-tune their delivery. This "dry run" is the dress rehearsal before the actual performance with the teenager present. A detailed discussion of this technique can be found in Chapter 5.

Parental Concerns

Parents may voice two concerns about this strategy. First, they may think that the adolescent will intentionally come up with the easiest possible consequences so that he or she can continue to break the rules. The counselor must point out to the parents that they are the judge and jury of the final set of consequences, not the adolescent. In addition, the parents can direct the conversation by intentionally "highballing" or "lowballing" the teenager with consequences they predetermine.

Second, parents may feel that this technique is a form of manipulation. The counselor can counter this claim by reminding the parents that this strategy not only mirrors real life but promotes the teenager's ownership of the consequences. The perceived victory will only increase the likelihood that the contract will be followed without future resistance.

Encouraging the Adolescent to Set Goals for Counseling

After consequences are discussed, the counselor and parents should take some time to encourage the adolescent to set his or her own goals for counseling. This often identifies previous conditions or periods of time in which the problem did not exist or was less prevalent.

The following solution-focused questions can be used by counselors and parents as a possible template:

1. If I followed you around with my video camera for the next week when you were on top of this problem, what would I see you doing when I played back the tape? How would it be different from what happened when the problem was in charge of you?
2. I need your help with something. I'm worried/concerned about [name the problem] and I know you are not happy with it either. How would you like things to go?
3. When was the last time you were able to make things the way you wanted them to be? Let's go back to times when the problem did not occur. Can you remember? I recall [parents come up with some examples to get the conversation started] . . . when you were able to . . . [examples of times the behavior stopped or lessened in severity]. (Metcalf, 1997, p. 54)

Each of these questions encourages the participation and collaboration of the adolescent in designing a customized treatment plan. When the teenager is allowed to set goals and to identify times when the problem did not exist, the probability of treatment success increases. In some cases, however, teen goal setting is unrealistic. The adolescent's behavior may be so extreme that until it is stopped or improved, the idea of future goals becomes difficult to address. When this happens, these severe behavior problems take priority and must be solved before other goals can be attempted.

Strategy 6: Facilitating Parental Consistency in Following Through

Before this process of determining rules and consequences is complete, the counselor should emphasize to the parents the importance of consistency in following through on a contract. The adolescent should not be present while the counselor covers this issue, since it would be detrimental for the adolescent to learn how the parents could be inconsistent. This would only serve to disempower the parents further or cause them to "lose face" by focusing a spotlight on their weaknesses.

For each rule and consequence, the counselor shows the parents how they could follow through either consistently or inconsistently. The counselor can use as an example something many parents do: saying "no" at first and then changing to "yes" for a particular reason, such as pouting or nagging by the teenager. This inconsistency gives the teenager the message that the parents can be manipulated. A counselor cannot assume that parents will follow a rule or consequence just because it is written and operationalized. Instead, the counselor must help the parents recognize their own inconsistent behaviors and collaborate to develop possible solutions. The counselor can give the parents the following "golden rule" to put on their bathroom mirror to look at before starting each day:

> "Do not say anything to your teen that you can't do or don't want to do, and do everything you say you are going to do."

Parents are also given a handout (Figure 4.6) listing the six potential pitfalls they should avoid when putting their contract into action.

Pitfall 1: Empty Statements

Parents can be coached not to say things that they cannot or do not intend to carry out (e.g., "I won't give you any money until you get a job," or "If you do not straighten up, pack your bags and leave"). Parents are encouraged to provide concrete examples of when they made empty statements in the past and of how this limited their effectiveness.

Pitfall 2: Overstatements

Overstatements often result when parents get angry and come up with a consequence that is too extreme (e.g., "You are grounded for 6 months," or "You cannot talk on the phone the rest of the school year"). The parents feel that they either have to save face and follow through with the stated consequence, or back-pedal and forget about what was said. Either way, the parents are disempowered. If they enforce the consequence, it will surely fail because it will be too difficult to follow and enforce. If they do not enforce the consequences, the adolescent will perceive them as being inconsistent.

---

1. Empty statements.
2. Overstatements.
3. Changing "no" to "yes" and "yes" to "no."
4. Not checking up on behavior.
5. Lack of one parental voice.
6. Different reactions to the same behavior.

FIGURE 4.6. Parent handout: Six potential pitfalls to avoid in following through on a contract. From *Treating the Tough Adolescent* by Scott P. Sells. Copyright 1998 by The Guilford Press. Permission to photocopy this handout is granted to purchasers of *Treating the Tough Adolescent* for personal use only (see copyright page for details).

Pitfall 3: Changing "No" to "Yes" and "Yes" to "No"

The first form of the third common pitfall occurs when parents say "no," but change their "no" to a "yes" after the adolescent harasses or irritates them long enough. This change gives the adolescent a clear message that the parents will give up their authority if pressure or harassment can be applied long enough. In contrast, if the parents tell the adolescent "yes" and then change it to a "no," this can send a clear message to the teenager that the parents cannot be trusted. When parents understand the possible long-term implication of these actions, they may be less likely to repeat either form of this particular error.

Pitfall 4: Not Checking Up on Behavior

Parents often tell their teenager to do something, but then do not check to see whether the task has been done. For example, parents may ask their daughter to clean her room. The next day the parents notice that the bedroom is not clean and yell at their daughter. This not only demonstrates inconsistency but also creates resentment, as the teenager gets in trouble because of a request that the parents failed to follow up on when originally issued.

Pitfall 5: Lack of One Parental Voice

In many cases, one parent may have a different parenting philosophy from the other. As a result, one parent may not check with the other before giving out punishments, or one may be consistent and the other may not be. If this type of discord exists, the counselor must give each parent concrete examples of how the adolescent will use these differences to play one parent off against the other. When this inconsistency is the result of underlying marital conflict, it is up to the counselor to convince the parents to put aside their differences temporarily to solve the teenager's problem. If this does not work, the counselor may have to suggest marital counseling in addition to the ongoing family counseling. (See Strategy 7, below.)

Pitfall 6: Different Reactions to the Same Behavior

A final type of parental inconsistency is treating the same behavior in different ways, depending on their particular moods. For instance, one day parents may lecture their son for not doing his chores, while the next day they may ignore it or ground him for the same behavior.

Once each pitfall is identified, the counselor asks the parents to write down how a particular pitfall occurs. This kind of self-monitoring helps the parents to identify where inconsistency problems exist and to decrease their occurrence. The counselor must reassure the parents that this assignment is not intended to criticize or judge their efforts. Instead, it is a way to determine whether there are areas that can be strengthened or improved over time.

CLINICAL EXAMPLE

The parents of 12-year-old Maya did not realize that they were consistently making overstatements whenever they became angry or extremely irritated. However, when they did the homework assignment, they realized that they were making overstatements at least three times a day and not following through. Once this was recognized, the parents stopped making overstatements and began to stick more consistently to the terms of the contract. They later reported that there was no longer a need to make overstatements once they consistently followed through on the contract.

Strategy 7: Consideration of Family Dynamics

The strategies described above will have limited effectiveness unless the counselor also understands how family dynamics influence the implementation of rules and consequences. For example, what happens when one parent is bitter toward the other and secretly takes satisfaction in undermining that parent's authority? Or when a single parent is enmeshed with the teenager and unable to get tough? Once rules and consequences become effective, other family dynamics may quickly surface, such as marital problems, alcohol or drug use, or depression. As stated earlier, these problems have a chance to surface because either the adolescent's problems are being solved or the parents are required to exert joint authority to administer the contract.

CLINICAL EXAMPLE

Twelve-year-old Noah was referred to counseling for threatening his mother with a knife, beating up his younger brother, and chronic truancy. Within the first few minutes of the session, it was apparent that there was extreme marital conflict between Noah's parents. Each time the counselor focused the session on setting goals and rules, the parents would start yelling and blaming each other for Noah's problems. As this was happening, Noah looked down at the floor and sank deeper into his seat; this indicated to the counselor that Noah had been at the center of this crossfire for quite some time.

The yelling and name calling got so bad that the counselor had to excuse Noah from the room. After Noah left, the parents reported that they had not slept in the same room for 2 years. The wife reported that they stayed together for economic reasons only. The husband said that the mother "babied" Noah and let him "get away with murder." The only times he was called to help were when Noah was totally out of control and hitting someone. Even then, his wife openly criticized his efforts in front of Noah.

The counselor then made the critical mistake of trying to establish rules and consequences without first addressing the marital problems or the mother's alleged overprotectiveness. As a result, the parents agreed in the office to put aside their differences, but in their subsequent actions they did not abide by this agreement. In the weeks to follow, each parent privately reported that the other was undermining his or her authority. Counseling seemed to only make matters worse. The father wanted to look good in front of the counselor, so he secretly began to tell Noah to come to him if he needed anything or if "Mom was too tough" on him. This behavior only exacerbated the marital problems further and made the mother even more protective of Noah. In response, Noah's behavior worsened, with increased truancy and threats of suicide. Subsequently, the parents told the counselor that therapy was not helping and ended treatment.

This case is a good example of what can happen if a counselor fails to address family dynamics and moves too quickly into contracting. In this example, the marital problems were so prevalent that they spilled over into other family issues. A prerequisite for constructing effective rules and consequences is the parents' ability to exert joint authority. This can only happen if the marital problems are manageable.

A Litmus Test of Parents' Ability to Work Together

On a case-by-case basis, the counselor must determine whether the parents have the ability to put aside their differences for the greater good of solving their teenager's behavioral problem. The parents' actions following the initiation of a contract can be considered a good litmus test of this ability. If the parents (or the teenager) report that the behavior has stayed the same or gotten worse over the course of several weeks, the family may be inadvertently telling the counselor that there are unresolved family dynamics blocking any change.

Even if change initially occurs, the counselor must always be ready to backtrack if a family member blocks change at a later point in the process. The counselor must pause and figure out what the family member is trying to say about an unresolved problem or issue. This problem must be removed or attended to before further change can occur. In some cases this may require breaking up the session into two parts: During the first part, the counselor may see the parents alone to conduct marital counseling, while the second part is devoted to the task of outlining clear rules and consequences. The counselor may even negotiate with the family members to see them twice a week on a time-limited basis, to work through specific family problems that hinder change in the difficult adolescent.

The Need for Respect on the Counselor's Part

It is important to remember that the counselor is an employee of the family, and as such must be respectful at all times. This includes receiving permission before launching into other family issues. The parents are usually initiating counseling to solve their teenager's problem, not their own marital, substance use, or other issues. The latter can only be dealt with after rapport and trust have been established and the counselor receives the family's permission to address the other problems. How quickly this trust and rapport are earned depends on the counselor, the family, and the severity of the particular problems.

Taking a "Wait and See" Stance

The counselor may need to begin with contracting and then take a "wait and see" stance to watch how the family responds. Only then may it be appropriate to hint to the parents privately that other family issues may be preventing change. After this possibility is brought to the table, the counselor will have to sit back and watch for the parents' response. If the parents are in agreement, the counselor can pursue the issue more deeply. If the parents are edgy or resistant, the counselor may need to step back and wait for another opportunity.

CLINICAL EXAMPLE

Sixteen-year-old Cindy was referred to counseling for issues of extreme disrespect. In the course of the first meeting, it was discovered that Cindy had tried to commit suicide on several occasions and had been sexually abused by her natural mother. Cindy was now living with her stepmother and father. The stepmother reported that Cindy's suicide attempts were not serious and only a form of manipulation. The stepmother also felt that since the sexual abuse had happened years ago, Cindy was using it as an excuse to get others to feel sorry for her.

When the counselor set up the contract, the stepmother agreed to try to follow through. However, the next week the stepmother and father reported that the contract had failed miserably. Privately, Cindy told the counselor that the stepmother would tell her to clean her room, but would then sabotage Cindy's efforts by saying that Cindy's room did not meet her standards. In addition, the stepmother yelled at Cindy so much that Cindy felt nothing would ever be good enough. At this point, Cindy "shut down," which only confirmed for the stepmother that this was a hopeless case.

With their actions, the family members were telling the counselor that setting rules and consequences was premature and that a contract could not be set up until the underlying dynamics between the stepmother and Cindy were resolved. In response to the feedback, the counselor asked the stepmother to come on her day off for an individual meeting. The reason given was that the counselor needed to gain insight into just how badly the stepmother had been treated. This meeting went extremely well. First, the stepmother was glad someone was taking the time to hear her side of the story. This helped build rapport with the counselor. Second, she revealed that Cindy was putting a great deal of stress on the marriage. Furthermore, the spouses were having marital problems. Finally, the stepmother reported that she was having bouts of depression and did not know where to turn. The counselor asked whether he could be of any help in these areas, and the stepmother asked to come in for individual counseling once a week. Over time, the husband joined in the counseling to work through marital problems.

As these issues were addressed, trust and rapport continued to build. Rules and consequences suddenly became effective. The stepmother became softer and more understanding with Cindy, who stopped "shutting down" and even began to tell her stepmother that she needed her love and guidance. Over time, the stepmother was able to help Cindy work through some of her sexual abuse issues, and the suicidal behavior stopped permanently.

Besides illustrating the importance of understanding family dynamics, this case also demonstrates that the family-based model is not a rigid set of procedural steps, but a sequence of guidelines to give the counselor a sense of direction. In this example, family issues emerged immediately in the first session, rather than later in Step 12 of the model. Counselors must therefore be innovative enough to rearrange the steps in response to the specific needs of their clients.

TROUBLESHOOTING

Troubleshooting is so important in treating difficult and defiant adolescents that it is highlighted in the family-based model as a separate and distinct step (Step 5). However, this step in practice is inseparable from Step 4, since it is an integral part of the "how to" portion of setting clear rules and consequences. Therefore, it is the last thing to be done before a written contract is initiated.

Taking Teens' Enhanced Social Perception Abilities into Account

As stated earlier, a difficult adolescent is often skillful when it comes to social perception (Keim, 1996). This means that for every rule or consequence initiated, the adolescent has the ability to think ahead and plot strategies to ensure victory.

CLINICAL EXAMPLE

One of 15-year-old Stephen's new rules forbade stealing. Yet soon after the rule was written, Stephen stole a credit card from a teacher's desk. He then used the credit card to buy $2,000 worth of sports equipment through a mail order catalog. After he was caught and brought to juvenile court, the judge asked Stephen why he did it and what he was thinking. Stephen made the following statement:

> "I knew the approximate time each day that the teacher went to the bathroom. I then pretended I was handing in an assignment and got the credit card. I knew I could use a pay phone to order from a catalog and avoid being traced. I then figured out that I could have the package delivered to the porch of a house that was for sale. I told the shipping company to leave the package at the door so that I could go by to pick it up unnoticed."

Stephen causally tossed out this rather complex seven-step process. He reported that he sat at school daydreaming and tested nine different scenarios in his mind before selecting what he thought was the best series of steps to steal the credit card and order merchandise without being caught.

Because of this skill, the counselor and the parents must brainstorm ways the teenager might use his or her social perception skills to unravel the written contract. For every action by the counselor or the parents, there is an equal and opposite reaction by the teenager. The counselor and the parents must anticipate the teenager's reaction and engage in careful preparation beforehand. If they do not, the teenager will win the battle and remain in a position of authority.

CLINICAL EXAMPLE

Neither the counselor nor the parents anticipated how 15-year-old Tiffany would react when a curfew was imposed with the consequence of phone restriction. The counselor failed to prepare the parents for any possible negative reactions when Tiffany was asked to come back in from the waiting room. As a result, when Tiffany heard the rule and consequence, she started swearing and telling her mother that she hated her and would "never speak to her again." The mother then became so flustered that she backed down and left the room crying. The daughter just smiled at the counselor as the mother left the room. The family never returned to counseling.

As in Tiffany's case, the lack of troubleshooting gives adolescents a distinct advantage and enables them to defeat the parents by pushing their buttons through inflammatory statements (e.g., "I hate you," "I will never speak to you again") or other tactics. This throws the parents off track and often causes them to back down and relinquish authority.

Use of Role Plays

To avoid this type of problem, the counselor should use role playing before any rules or consequences are actually initiated. The counselor prepares the parents by describing some of the negative ways in which the adolescent might react when rules and consequences are initiated. The counselor then plays the part of the adolescent and tries to derail the parents in any way possible. If the parents are derailed, the counselor temporarily stops the role play to inform the parents how to get back on track and avoid having their buttons pushed. This technique has been extremely helpful in getting parents ready to battle an adolescent's negative reactions and provocations.

Use of "What If" Scenarios

In addition to role plays, "what if" scenarios are helpful in coaching the parents on troubleshooting techniques. The counselor asks the parents to answer the following three key questions for each rule and consequence on the contract:

1. "What are two or three things that could go wrong with this plan?"
2. "If these two or three things go wrong [name them], what is your backup plan or strategy?"
3. "What do you think your teenager will say or do when this rule and consequence are presented?"

Parents and counselors must go through as many "what if" scenarios as possible before the contract is initiated. The counselor also lets the parents know that he or she is on call 24 hours a day if something unanticipated happens. The rationale for 24-hour-on-call duty is to solve problems as they happen rather than waiting until the next session, when the situation may be beyond repair. If the counselor can convince the parents of reasoning, they will be more likely to call when problems arise.

Two parent handouts (Figures 4.7 and 4.8) are provided to illustrate how "what if" scenarios can be applied to the examples of running away and problems with doing household chores. These handouts are used to educate parents on the thought processes required in troubleshooting and the basic mechanics involved in designing "what if" scenarios.

Using these handouts as guidelines, the parents and counselor then cus-

Fifteen-year-old Tamara ran away each time her parents grounded her or took away her phone privileges. Here are the "what if" scenarios her parents generated after brainstorming with the counselor:

What happens if:
1. Tamara tries to leave after we say she is grounded?
    A. We will physically try to stop her.
    B. However, then she may try to push or strike us.
    C. If that happens, we will dial 911 and state that we have been physically assaulted. If she is arrested, we will not answer the phone when the police call for us to pick her up at the station. Then she may have to stay overnight in detention, in order to get the message of how serious her behavior was.
    D. When Tamara comes home, she will be under 24-hour watch until we feel more comfortable that she is not at risk.
    E. If she tries to leave again, we will repeat the same steps above over again.

2. Tamara gets away from us and leaves?
    A. We will file a missing-person report with the police.
    B. We will post flyers with her picture all over her school the next day and offer a small reward on the flyer for information on her whereabouts.
    C. We will harass her friends' parents and let them know that we will pursue legal action if they are harboring our daughter without permission.

3. Tamara calls us names and starts throwing a temper tantrum at home or when we pick her up from the police station?
    A. We will remain calm and not "pour gasoline on the fire" by shouting or yelling back.
    B. If she continues after one warning to stop, we will simply walk away as we control the mood and flow of the argument and refuse to allow our buttons to be pushed.
    C. If she follows us around the house, we will go to our bedroom and lock the door very calmly.

4. Tamara calls child protective services (CPS) and claims abuse?
    A. We will remain calm and try not to take it personally, as we know she is just trying to do whatever it takes to regain her power.
    B. We will cooperate and realize that the CPS worker is just doing his or her job.
    C. We will contact our counselor to advocate for us.
    D. We will tell our daughter that she can call CPS, but that we are not buckling under this pressure and that we will still be in charge.

FIGURE 4.7. Parent handout: "What if" scenarios for running away. From *Treating the Tough Adolescent* by Scott P. Sells. Copyright 1998 by The Guilford Press. Permission to photocopy this handout is granted to purchasers of *Treating the Tough Adolescent* for personal use only (see copyright page for details).

Sixteen-year-old Kevin's new rule was that his chores must be done by 5:30 P.M. or he would have to pay a $5 fine. Here are the "what if" scenarios his parents generated after brainstorming with the counselor:

What if:
1. Kevin refuses to give us any money he may owe us at the end of the week or does not have the money?
    A. We tell him ahead of time that if this happens, we will confiscate his personal property (whether he paid for it or not) and hold on to it for 7 days. If at the end of 7 days the debt is still not paid, we will pawn enough items to equal the amount of money owed. If Kevin wants his things back, he will have to go to the pawn shop and buy them back, plus pay whatever interest is owed. We will not replace any items that are pawned.
    B. If Kevin runs out of items, then his car will be impounded at $5 per day with its distributor cap removed until the money and the impound fees are paid.

---

2. Kevin is late completing the chores?
    A. Kevin is told ahead of time that official time is kept by the kitchen clock, and that completing the chores even 1 minute past 5:30 P.M. will incur a fine of $5 unless he has documentation of a medical emergency, evidence that the car or bus broke down, or a note from his boss saying Kevin had to work late. The burden of proof lies with Kevin, not us.

---

3. Kevin completes the chores before the deadline, but they are only partially done or not done well?
    A. Kevin will be told ahead of time that chores must be done to our satisfaction. We will describe to him what our expectations are for each chore. If those standards are not met, we will give Kevin one warning and tell him specifically what needs to be done to complete each chore to our satisfaction. If the chores are not done to our satisfaction on the second try, the fine will be enforced.

FIGURE 4.8. Parent handout: "What if" scenarios for problems with doing household chores. From *Treating the Tough Adolescent* by Scott P. Sells. Copyright 1998 by The Guilford Press. Permission to photocopy this handout is granted to purchasers of *Treating the Tough Adolescent* for personal use only (see copyright page for details).

tom-design their own "what if" scenarios for the teenager. The counselor should not wait until the last 10–15 minutes of the session to start this troubleshooting process. If time is running out, he or she should ask the parents to bring the contract to the next meeting but keep it out of the adolescent's sight. The counselor should explain to the parents that the contract cannot be implemented until troubleshooting has been fully discussed. If the contract is initiated without adequate preparation, more harm than good can be done, and the adolescent may easily defeat the plan before it has a chance to succeed.

SUMMARY

Setting clear rules and consequences is not only the basic work of therapy, but also the foundation for all subsequent treatment steps. For example, parents cannot regain their authority unless they can respond more appropriately to confrontations and provocations. This can only be accomplished when rules are clearly stated and consequences are determined before a particular rule is broken.

In addition, a difficult adolescent has enhanced social perception abilities and can easily think several steps ahead to outmaneuver the parents and render seemingly effective rules and consequences futile. Therefore, the counselor must engage in troubleshooting—that is, anticipate problems with the parents beforehand, and utilize "what if" scenarios and role plays to plan strategies to neutralize future difficulties.

The following is a summary of the major points contained within this chapter:

1. Counselors must understand that every great battle is won before the first shot is ever fired; victory depends on thorough preparation beforehand. Therefore, the key is to establish clear rules and consequences in a written contract format before the treatment begins.

2. Before rules and consequences can be determined, a counselor must help parents prioritize the behaviors needing the most improvement. Parents are taught to ask themselves key questions, such as "Is this behavior really important?" and "Could I let this behavior go for now?" Parents must realize that if they try to confront every behavior, they will burn out more easily, and the adolescent will defeat them.

3. Parents must understand that a difficult adolescent is extremely literal and must have rules and consequences clearly written down beforehand. If this does not happen, the chances for provocations and confrontations increase as the parents try to think "off the cuff" and justify their actions. Unfortunately, the longer the argument goes on, the greater the chances are that both parents and teenager will lose emotional control.

4. Parents must limit their rules to no more than three at a time. In this way, the family members can address important issues without becoming overwhelmed by too many rules at one time.

5. Whenever possible, it is important to establish for each rule a negative consequence for noncompliance and a positive consequence for adher-

ence. This mirrors the real world and avoids a strictly negative focus. Exceptions to this principle are made for extreme behaviors, such as running away, chronic truancy, suicide threats, or violence. In these cases, negative consequences must be used alone to stop the extreme behaviors before positive consequences can be implemented with the desired impact.

6. Counselors must model patience. Parents need to understand that the treatment process will be trial-and-error experimentation until they hit on the right combination of rules and consequences. If a consequence does not seem to be working, a good rule of thumb is to wait at least 1 to 2 weeks before switching to new ones. Consequences must be given time to "kick in."

7. Initially, an adolescent should not be in the room when parents are struggling to write their first working contract of rules and consequences. This is because the adolescent will often argue, complain, and demand numerous explanations. This interference can throw parents off track and prevent them from completing the initial contract. After the preliminary contract is drafted, the adolescent is then invited back into the room to provide his or her expertise. However, it must be clear that the parents are still in charge and therefore have the final word on what will be in the final contract.

8. The counselor's strategies will have limited effectiveness unless he or she also understands how family dynamics influence the implementation of rules and consequences. In addition, as rules and consequences become effective, other family problems may quickly surface.

9. Troubleshooting is an underutilized but critical step in treatment effectiveness. After the parents establish rules and consequences, the counselor must coach them to determine at least two or three things that could go wrong with their plan, to develop a backup plan, and to anticipate their teenager's reactions when each rule and consequence are presented. Counselors and parents must anticipate all the possible things that adolescents might say or do in reaction to new rules and consequences.

10. After the rules and consequences are written and implemented, the counselor should keep the contract on file and go over the contract again at the beginning of each session. This is done to ensure that the contract is followed and that there are no problems. This is a critical procedure in the overall therapeutic process.

CHAPTER 5

Changing the Timing and Process of Confrontations

Parents and adolescents perceive confrontation differently. Parents are outcome-oriented; they only care about the end result (i.e., rules followed and consequences obeyed). Difficult adolescents are process-oriented; they are concerned with controlling the mood or direction of the argument itself—that is, pushing the parents "buttons" or "hot spots" so that they will lose control of their emotions and their ability to enforce rules.

CLINICAL EXAMPLE

Fifteen-year-old Latisha would yell each time her parents enforced the rule of not going out on school nights. The parents got so upset by the yelling and screaming that they lost control of their emotions and got into a bitter argument. In turn, they became so frustrated that they gave in and let Latisha leave. Latisha thus proved that she could skillfully use the tactic of yelling to change her parents' mood and control the direction of the argument.

Rules and consequences may look good on paper, but they are ineffective unless parents are first shown how their buttons are pushed and then taught techniques for responding to conflicts differently. Adolescents are typically more skillful than their parents in the art of confrontation. A counselor must help parents realize that their teenager is not inherently mean or chemically imbalanced, but merely more adept at making use of their vulnerable points. Consequently, parents must learn to "play the game" as well as or better than their teenager—in other words, to change the timing and process of confrontations.

Once the counselor reframes how and why the teenager wins by outmaneuvering the parents, it becomes necessary to show the parents new techniques so that they can outmaneuver their teenager. This is accomplished by means of the following three strategies:

1. Parents are shown how to identify the buttons or hot spots pushed by their teenager and the buttons they push on their teenager during confrontations.
2. Parents are shown how to find examples of when they did not allow their buttons to be pushed and times they did not push their teenager's buttons.
3. Parents are shown how to respond differently by using one or more of the following 11 techniques:

   - Exiting and waiting.
   - Staying short and to the point.
   - Using deflectors.
   - Creating secret signals.
   - Speaking in one parental voice.
   - Asking whether a behavior is relevant.
   - Energizing and recharging.
   - Staying in the present.
   - Separating misbehavior from personal attacks.
   - Restoring good feelings.
   - Understanding the five levels of teenager aggression.

STRATEGY 1: FINDING AND NEUTRALIZING BUTTONS

First, parents must identify through concrete examples all the possible buttons they allow their teenager to push. As defined in Chapter 3, "buttons" are words or actions adolescents use (e.g., "You don't love me") to get the parents to lose control of their emotions and become angry, frustrated, or defensive. The counselor should first see the parents without the adolescent present. The rationale here is that the adolescent is already skilled in this area and may try to sabotage this step if he or she is present.

How Adolescents Push Parental Buttons

To identify the parents' vulnerable points, the counselor asks each the following question:

"If you had big red buttons with names on them all over your body that your teenager pushed to make you lose control of your emotions, what would they be called or look like?"

To make the point clearer, parents can be given the metaphor of a fishing expedition in which the teenager casts a line into the water and says or does something to hook the parents and reel them in. Each parent is then asked to take a few minutes and individually write down all their buttons ("I hate you," "You never let me do what I want," etc.). Each parent is then asked to read them to the counselor and the other parent (if present).

Parents are often surprised to recognize the types of buttons that make them feel angry, defensive, guilty, sad, or manipulated. They usually smile or laugh at this exercise, because they have never thought about confrontation in this way. This change in perception creates flexibility within the parents and empowers them to change their reactions and confrontational styles. The counselor then gives the parents a handout (Figure 5.1) that lists 10 common adolescent button-pushing tactics. These "top 10 tactics" are discussed with the parents as follows:

1. *"You never let me do anything."* This statement invites the parents to point out specific times that they have let the teenager do what he or she wanted. This forces the parents off the real issue at that moment and gives the adolescent the upper hand in the discussion.

2. *"You don't love me."* This statement is intended to induce guilt and make the parents question their self-worth. Unfortunately, many parents take

---

1. "You never let me do anything."

2. "You don't love me."

3. "I hate you" or "You're a liar/asshole/bad parent."

4. "You're not my real mother/father. I don't have to listen to you."

5. A disgusted look, improper gesture, or whiny voice.

6. Finding a parent's most vulnerable area and preying on it.

7. "I'm gonna kill/hurt you/myself/others."

8. "I am gonna lie, lie, lie."

9. "I hate school."

10. "I'm going to leave."

FIGURE 5.1. Parent handout: The top 10 adolescent button-pushing tactics. From *Treating the Tough Adolescent* by Scott P. Sells. Copyright 1998 by The Guilford Press. Permission to photocopy this handout is granted to purchasers of *Treating the Tough Adolescent* for personal use only (see copyright page for details).

this bait instead of recognizing that asking the adolescent to do something he or she does not like has nothing to do with love. Parents often have to administer medicine that may taste bad but is necessary for health.

3. *"I hate you"* or *"You're a liar/asshole/bad parent."* These statements are meant to get the parents to lose their tempers through personal character attacks. This clouds the parents' thought processes and limits their ability to enforce consequences effectively.

4. *"You're not my real mother/father. I don't have to listen to you."* This statement really unnerves stepparents, but it rarely has anything to do with a parent's not being a biological one. It is a merely another tactic designed to get the parent flustered and angry so that the real issue is not addressed.

5. *A disgusted look, improper gesture, or whiny voice.* Body language, gestures, and tones of voice are some of the most powerful tools an adolescent may use to play with parents' emotions. Unfortunately, if the parents respond to these barbs by losing control of their emotions, it gives the adolescent a great deal of power, as he or she now knows how to get under the parents' skins.

6. *Finding a parent's most vulnerable area and preying on it.* Adolescents have an uncanny ability to find the areas that bug their parents the most and to apply pressure to those areas. For example, some adolescents will intentionally keep their rooms messy because of their mother's emphasis on cleanliness. Again, this behavior is not a personal attack, but just a clever way of throwing the parents off balance.

7. *"I'm gonna kill/hurt you/myself/others."* Such statements are meant to scare the parents so that they will back off and remove pressure from the adolescent. Teenagers usually use threats of violence as a last resort when nothing else has worked.

8. *"I am gonna lie, lie, lie."* Parents do not like lying and will often lose control of their emotions quickly when a teenager lies or threatens to do so. Adolescents know that lying is a pet peeve of most parents, and they will play on this peeve so that they can win, win, win.

9. *"I hate school."* Most parents value education, so this statement invites a lecture on how a teenager is throwing away his or her future. Teenagers normally cannot see past tomorrow, so they do not see failing school as a problem in the immediate future. However, they do know that education is important to their parents, and they use this knowledge to their advantage.

10. *"I'm going to leave."* This statement gets parents to back off from exerting their authority, because they fear what might happen if the adolescent runs away and lives on the streets. Adolescents know this and use this statement as another effective tool to keep their parents from taking action or enforcing a rule or consequence.

After reviewing and discussing the handout, parents are asked whether they can add some of these buttons to their original list. Most parents will add some and will begin to realize for the first time just how skillful their teenager has been in knowing what buttons to push.

How Parents Push Adolescents' Buttons

Once the parents' buttons have been reviewed, the counselor explains to the parents that "it takes two to tango." This means that while the adolescent is pushing the parents' buttons, the parents are often pushing the adolescent's buttons at the same time. It is important to help the parents recognize how they help their adolescent lost control of his or her emotions by identifying possible buttons that they push during an argument. The parents should model self-control and control the mood of the argument by not reacting to the adolescent's attack or attacking the teenager's areas of vulnerability.

The parents are asked to brainstorm all the possible buttons that they inadvertently push on their teenager. Parents often have trouble with this exercise; it is easier for them to see how they have been attacked by their teenager than to see how they often unintentionally attack the teenager themselves. The counselor then gives the parents a handout (Figure 5.2) listing eight common parental button-pushing tactics, and discusses these with the parents as follows:

1. *Preaching or using cliches.* As soon as adolescents hear lectures beginning with cliches like "When I was your age," they instantly go deaf. Adolescents do not want to hear how bad they are or how good other family mem-

---

1. Preaching or using cliches.

2. Talking in chapters.

3. Labeling.

4. Futurizing.

5. Instant problem solving.

6. Questioning a teenager's restlessness and discontent.

7. Not tolerating experimental behavior.

8. Collecting criticisms.

FIGURE 5.2. Parent handout: Eight common parental button-pushing tactics. From *Treating the Tough Adolescent* by Scott P. Sells. Copyright 1998 by The Guilford Press. Permission to photocopy this handout is granted to purchasers of *Treating the Tough Adolescent* for personal use only (see copyright page for details).

bers are in comparison. They will usually get angry, walk away, or ignore their parents. In turn, the parents get angry and the argument escalates. The counselor can request that the parents close their eyes and remember a time when their parents gave them lectures. When they have that image in mind, the counselor asks whether the lectures helped them or caused them to "shut down." A majority of parents will say that lecturing did not help in the long run and only made things worse. Parents are reassured with the understanding that it is hard not to lecture when lecturing was role-modeled by their own parents. However, since it did not work for them when they were teenagers, it will probably not work any better with their own children.

2. *Talking in chapters.* Adolescents may ask a short question but not receive as short an answer from the parents. For example, instead of simply saying, "Take out the garbage," parents often talk in chapters and state: "I have told you for weeks and weeks to take the garbage out. How many times do we have to go through this? I am sick and tired. . . ." When this happens, there is a greater chance that an adolescent will become angry; because the long speech contains many negative elements, he or she may feel personally attacked.

3. *Labeling.* Adolescents hate it when parents label them as "always" being this way or that way. This can be an especially dangerous practice, because adolescents will eventually live up to these labels; in other words, they become permanent self-fulfilling prophecies.

4. *Futurizing.* "Futurizing" is parents' talking about their teenagers' future within a negative framework. Typical futurizing statements include "You'll never get into college," "No one will hire you," or "You'll never get a date for the prom with that attitude." Futurizing often results in a teenager's shutting the parents out, as well as in hurt feelings, resentment, and anger.

5. *Instant problem solving.* Adolescents do not want instant understanding and problem solving when they come to their parents with a problem. When troubled by conflicts, teenagers feel different from everyone else; they believe that their emotions are new, personal, and unique. Parents mean well by saying that they understand just how the teenager feels and offering instant solutions, but the teenager's real need is often just to feel listened to.

6. *Questioning the teenager's restlessness and discontent.* Developmentally, adolescence is a time of uncertainty, self-consciousness, moodiness, and suffering. These feelings usually pass over time. However, until they do pass, parents only aggravate the situation when they ask questions such as "What is the matter with you?" and "What has suddenly gotten into you?" These are unanswerable questions for a restless and discontented teenager. Even if he or she did know what the problem was, the teen could not say, "Look, Mom or Dad, I am torn by conflicting emotions, engulfed by irrational urges, and confused by raging hormones." The parents should accept the behavior in the

most supportive but unobtrusive way possible, unless it continues over a prolonged period of time or seems severe.

7. *Not tolerating experimental behavior.* Parents can be shown how to tolerate certain behaviors without accepting them. Changes in clothing and hairstyles are part of a teenager's attempts to find an identity. If the parents constantly focus on these changes rather than simply expressing their disapproval once and letting things work themselves out, the teenager may rebel further, and a power struggle between parents and teenager may ensue. The counselor should encourage parents to save their energy for bigger issues (drug or alcohol use, skipping school, curfew, etc.).

8. *Collecting criticisms.* Insults and criticisms cut deeper when they come from parents. They can damage a teenager's inner spirit and, unlike physical bruises, can often take years to heal. When parents push this type of button by focusing on unpleasant facts about the adolescent's behavior again and again or by pointing out defects, no one benefits. Parents also often keep a mental scorecard handy for rehashing past behavior problems during current arguments. This shuts down communication and reinforces the behaviors until they become permanent fixtures within the adolescent's personality.

After reviewing and discussing the handout, parents are asked whether they can add some of these buttons to their original list. Many parents will begin to see how they have inadvertently pushed their teenager's buttons. This realization can lead to changes in perception, which can then lead to changes in how the parents act in future confrontations.

STRATEGY 2: UNCOVERING EXCEPTIONS AND POSSIBILITIES FOR FUTURE CHANGE

In Strategy 2, parents are asked to provide recent and past examples of times when they had a confrontation with their teenager that did *not* intensify. These "exceptions" are used to show parents how they achieved past success. The parents and the counselor can then build on these achievements rather than starting from scratch.

CLINICAL EXAMPLE

A father was able to identify two situations in which he remained calm and left the room before he became angry and said things to 13-year-old Stacy that he would regret later. These confrontations differed from others because he did not persist until he got the "last word." In this way, the father was able to identify specific instances when he was able to block Stacy's button pushing. The counselor was able to expand on this success by finding out what was different about the times he remained calm versus the times he did not. The father reported that during the calm times, he was able to take a deep breath and tell himself not to take the yelling as a personal attack. From this description, the counselor asked the father to experiment by doing more of the same in the weeks following. After several experiments, the father became much better at confrontations with Stacy.

If parents cannot find any exceptions, the counselor can ask them the following question: "If a miracle happened in the future, what would you be saying or doing differently during the next argument, so that someone watching would instantly recognize that your buttons were no longer being pushed and you were not losing control of your emotions?" In response to this question, many parents will begin thinking up ways they can be more skillful than their teenager during confrontations in the future. The counselor can then take these ideas and refine or expand upon them. In this way, the parents and the counselor are collaboratively constructing solutions for future confrontations. The likelihood that these solutions will be followed increases if the parents come up with the ideas rather than the counselor.

CLINICAL EXAMPLE

The mother of 14-year-old Kent answered the "miracle question" by saying that in the future, she somehow would have to find a way not to stay in the argument. In response, the counselor introduced the technique of staying short and to the point (see below), and demonstrated through role plays how the mother could put this idea into practice. The counselor played the part of Kent and pretended to do everything in his power to keep the mother in the argument and throw her off track, while the mother practiced staying short and to the point. After the role play, counselor and parent collaborated to come up with strategies that custom-fit the mother's needs.

STRATEGY 3: SHOWING PARENTS HOW TO RESPOND NONREACTIVELY AND CALMLY

At this point, the counselor is ready to teach the parents specific techniques for responding nonreactively and calmly during confrontations. These techniques include (1) exiting and waiting; (2) staying short and to the point; (3) using deflectors; (4) creating secret signals; (5) speaking in one parental voice; (6) asking whether a behavior is relevant; (7) energizing and recharging; (8) staying in the present; (9) separating misbehavior from personal attacks; (10) restoring good feelings; and (11) understanding the five levels of teenager aggression. After the counselor describes each technique, he or she can use videotaped vignettes to show what can happen if the technique is not implemented. In addition, the counselor can role-play the adolescent while the parents practice implementing a particular technique. Glitches are located and solved before the adolescent is asked back into the room.

Technique 1: Exiting and Waiting

Rationale

Parents are told that sometimes it is possible to act more calmly and more in control than they feel, but that such occasions are exceptions to the rule. For this reason, the most important instruction they can give themselves when they are angry or thrown off track is this: "Exit and wait." The best thing about this technique is that when they say nothing, parents never have to take back or regret harsh words or criticisms said in anger. The counselor asks the parents to take a leadership role by exiting a heated confrontation before harsh words are said in anger, and by waiting until they are calmer to continue the discussion.

Some parents may express reluctance to experiment with this approach. Many parents feel that if they leave the room first, their teenager wins. These parents must be convinced that just the opposite is true. Exiting calmly is a quiet but powerful way of demonstrating how serious the situation is while simultaneously role-modeling self-control. In addition, if the adolescent is yelling and swearing, a calm exit takes the wind out of his or her sails. Without an audience, the adolescent quickly learns that he or she cannot get his point across by using disrespectful or abusive language. The teenager is then faced with the choice of either changing the behavior or being ignored. The adolescent will usually choose the former.

Hesitant parents may also feel that it is the teenager's duty to exit and wait in a heated confrontation, not theirs. Depending on the particular adolescent, this is a possible option. Some adolescents can be encouraged to take time outs when they lose control of their emotions.

Implementation

After obtaining a commitment to this technique and addressing any concerns, the counselor describes how to implement this procedure. First, he or she must explain that this technique should be predetermined and explained to the adolescent beforehand. This is done so that the adolescent does not think the parents are exiting from the confrontation because they do not want to listen to what the teen has to say. It also sends one or more of the following messages: (1) The argument is getting too heated to be productive; (2)

the adolescent is disrespectful; and/or (3) the adolescent is using language and a tone of voice that are unacceptable.

First, the parents should tell the adolescent that they will talk with him or her later that day, but only after everyone has calmed down. Sometimes the parents and adolescent have to agree to disagree. Even when calm, the adolescent may not like a particular decision, rule, or consequence, when this happens, the discussion need not continue, as no explanation will be good enough. However, this does not mean that communication stops on other issues. It just means that on this particular issue there is disagreement, and thus there is no need for further discussion at this time. It is important for the parents to make this distinction and communicate it to the adolescent. Otherwise, the adolescent and parents may generalize disagreements to all communication and stop talking with one another.

Second, the counselor asks the parents to define clearly what future behaviors will create the need for exiting and waiting. The parents are asked to explain these target behaviors to the adolescent beforehand. However, the parents also reserve the right to exit and wait any time they need to gather their thoughts or calm themselves down. Most adolescents will agree with this rationale. They would rather have a break in a confrontation before a parent lectures or uses harsh words or criticisms. This benefit should be pointed out to the adolescent by both the parents and the counselor.

Third, the parents and adolescent discuss whether or not the adolescent should also be able to use the technique of exiting and waiting. This decision should be made on a case-by-case basis and should be made by the parents. If the parents decide to let the adolescent use this technique, a parent, not the adolescent, should determine when the adolescent needs to take a time out. This is because the parents, not the adolescent, should determine the mood and direction of arguments. If the adolescent is allowed to exit at will and wait for as long as he or she wants, the teen may abuse this privilege by leaving discussions any time he or she does not agree with the parents. It is important to note that although the parents are in charge of determining time outs, the adolescent is encouraged to ask for a time out if he or she feels one is needed. If it seems like a reasonable request, given the particular circumstances, the parents can grant a time out. In this way, the adolescent is encouraged to ask appropriately for time outs while the parents remain in charge.

The parents should explain to the adolescent beforehand that a time out becomes mandatory rather than optional when a discussion gets too heated. If the teenager refuses to exit into time out, the parent will still exit. There will be consequences later after both parties have cooled off. In addition, the teenager is not allowed to follow the parents when they exit from conversations. These consequences are to be clearly stated beforehand in a written contract and should be severe.

Finally, the parents and adolescent practice exiting and waiting together through role plays with the counselor present. The counselor shows videotaped scenarios of families that have used this technique successfully and unsuccessfully, and pauses the video to highlight critical points. The family members should critique each other's performance and offer possible solutions. The parents practice what they will say to the adolescent immediately prior to exiting from a confrontation. Each parent should come up with a statement that works best for him or her. The statement can sound something like this:

> "What you are saying [name the statement] and/or doing [name the behavior] is not respectful, so I am going to leave right now and talk to you later."

This statement signals inappropriate behavior and is short and direct. It also makes it easier for the parents to exit and wait without feeling guilty, because they have given the adolescent a quick explanation instead of just walking out on him or her.

CLINICAL EXAMPLE

Fourteen-year-old Monica was particularly adept at pushing her parents' buttons whenever they tried to enforce a rule. When this happened, Monica would swear, call the parents names, and cry uncontrollably. The mother would then placate her and give in, while the father became extremely angry and lectured. The parents only served to help the daughter's negative behavior escalate further.

Because of the severity of the problem, the counselor decided to go through a number of role plays with the parents before Monica came back into the room. The counselor played the part of the daughter as the parents practiced exiting and waiting as soon as Monica started to yell. When the parents felt confident, Monica was asked back into the room. As predicted, Monica began to scream and cry as soon as her parents told her she was grounded for missing school. However, this time the mother told her to stop in a firm voice, instead of placating Monica and giving in. When Monica refused, the mother stated:

> "Yelling and talking to me in that tone of voice are not respectful, so I'm going to leave right now and talk to you later."

After this statement, the mother quickly exited, and Monica sat back speechless and stunned. She immediately calmed down. The next week both the mother and father experimented with this strategy, and the daughter stopped these behaviors. Later in treatment, Monica was asked why she had suddenly stopped yelling, swearing, and crying. She answered that she did not like to be ignored, and that when her parents were calmer, it was easier for her to be too. Monica also noticed that when she was calm she could get her points across more effectively, because her parents were listening instead of reacting.

In this way, the technique of exiting and waiting interrupted and changed the confrontation style between parents and teenager by giving the parents specific tools to change the mood and direction of the argument.

Technique 2: Staying Short and to the Point

Rationale

"Staying short and to the point" means that a parent will state a particular rule or consequence and then exit from the conversation, instead of lecturing or offering long explanations. This is extremely difficult for parents, because many times they feel must justify their actions for the teenager. However, the longer an argument goes on, the more the parents regress toward behaving just as their teenager is. For every 2 minutes they stay in an argument, parents should deduct 5 years from their chronological age. For instance, a parent who is 45 years old will regress to age 30 after only 6 minutes in an argument with a teenager. One can see that it will soon be difficult to distinguish who is the parent and who is the child. Most parents are amused at this example, because they know the transformation to be true.

Implementation

Once the groundwork is laid, the counselor asks the parents to experiment with this technique when delivering rules and consequences or making decisions that the teenager may dislike. The counselor uses concrete examples to illustrate the price the parents have paid for not staying short and to the point. The counselor should either show videotaped vignettes or role-play both the adolescent and the parent to illustrate this technique. Parents need to know how to get in and out of a conversation quickly.

CLINICAL EXAMPLE

COUNSELOR: I'm going to play the part of your daughter, Annie, and try to reenact what she did to you yesterday when you asked her to clean up her room before she went out with friends. [It's important to mirror a real-life scenario as closely as possible and to set up the role play in a clear, concrete manner.]

MOTHER: What do you want me to do? [The mother sought clarification.]

COUNSELOR: Just do what you did yesterday, and I want you to critique how well I play Annie's part and let me know if I leave anything out. [The counselor provided clarification.]

MOTHER: OK.

COUNSELOR: Let's begin. I am now Annie. . . . Mom, can I go over to Deirdre's house?

MOTHER: Not until your room is cleaned up.

COUNSELOR: Why? I'll do it later. You never let me do anything!

MOTHER: This is not true. I let you go out sometimes without cleaning your room, but this time I need you to clean it now. [The mother thought that she had to explain and defend her directives, instead of staying short and to the point. This opened the door and allowed the teenager room to maneuver and begin to wear the mother down.]

COUNSELOR: I disagree. Andrea doesn't have to do chores, and she still gets to go out. It's not fair! [Again, the longer the mother stayed in the argument, the more opportunities the daughter had to push the mother's buttons and throw her off track from the real issue—the fact that she told Annie to clean her room before she could go to a friend's house.]

MOTHER: Andrea was sick on those days, and she does her share. [Again, the mother tried to justify her actions, but failed to realize that no justification would be good enough if her daughter wanted to avoid cleaning.]

COUNSELOR: Well, when Andrea picks up her room, then I will pick up mine. [The daughter still would not back down and was fast controlling this conversation by wearing the mother down and keeping her preoccupied with explaining her actions, so that Annie would understand and agree with her decision.]

MOTHER: (*Exasperated and frustrated*) I am too tired to argue. Just go! [Annie won by pushing her mother's buttons until the mother gave in.]

After the first part of the role play, the counselor and parent collaboratively brainstormed how the daughter derailed the mother. In this case, the mother began to see her part in helping the daughter win the confrontation.

COUNSELOR: Mom, what are all the ways I, playing your daughter, was able to throw you off track and win this argument? [The counselor asked the mother's opinion before offering his own, thereby making this process more collaborative in nature.]

MOTHER: I think she was able to get me off track by hooking me, as you have said before, like a fish. She knows that I like to justify my actions so that I will feel better. She also knows that if she can keep me in the argument longer, I will get more and more frustrated and usually give in. [The mother began to gain insight and change her perceptions on how the daughter defeated her. This change in perspective opened the door for the mother to try new approaches.]

The counselor then carefully went over the technique of staying short and to the point, and asked the mother to play the daughter while he played her to demonstrate this technique. The counselor paused to highlight key points in the process.

COUNSELOR: This time let's switch roles. Let me play you, the mother, and reenact the same scene over again, only this time I will show you how it might have gone if you had stayed short and to the point.

MOTHER: (*Playing daughter*) Mom, can I go over to Deirdre's house?

COUNSELOR: Not before your room is cleaned up.

MOTHER: Why? I'll do it later. You never let me do what I want!

COUNSELOR: The rule still stands. You now have a choice to make: Either the room is cleaned up in the next half-hour and I check to make sure that it is clean so you can go to Deirdre's, or you choose not to do it and you cannot go out the rest of the night. [Here the counselor modeled staying short and to the point in the following manner: (1) He demonstrated how to be concise instead of being taken off focus by the daughter; (2) he modeled being calm and nonreactive; (3) he put the choice back on the daughter's shoulders; and (4) he modeled the stance that the mother did not have to give Annie any explanations.]

MOTHER: I disagree. Andrea doesn't have to do chores, and she still gets to go out. It's not fair! [The daughter still tried to push the mother's buttons and throw her off track.]

COUNSELOR: That is all I have to say on the matter. I am leaving now and will check back with you in a half-hour to see what you decided. [Rather than offering explanations, the mother continued to stay focused, delivered the message again, and then left before the daughter had a chance to push her buttons.]

Here, the technique of exiting and waiting was combined with that of staying short and to the point: The counselor, playing the parent, delivered the message in clear, concise terms without explanations and then exited before the adolescent could continue to be disrespectful or difficult. As in this case, doing this takes practice, because parents are in the habit of doing completely the opposite. This is another reason why it is crucial to have preplanned consequences and rules that are well defined. If rules are broken, the parents simply have to remind the teenager what the consequences are and enforce them, instead of trying to offer explanations. The parents can repeat the message once, but if the adolescent continues to argue with or question the parents, the parents can say that the discussion is over and exit quickly yet calmly.

Technique 3: Using Deflectors

Rationale

Along with staying short and to the point, the counselor can teach the parents how to use deflectors. "Deflectors" are words or phrases like "nevertheless," "regardless," "that is the rule," and "no exceptions," which help the parents stay on track rather than getting drawn into long explanations or discussions. They are called "deflectors" because they are used by the parents to deflect or direct the conversation back to the issue at hand, instead of allowing it to be led by the adolescent in some other direction.

Implementation

The parents can help themselves stay short and to the point by using these key deflectors to keep on task and get the central message delivered. As described earlier, the counselor engages in role plays or dry runs until the parents have achieved mastery over this strategy. The following short transcript illustrates how this works. Deflectors are underlined.

CLINICAL EXAMPLE

BRANDON: I want to go out with my friends to a concert next week, so I will need to extend my curfew from 11 P.M. to 2 A.M.

FATHER: <u>The rule is</u> 11 P.M., <u>no exceptions</u>. [Rather than try to argue with Brandon, the father used "the rule is" and "no exceptions" to let the adolescent know immediately that there would be no negotiation on this rule. This would prevent the adolescent from thinking that the father could be manipulated. In this particular case, the adolescent had run away a week earlier. To negotiate a change in rules at this point in time would have been counterproductive. However, to try to explain this reasoning would only have resulted in a bitter confrontation on the issue of trust and taken the focus off the issue being discussed.]

BRANDON: You never let me do anything! [Here, Brandon was still trying to test the waters by seeing whether the father would take the bait and explain times when he did allow Brandon to do things he wanted. If this occurred, Brandon would control the direction of the discussion by taking the father off focus. This would begin to unravel the father's authority, because he would be unable to control the focus of the discussion.]

FATHER: <u>Nevertheless,</u> you may not go. [The father did not take the bait, but used the deflector of "nevertheless" to stay focused, thereby controlling the direction of this confrontation and maintaining his authority.]

BRANDON: I hate you! [Brandon refused to give up and shifted his tactics to personal attacks.]

FATHER: I hear that you are angry, but <u>regardless,</u> the rule still stands as written in the contract. [The father acknowledged that Brandon was angry, but used the deflector of "regardless" to return the discussion to the issue at hand.]

BRANDON: Screw the contract! [When all else failed, Brandon tried to push the button of swearing as a final attempt to get the father angry.]

FATHER: I will not let you talk to me that way, so I am exiting like we talked about. Goodbye. (*Father exited*) [As Brandon continued to become disrespectful and swear, the father employed exiting and waiting to control the mood of the confrontation and not provide an audience for the adolescent. This is a good example of combining the strength of several techniques into one in order to maintain parental authority.]

Technique 4: Creating Secret Signals

Rationale and Examples

When both parents are involved in counseling with the teenager, the counselor can show them how to help each other when one parent appears to be losing control of his or her emotions during an argument. Parents are shown how to develop their own secret signs or "Morse code" as signals to each other that the teenager is pushing buttons, that the discussion is becoming too heated, or that another predetermined behavior is occurring. Parents' signs should be individual and kept private from other family members. Examples include the following:

- Every time one parent was losing control, the other walked over without saying a word and kissed her on the cheek to remind her in a playful and fun way to calm down. This also modeled nurturance between the parents for the teenager.
- One parent held up the word "Stop" on a sign, while another used a cutting motion across the throat as a sign to exit and wait.
- One mother pretended to be pushing buttons on an appliance to signal the father that the teenager was pushing his buttons.
- When one father wanted to encourage his wife to get firmer with their teenager, he drew a line in the air with one finger, to remind her to "draw the line" with the adolescent.

In a single-parent family, the counselor can help the parent create a system of signs between the parent and an older sibling or other family member.

Implementation

This strategy is helpful because it encourages parents to work together as a team in a playful, lighthearted manner. Often parents criticize each other's parenting skills in front of the adolescent. However, this strategy gives the parents specific signs that are supportive and often humorous.

The counselor asks each parent to come up with a sign, a word, or a very short phrase that will immediately point out that the other parent is falling victim to one of his or her weaknesses, but at the same time will make the other parent feel supported. If parents cannot come up with signs or words on their own, the counselor offers suggestions to make the parents laugh and get them thinking in this direction. Often the parents will take a sign offered by the counselor and modify it slightly to fit their needs.

CLINICAL EXAMPLE

Sixteen-year-old Kristin constantly pushed her stepfather's buttons by swearing and telling him that he was not her real father. The mother would take Kristin's side by telling the husband that he was too hard on her. This infuriated the stepfather until he stopped talking to the daughter completely. The mother consistently allowed Kristin to do as she pleased without enforcing consequences. When this happened, the stepfather yelled at his wife in front of Kristin and criticizes her parenting skills. In turn, this angered Kristin, put the mother on the defensive, and made her want to defend the daughter all the more.

Discussing the technique of creating secret signals, the counselor asked the stepfather for a sign that his wife could give that would be light and playful but at the same time would let him know that Kristin was pushing his buttons. In turn, this would signal the stepfather to exit and wait until the mother was able to support him and enforce predetermined consequences for disrespect. The stepfather asked his wife to pretend that she was casting out a fishing line and reeling in a big fish. In turn, the wife asked her husband to pretend that he was turning up the burners of the stove, to signal her to get firmer and stay short and to the point. Both parents laughed as they practiced these signs and discussed how to use them during the upcoming week.

The counselor then role-played the part of Kristin by trying to push each parent's buttons while the parents practiced their new signs. Suddenly the mood in the office shifted from one of criticism and blame to one of playfulness, cooperation, and support. The next week, both parents and teenager reported a big improvement in communication. Kristin stated that her parents made these "weird signs," but admitted that whatever they were doing seemed to work.

The adolescent should not be present during the creation of these signs. Parents are told that they should remain secret as a sign of parental unity and togetherness. If the adolescent persists in wanting to know, the parents can simply say that these are ways to help them be better parents.

It is important to note that this technique can be combined with other techniques to produce an optimum effect. For one parent, as noted above, a cutting motion across the throat signaled that it was time to exit and wait. For Kristin's mother, the gesture of turning down the burners of the stove signaled her to keep the conversation short and to the point.

Technique 5: Speaking in One Parental Voice

Rationale

Often an adolescent will try to take advantage of the parent who is softer or more inconsistent. The adolescent will frequently wear that parent down with button-pushing tactics, such as guilt induction, personal attacks, threats, or disrespect. Or, when the other parent is not around, the teenager will try to persuade the more lenient parent to overturn consequences or award special privileges. If the parents fail to work together or have different parenting philosophies, the adolescent will remain in a position of authority.

Implementation

The counselor must take charge and convince the parents that none of the strategies and techniques they have spent so much time learning will work unless they agree to put aside their differences or unite in all disciplinary matters. It is critical not to give in or change the rules in the middle of a discussion with the adolescent; the parents need to discuss these issues privately. If the adolescent tries to "corner" a parent and demand an answer, the parents should stick to statements such as "That is the rule," or "I will discuss this with your father/mother first and we will make a decision together." If the adolescent tries to divide and conquer by stating that the other parent told him or her it was OK, the parent should immediately confirm this with the other.

CLINICAL EXAMPLE

Fourteen-year-old Nancy always went to her mother when she wanted something. Nancy would nag her mother until she gave in, and then tell the mother that she was the only parent she could talk to because the father was too strict. The mother agreed and spent extra time with Nancy to make up for the poor relationship with the father. As time passed, the father observed this coalition and became resentful of their exclusive relationship. He then began openly criticizing the mother for always giving in to the daughter. He felt that he had to be overly strict to compensate for his wife's lack of discipline. This reinforced the wife's perception that he was too strict. A vicious cycle was created, with the father and mother maintaining different parenting philosophies; this enabled Nancy to play one parent off against the other very effectively.

Technique 6: Asking Whether a Behavior Is Relevant

Rationale

To lessen the amount of conflict and confrontation in the family, parents should always ask themselves whether the behavior they are fighting is really one they want to take a stand on or one they should let go. If parents choose to make every misbehavior an occasion for a battle, they will burn out and be in a constant of emotional upheaval.

Implementation

To get parents to accomplish this goal, the counselor must review the parents' combined checklist of relevant behaviors. The parents should have identified their teenager's three worst behaviors on this checklist, and they should have agreed to postpone addressing other behaviors (noted on their individual lists) until a future date. Parents are then asked to rate on a scale from 1 to 10 (with 1 being the worst and 10 the best) how well they are focusing on the relevant behaviors. Regardless of the number given, the counselor asks them what would have to be done to move to the next highest number.

CLINICAL EXAMPLE

Using the technique above, a mother of two teenagers rated herself a 3 on a scale of 1 to 10. She reported that she was not at a 2 or a 1 only because there were some days when she was not stressed at work. This allowed her to approach conflict more calmly and not "jump on the kids for every little thing." However, to improve from a 3 to a 4, she would have to remind herself on the way home from work what misbehaviors she would focus on and forget the others. The counselor and mother came up with a plan that included sticking a list of relevant behaviors to the dashboard to review while she was driving home from work. This custom-built plan moved the mother's rating rapidly up the scale and allowed her to choose her battles carefully. In turn, this greatly reduced her stress level, and she was able to punish less but more effectively.

Before parents enter into an argument, they must be taught to ask themselves this question: "Is this worth a fight, and is it relevant to the big picture?" The counselor can then play the part of the adolescent and create role-play scenarios that contain both relevant and irrelevant misbehaviors. Parents are told to practice asking themselves whether the behaviors are relevant. The counselor or parents can stop the role plays at any time to ask questions, focus on weaknesses, and highlight strengths.

Technique 7: Energizing and Recharging

Rationale

Unlike the Energizer bunny, parents cannot be expected to keep going and going without recharges. If they do not occasionally take the time to relax and refocus, parents will be overstressed and will have no outlets to relieve some of this stress. As a result, they can become hypersensitive and unable to handle conflicts properly. Methods of recharging are very individualistic and can be anything that the parents enjoy separately or together. Examples include romantic or fun dates, exercise, travel, or simply quiet times away from everyone.

When the parents are taking part in an energizing activity, it is important that they completely remove themselves from the problems occurring at home. Many times when parents are out alone enjoying a nice dinner, for example, their conversation somehow tends to keep turning back to the problems in the family. This clearly defeats the entire energizing experience, and it leads over time to burnout and resentment on the parents' part. The counselor must again take charge and convince the parents to stop changing their lifestyle to accommodate the teenager. This is not an easy task. Parents are likely to say that they do not have the time or that they cannot trust their teenager enough to leave him or her alone or in the case of someone else.

Implementation

First, the counselor must outline the long history of the parents' accommodation of the teenager. Many parents will be surprised at how much their lives have changed since the behavioral problems began. They may not even have been aware of this until it is pointed out. The counselor can then ask the parents whether changing their lifestyle has helped the teenager change his or her behavior. Once the parents answer "no," the counselor can suggest trying something different.

Second, even if they agree with this idea, parents will say that they still cannot trust the adolescent long enough to leave the house. The parents can be reminded that they already leave the adolescent at home when they go to work, to the store, or to visit a friend. Therefore, to make the parents feel more secure, they must have predetermined rules and consequences for any time they are away. These may include calling the police if there are any problems, having neighbors watch the house, grounding, taking away privileges, and so on. Parents are told that with firm parameters, the teenager will have the opportunity to regain their trust slowly. However, confining themselves to prisoners in their own home will never give the parents piece of mind or allow the teenager to rebuild trust.

Third, parents will say that they do not have enough time in their schedules for energizing activities. At this point, the counselor can ask the parents whether they want to be the best parents possible. Most parents will answer affirmatively. Then the counselor can point out examples of how their stress has contributed directly or indirectly to the extreme conflict in the family. To be better parents, they must sometimes be selfish and make the time to reduce tension. Research shows that just 10 minutes a day spent walking around the neighborhood before or after work can reduce stress significantly. Parents are asked to experiment with recharging themselves consistently for 1 month. If the parents do not see results, they can then return to the way things were. When the idea is framed in this manner, it becomes increasingly difficult for the parents not to agree to try this approach.

Finally, when pressed, parents will frequently be unable to come up with ways that they can energize themselves. It has usually be a long time since they have given themselves permission to have fun or relax. Or they may have received messages from their parents that such "overindulgence" is selfish and unnecessary. If the latter is the issue, the counselor must use his or her rapport with the parents to convince them otherwise. For example, one mother wanted to exercise at a gym to energize herself but was hesitant. The counselor helped her create a schedule of going just 1 day a week, and even went down to the fitness club with the mother when she signed up. This kind of commitment by the counselor gave the mother the support and encouragement she needed to begin the exercise program.

CLINICAL EXAMPLE

The parents of two difficult teenagers promised that they would take a walk together the following week. However, at the next session they reported that they had failed to carry out this plan, because neither knew when the other was available. In addition, the kids wanted to come on the walk. This time, the counselor persuaded them to set an exact day and time for the walk. He also coached them on what they would say to the kids so that they could walk alone. Because of this attention to detail, planning, and troubleshooting, the couple was able to carry out the plan.

Technique 8: Staying in the Present

Rationale

Parents often make the mistake of using current conflicts as a basis for forecasting gloom or dredging up ancient history. For example, instead of saying that they are disappointed with the teenager's current report card and stopping there, parents commonly add such statements as "Your report cards are always bad," or "At this rate, you'll never amount to anything." When parents keep a scorecard of all past transgressions and predictions of future failures, the teenager begins to think that nothing he or she does will ever be good enough. Eventually, the teenager will rationalize that he or she can avoid failure by never trying. When this happens, the parents lecture about past failures even more, which only reinforces the teenager's unwillingness to try. As this destructive cycle repeats itself, the confrontations get more and more frequent until the teenager completely shuts down all communication. The parent responds by giving even more sermons or lectures.

If parents continue to dredge up the past, their conflicts with the adolescent will continue to be extremely bitter, and they will ruin the chance to restore good feelings. Often the counselor must locate and bring to the surface unresolved issues that keep revealing themselves in the form of present-day conflicts.

CLINICAL EXAMPLE

Sixteen-year-old David had been abandoned by his mother at an early age. When they were eventually reunited, neither one could maintain a civil conversation. The unresolved issue of abandonment repeatedly presented itself in the form of anger, resentment, guilt, and blame. It was not until the mother apologized on her knees to the son that David received the closure necessary to heal his deep wounds. The parent and teenager could now keep conflict in the present and develop a much stronger relationship.

Implementation

When the parents and/or the teenager bring up issues from the past, the counselor can initiate the following procedures. First, he or she must make the parents and adolescent aware that they are doing this during conflicts, and must provide concrete examples. Many parents and teenagers have no idea that they do this or that it can have devastating effects on others.

Second, unresolved issues must be brought to the surface and worked through. Otherwise, staying in the present will be futile. The counselor can also use role playing to illustrate each person's feelings and the differences between dredging up the past versus staying in the present.

Technique 9: Separating Misbehavior from Personal Attacks

Rationale

The counselor must help the parents separate the teenager's behavior from his or her inner feelings. Any time the parents say to themselves, "Why is my child doing this to me?," their feelings are automatically involved and they are taking the misbehavior as a personal attack. Parents can then lose control of their emotions quickly. When the parents are unable to separate the behavior from the child, conflicts will be bitter, and the parents will be unable to show any tenderness or affection.

CLINICAL EXAMPLE

Sixteen-year-old Lisa's father reported to the counselor that Lisa never did what she was told. He seemed to take this behavior very personally. The father described Lisa as mean, spiteful, and ungrateful. However, Lisa reported that she merely pushed her father's buttons so that she would be left alone and not bothered. She said that she had never meant her arguments as personal attacks, but over the years her father had interpreted them that way, so they'd stopped talking. Furthermore, she reported that it had been years since they had done anything special as father and daughter. When Lisa tried to explain that she loved him and that she was just trying to get her way, he saw this as another form of manipulation. The father was unable to separate the teenager's behavior from her feelings. As a result, the father was unable to change his behavior or show any acts of tenderness or affection in the future.

Implementation

To counter the parents' perception that the teenager's misbehavior is a personal attack, the counselor must get the parents to accept the reframe that the problem behavior simply reflects the teenager's attempt to regain or maintain control. If the parents accept this reframe, there can be tremendous positive changes in their confrontational styles. Often just getting the parents to *try* to accept this new perception constitutes major progress in therapy. Years of bitterness and resentment can make it difficult for parents to stop taking attacks personally.

A good place to start is with a daily log. The parents divide each page into two columns. In the left column, the parents write down what the teenager said or did that day that made them angry or upset. In the right column, the parents record whether or not they believe this behavior was a personal attack, as well as their reasons for this belief. The counselor can look at the log and identify the particular themes or patterns that makes the parents more likely to feel attacked. The counselor then shows the parents that what appears to be a personal attack is just the teenager's skillful way of pushing their buttons and throwing them off track. This simple exercise often helps the parents to change their perceptions.

Technique 10: Restoring Good Feelings

Rationale

It is crucial for the counselor to explain to the parents the importance of making peace with the teenager in the aftermath of an explosive confrontation. Without reconciliation after each conflict, bitterness and resentment will continue to build, and communication will be even more difficult. Every time there is an argument, old wounds that have never healed reopen. Increasingly bitter confrontations only make the wounds deeper and more difficult to heal. Another negative side effect is that many parents will give their teenager the "cold shoulder" after a bitter confrontation. Unfortunately, this only adds to the bitterness and increases the chances that even more explosive arguments will occur in the future.

It is often an extremely difficult task to convince the parents to reconcile with their teenager. It requires good rapport with the clients, as well as considerable finesse. It is also difficult to make the teenager understand that the parents can dislike the child's behavior but still love the child. The restoration of good feelings between parents and child communicates this message clearly to the teenager and demonstrates unconditional love.

Parents may say that they cannot reconcile with the adolescent because of these concerns: (1) They have been hurt in the past by the teenager and do not want to go through it again; (2) they think that the teenager will take advantage of reconciliation; and/or (3) they are afraid that the teenager will push them away. To address the first concern, parents are told that the hurt they feel now and felt in the past can only be healed with a better future. In other words, if the relationship becomes more nurturing in the present, past wounds can and will heal. The only problem is that this cannot happen if someone does not make the first move. The best persons to make this move are the parents, because they are older, wiser, and more mature; hence, they are able to see the "bigger picture." In addition, if the teenager does not receive positive interaction within the family, he or she will look for this nurturance within a "second family" of peers. However, this may backfire in the form of abusive boyfriends, drugs, gangs, or the like. If the parents do not take the lead, someone outside the family will.

To address the second concern, the counselor must make a clear distinction between behaviors and feelings. Parents who are trying to restore tenderness and good feelings do not stop enforcing rules and consequences. The parents enforce the rules without getting emotionally involved in the process, but they still communicate loud and clear that they love the teenager whether he or she misbehaves or not. Parents are warned that their teenager may be thrown off balance the first few times the parents attempt to restore good feelings. This is because the teen is looking for the "catch" in the parents' softer behavior. However, if reconciliation is attempted consistently, the teenager will begin to trust this behavior as genuine and unconditional.

CLINICAL EXAMPLE

A father had given his son the cold shoulder for years and was afraid to show any softness. The father was convinced that 15-year-old André would take advantage of him as he had in the past. After explaining the bigger picture, the counselor persuaded the father to give his experiment just one try. The counselor predicted that André would initially take advantage of his father's reconciliation attempts, because he would not initially trust his sincerity. Therefore, the father should ignore any negative reactions by André and persist with his reconciliation efforts.

Over the next 3 months, the counselor had to keep encouraging the father to go on trying, since (as predicted) the son continued to reject him. However, the father liked the counselor and trusted his judgment, so he continued to try. With more time, the son started to soften up and stop running away so much. When asked for the reason months later, André simply stated that he really "felt Dad's love for the first time, without conditions or strings attached."

To address the third potential concern, the counselor prepares the parents for the possibility that the teenager will push them away because restoration of good feelings is initially uncomfortable. The teenager, like the parents, does not want to risk getting hurt again. Furthermore, physical and emotional affection from the parents is often a new experience for the teenager, who has to adjust to the hugs and softness. If the teenager initially pushes the parents away, the coaching they receive from the counselor will help them continue to try, realizing that the teenager's strong reaction itself indicates the need for reconciliation. If parents are still hesitant, the counselor can point out the results of a research study involving infants and touch. The babies who were frequently touched and held thrived, but those who were rarely held either developed serious medical problems or died (see Skeels, 1966). This example helps drive home the point that the teenager needs the parents' nurturance to survive. The only times hugs are not appropriate are in front of the teenager's friends (because it creates embarrassment), and in cases of suspected sexual abuse.

Implementation

Once all initial concerns are covered, the counselor asks the parents to brainstorm ways they can restore good feelings. Some parents will already have success stories that the counselor can refine and expand upon. For example, one parent said he could remember a time when he just hugged his son and told him he did not like his son's behavior but still loved him. Since this had worked before with this particular family, it was incorporated into the treatment plan.

If exceptions cannot be found, the counselor asks the parents to guess at possible things they could do in the future that would restore good feelings. If the parents cannot come up with ideas, the counselor intervenes with possible suggestions. Some examples include (1) writing the teenager a letter or note explaining why they are proud of the teenager, or apologizing for something they said or did that hurt the teenager; (2) as described above, giving the teen a simple hug and saying that even though the parents do not like the teen's behavior, they still love him or her; (3) making a simple statement of apology; and (4) making time for a special outing together, regardless of how good or bad the teenager was that week (thus separating the misbehavior from the unconditional love).

The counselor must communicate to the parents how extremely important it is that their attempts at restoration of good feelings should begin as quickly as possible. The longer they wait, the more likely it is that bitterness or resentment will gain a stronghold in the relationship. Some parents may want the teenager to make the first move, but this is not likely to happen. The teenager does not see the bigger picture and therefore will not understand the benefits of or purpose behind restoration of good feelings. Therefore, the parents must take the lead and hope that the teenager will follow.

Technique 11: Understanding the Five Levels of Teenager Aggression

Finally, it is imperative that the parents understand the five levels of teenager aggression. After the counselor describes each level, the parents are taught how the 10 techniques described above can be employed to reduce the adolescent's aggression level quickly. However, if the behavior reaches a dangerous level of violence, the counselor should intervene to provide specific methods for handling these potentially volatile situations.

Level 1: Whining and Complaining

Description. When asked to do something like pick up clothes or do household chores, a teenager will begin to whine or complain. The teen does this to annoy the parents and get them to back down. When tired or overstressed from work, parents will often give in rather than continue to listen to a whiny teenager.

Possible Solutions. The counselor should inform parents that the best solution is to ignore the whining and enforce the consequence if a rule is not followed. Parents can also be playful and whine right back, making the teenager laugh and thus disarming him or her. For example, one parent said in a whiny voice, "I know it is hard to do," and then hugged the teenager. This made the teenager laugh, disarmed him, and closed the incident with reconciliation. However, if the parents start to lecture, get angry, or lose control of their emotions, the teenager's aggression can escalate from whining to stubborn refusal.

Level 2: Stubborn Refusal

Description. At the second level, the teenager stubbornly refuses to follow directions or listen to authority. The teenager says that he or she is too busy or will perform a task later. In addition, he or she may try to globalize the situation through exaggerated statements (e.g., "You never give me a break," "You're always on my case"). This stubborn refusal is intended to place the teenager, not the parents, in charge.

Possible Solutions. The parents should stay short and to the point by simply repeating what the consequence will be and enforcing it if the refusal continues.

CLINICAL EXAMPLE

Twelve-year-old Michelle would stubbornly refuse to complete chores. The mother begged, threatened, and bribed, but Michelle would still refuse to comply. Then the mother would start yelling and swearing while Michelle countered with the same. It was usually not long before they were actually throwing punches at each other.

After counseling began, the mother learned to stay short and to the point. She told Michelle that she had 5 minutes to complete the chore, or the pre-planned consequences of 1 day of grounding would be enforced. When Michelle refused, the mother simply exited and waited 5 minutes to enforce the consequence. In this way, the mother was able to control her emotions and the direction of the argument. This prevented Michelle from proceeding to the next level of teenager aggression.

Level 3: Verbal Abuse and Personal Attacks

Description. The teenager begins to swear and call the parents names. He or she may appear to be on the verge of violence, but instead is probably trying to intimidate the parents and push their buttons. In other words, "the bark is much worse than the bite." Nevertheless, this level is potentially dangerous, because by now the adolescent has begun to lose control of his or her emotions and is very agitated or angry. If this continues, the teenager can quickly work himself or herself into a frenzy, saying and doing things that the teen would never say or do in a calmer state. Therefore, parents must act quickly before the teenager loses control altogether.

Possible Solutions. At this level, parents should follow the techniques of using deflectors, staying short and to the point, and exiting and waiting. It is important not to give the teenager an audience by staying too long in the argument and allowing him or her to become verbally abusive. If this happens, the teenager can quickly move up to threats of violence (see below). Parents must also learn not to personalize these attacks. Instead, they must see that this is the teenager's best way to regain his or her authority. Once parents accept this reframe, they can remain calm and increase their effectiveness.

CLINICAL EXAMPLE

Thirteen-year-old Katie would quickly jump to Level 3 any time she was asked to do something that she did not like. Immediately she would start swearing and calling the parents "assholes." Both parents took this very personally and lectured Katie as to why she should not swear. This only angered Katie more until the parents got scared and left the room without enforcing the consequence.

This cycle repeated itself again and again until the parents drastically changed tactics. Their new techniques included using deflectors and exiting and waiting as soon as Katie became verbally abusive. After things were calm, they enforced preplanned consequences. The personal attacks and verbal abuse stopped soon thereafter.

If the parents take these attacks personally or stay in the argument too long, the risk increases that the teenager will quickly go to Level 4 and begin to threaten violence.

Level 4: Threats of Violence

Description. The adolescent threatens to kill or injure the parents, another sibling, animals, property, or other people. Most teenagers usually have no intention or desire to commit acts of violence. Instead, they want to see their parents' reaction and scare them into submission. In the past, these threats have been successful in getting parents to back off; for many teenagers, they have become their "big guns" and are used as a last resort if the previous three levels are ineffective. This level immediately precedes acts of violence, so it is a very dangerous area. Threats must be dealt with swiftly yet carefully, before the teenager's behavior has a chance to escalate into acts of violence.

Possible Solutions. At this level, the temptation is very high for parents to get aggressive, lecture, and lose control. However, if parents get agitated, they will quickly help push the teenager into acts of violence.

It is critical to exit and wait until the teenager calms down. No explanation or reasoning will be successful at this point and will only serve to agitate the teenager further. The parents should immediately tell the teenager that this behavior is not acceptable and that if he or she continues, the consequence will be severe. The parent then immediately walks away from the situation. The teenager can be required to go to a specified time-out or "cooling-off" area in the house. The goal here is for the parents to model self-control and remove themselves or the teenager from the situation as quickly as possible.

If the teenager is intoxicated on drugs or alcohol, these techniques rarely work, and violence is likely to occur regardless of what the parents do or say. The police should then be immediately called, and the parents should leave the situation for their own safety. Under special circumstances, an intoxicated teenager can be placed in the bathroom if this option has been planned ahead of time. If the parents lose control of their emotions or are unwilling or unable to exit and wait, the teenager will proceed to the final and most dangerous level—acts of violence.

Level 5: Acts of Violence

Description. At Level 5, the teenager actively attacks objects or people. He or she may knock holes in walls, throw and break valuable objects, or smash windows; the teenager may even attack another family member or attempt suicidal or suicidal gestures in a fit of rage and frustration. The adolescent may have reached such a state of emotional frenzy that he or she is not aware of these actions or is unable to recall them later. Behavior at this level is extremely dangerous and must be terminated quickly.

Possible Solutions. At this point, there is no more talk. Action must be taken quickly and decisively to ensure the safety of the teenager and those around him or her. Physical restraint in the form of a "takedown" can be used if the teenager is smaller than a parent and the parent is able to retain emotional control. After the teenager has calmed down to a certain extent, he or she can be placed in the bathroom for a specified period of time. These procedures are explained in detail in Chapter 6.

If the teenager is physically stronger than the parents, they must immediately dial 911 and have the police come to the house. The parents should leave the house and wait for the police to arrive. Physical assault or property damage charges must be filed at the time of arrest; otherwise, the teenager will get the message that violence is an acceptable behavior. The parents should avoid hospitalization at all costs, because the teenager is not mentally ill but behaviorally out of control. In our society this type of behavior warrants prison, probation, or detention, not hospitalization for the mentally ill. If hospitalization is used, it communicates to the teenager that he or she is not responsible for violent acts because he or she is mentally ill. This is the wrong message to send and may increase the probability that this behavior will occur again. Hospitalization should only be used if a teenager tries to commit suicide, and then only under the special circumstances explained within Chapter 6.

When the violence is over and things have calmed down, the teenager must pay for any damage done. The value of the damage should be assessed, and the teenager should be required to pay it off with hard labor, wages from a job, or possessions that are taken away and sold if repayment of the debt is not received within a specified time period. Details of this procedure are also outlined in Chapter 6.

SUMMARY

Difficult adolescents have an uncanny ability to push parental buttons so that the parents will lose control of their emotions and their ability to enforce rules. This ability makes adolescents more skillful than their parents in the art of confrontation. A counselor must help parents realize that button pushing is not a personal attack, but rather a skillful game by their teenager to gain control of the mood and direction of the argument. Consequently, parents must be shown how to "play the game" as well as or better than their teenager. This is accomplished via the following three strategies: (1) Parents are shown how to identify the buttons they and their teenager push on each other during confrontations; (2) parents are shown how to find examples of when they did not allow their buttons to be pushed and times they did not push their teenager's buttons; and (3) parents are shown how to respond differently by using a combination of 11 different techniques.

The following is a summary of the major points contained in this chapter:

1. The counselor must help parents identify through concrete examples all the possible buttons (e.g., "I hate you," "You don't love me," "You asshole") they allow their teenager to push.

2. The counselor explains to the parents that "it takes two to tango." This means that while the adolescent is pushing the parents' buttons, the parents are often pushing the adolescent's buttons (e.g., preaching, talking in chapters, labeling). It is important to help the parents recognize how they help their adolescent lose control of his or her emotions by identifying possible buttons that they push during an argument.

3. Once parents understand the concept of button pushing, the counselor teaches parents the 11 specific techniques for responding in a nonreactive and calm manner during confrontations: exiting and waiting; staying short and to the point; using deflectors; creating secret signals; speaking in one parental voice; asking whether a behavior is relevant; energizing and recharging; staying in the present; separating misbehavior from personal attacks; restoring good feelings; and understanding the five levels of teenager aggression. After the counselor describes each technique, he or she can use videotaped vignettes to show what can happen if the technique is not imple-

mented. In addition, the counselor can role-play the adolescent while the parents practice implementing a particular technique. Glitches are located and solved before the adolescent is asked back into the room. The parents can now play the game and its rules like master chess players, using these new techniques and tools.

4. Parents must be educated that they do not owe their teenager an explanation or justification for their actions. Later and in a calm situation, an explanation may be given, but not during an argument. In the heat of the moment, no explanation will ever be good enough and can only lead to further escalation.

5. The counselor helps parents to keep their explanations short and to the point. This is because the longer they stay in the argument, the more the parents regress in chronological age.

6. After a heated confrontation, it is important for the parents to try to make the first move and restore good feelings with their teenager. The longer they wait, the harder it will be to accomplish this goal. A teenager who does not receive positive interaction within the family will look for this nurturance within a "second family" of peers; however, this may backfire in various ways. If the parents do not take the lead, someone outside the family will.

7. It is imperative that the parents understand the five levels of teenager aggression. After the counselor describes each level, the parents are taught how the 10 other techniques can be employed to reduce the adolescent's aggression level quickly. However, if the behavior reaches a dangerous level of violence, the counselor should intervene to provide specific methods for handling these potentially volatile situations. Chapter 6 describes these methods in detail.

Neutralizing the Adolescent's "Five Aces"

When parents try to restore their authority, the difficult adolescent will often use one of the "five aces"—running away, truancy/poor school performance, suicidal threats or behaviors, threats or acts of violence, and disrespect—to intimidate the parents into giving their newfound authority right back to the adolescent. These "aces" cause traditional methods to fail and lead to a high relapse rate. Parents and counselors are unable to create consequences that will cause the teenager to give up his or her extreme behaviors long enough to let the parents remain in charge and to result in permanent change. To neutralize these "aces," the parents and counselor must establish consequences that are severe enough that the adolescent would rather give up the extreme behavior than continue to suffer the punishment. The challenge is finding the right consequences.

CLINICAL EXAMPLE

Thirteen-year-old Kareem chronically ran away. When the counselor asked the boy why, he stated that he loved his freedom. He had houses to stay at all over the neighborhood that his parents did not know about. Why would he ever want to give this up? No current bribe or punishment would be strong enough to make Kareem want to give up staying out all night. Even if his parents grounded him, he would just walk out the front door.

Coming up with an effective consequence is only one part of the overall process; the consequence must also be administered without any verbal or physical abuse. Without a clear road map, many parents will grow weary, lose hope, and then resort to physical or verbal abuse. Therefore, the counselor must not only construct an effective consequence, but also show the parents how to administer it effectively so as to eliminate the risk of abuse.

CLINICAL EXAMPLE

One single father was known by protective services as extremely abusive. Each time 13-year-old Markel skipped school, he was severely beaten by his father with a belt. Over time, the beatings got so bad that Markel stopped coming home for weeks at a time. This only angered the father more, and the cycle of abuse continued when Markel returned home.

As the counselor talked with the father, it became clear that the father loved Markel very much and that he felt "out of control" because nothing he had tried before worked. The father did not want to hit Markel but needed a better road map to follow. In addition, Markel would push his father's buttons by swearing and calling him a "shitty father." Naturally, the father took this personally and lost control of his temper each and every time until he became physically violent. The cycle of violence was inevitable because of the lack of effective consequences and the son's ability to goad his father. However, the violence immediately stopped when the counselor addressed these issues on the following two levels.

First, the counselor helped the father construct a set of nonviolent consequences and write down all the procedural steps in a contract format. If Markel refused to go to school, the father would take him to his construction site in the hot desert sun, and Markel would sit on a woodpile and do nothing. The father knew that Markel would dislike this consequence to such a degree that a nice air-conditioned school would be the better alternative. In addition, if Markel chose to go to school, he would earn coupons each day for up to 1 extra hour on the weekends to be with friends. This was an incentive, because Markel valued his freedom.

Second, the counselor helped change the father's perceptions of Markel's verbal aggression as personal attacks. Once the father understood that the son was just skillful at throwing him off track, he was more than willing to use the technique of exiting and waiting. The father soon became able to ignore the son and exit from the argument until he regained his composure. Since the father now saw Markel's behavior as a game rather than a personal attack, he was able to change his style of confrontation.

After these two areas had been addressed, the verbal and physical abuse immediately stopped, as did Markel's extreme behaviors of running away and truancy. The father reported that things had improved because he had a set of step-by-step procedures that he could refer to and read each day until it became second nature.

It is important to note that many parents who appear to be abusive are this way because, like Markel's father, they feel helpless and "out of control." However, once the parent has a clear set of procedures and a new format for confrontation, the violence suddenly stops and the household becomes less chaotic.

The aim of this chapter is to give counselors treating difficult adolescents a set of effective consequences for each of the "five aces." These interventions are assembled within one chapter so that a counselor can refer to them easily when determining consequences and interventions for extreme behaviors with which a family is struggling. I have also found it helpful to have parents read this chapter themselves, so that they are better prepared for counseling. Before lending parents the book or encouraging them to purchase it, however, the counselor must state clearly to the parents that none of these interventions should be initiated until they have been thoroughly discussed in treatment sessions.

The chapter discusses specific consequences for stopping the extreme behaviors of running away, truancy/poor school performance, suicidal threats or behaviors, threats or acts of violence, and disrespect. Each consequence is described in detail, and the steps for its implementation are outlined. Some of the same consequences can be used for several different extreme behaviors. Special circumstances are noted within each consequence. Each of the consequences has been used with many different types of families at every socioeconomic level.

These interventions are proposed to the parents without the adolescent present. The parents and counselor must work out the details and then troubleshoot how the adolescent might try to sabotage the plan; no intervention should be initiated until this process is completed. Consequences are always predetermined, and their exact procedures are written down in a contract format so that the parents can refer to it as a handbook. The counselor must modify each consequence to custom-fit each particular family's needs. Finding the strategy or combination of strategies that works best for a particular teenager can be a trial-and-error process.

It is important to note that threats of suicide and acts or threats of violence fall into a special category. These behaviors are potentially lethal and therefore more difficult to control. The threat or act of hurting oneself or others is serious and must be dealt with immediately. Preparation is the key to success. The roles of parents and outsiders (e.g., police, probation officer, foster care agency) must be clarified beforehand. Each person must be asked "what if" questions and use dry runs to role-play what they would do and how they would react in any given situation. The counselor must be available 24 hours a day until these behaviors are neutralized. He or she must be ready and willing to conduct home visits if necessary. The consequences must be harsh and applied as quickly as possible. If not, these behaviors will quickly escalate out of control and become lethal. Examples of such scenarios are outlined in the upcoming sections on violence and suicide.

Each of these strategies may initially provoke an extreme reaction from the teenager. Parents should be warned about this fact beforehand and told that this is normal. The reason for the escalation is that the teenager senses that his or her most powerful behaviors may be threatened. This initial escalation is the teenager's best way to get the parents to back off and leave his or her "ace(s)" intact. Parents can be told that an adolescent in this situation can be compared to an army that is on the brink of defeat but uses the last of its arsenal in a last-ditch effort to defeat the enemy. The escalation means that the parents are turning the tide of battle and winning the war. However, to win they must endure and not waver. To address this concern, counselor and parents must troubleshoot each possible escalation and develop a subsequent plan of action. The counselor needs to be available on a 24-hour basis, and he or she should anticipate emergency phone calls, home visits, or additional therapy sessions throughout the week. Finally, the counselor needs to be able to think quickly and to change tactics rapidly if an intervention really appears to be ineffective. The window of opportunity for working with an adolescent and family is often small, and flexibility is thus essential.

ACE 1: RUNNING AWAY

Running away occurs most often when the teenager seeks escape from something negative in the family environment. These issues must be worked through if the cycle of running away is to be broken permanently. (Note that although these points are made here in regard to running away, they are very often pertinent to the other four "aces" as well.) Before interventions are proposed, the counselor should ask each parent the following questions:

1. "What are all the reasons why your teenager would want to run away?"
2. "What is happening within the household that is potentially poisonous?"
3. "What are all the things that would need to change to make your teenager want to come back and stay at home?"

The teenager should be asked these same questions away from the parents. Some of the potentially poisonous issues might include the following:

• One or both parents are overly strict, harsh, or punitive, or they focus on the negative to the extent that the teenager feels that nothing he or she does will be good enough. In essence, the teenager feels that he or she can never live up to the parents' expectations.
• One or both parents constantly push their teenager's buttons, so that the confrontations become so negative or violent that the teenager runs away or is asked to leave.
• At least one parent is an addict of some type (alcohol, drugs, gambling, etc.). Because of an addiction, a parent can be violent or extremely verbally abusive.
• Undisclosed sexual abuse is occurring or has happened in the past within the home environment. When there is ongoing sexual abuse between a

parent and teenager, the teenager will usually choose to leave rather than reveal the secret of incest or continue to be abused.

• There is physical violence in the home, such as spouse/partner or child abuse.

• Marital conflict and/or parental depression exists. In some cases, the teenager protects the parents by keeping the focus on his or her running away. As long as the parents are concerned about the teenager's problems, they do not have time for their own pain.

• A boyfriend, girlfriend, gang, or other peer or group of peers is pulling the teenager away from the family. For example, in one case the teenager's boyfriend told her that she had to skip school and come to his house, or he would end the relationship. Teenagers would rather suffer the consequences for running away than risk losing a boyfriend, girlfriend, or other peer relationship.

The consequences described below are merely "Band-Aids" to stop the behavior long enough that the issues above can be addressed and solved. That is, these consequences are designed to "stop the bleeding" long enough for the counselor to help make the family environment less toxic and more livable. The following seven strategies are suggested to stop a teenager from running away: (1) atom bomb interventions; (2) the bathroom strategy; (3) the Gandhi strategy; (4) poisoning the adolescent's safe houses; (5) using positive reinforcers; (6) trust building, when possible; and (7) predicting relapse.

Strategy 1: Atom Bomb Interventions

The methods I call "atom bomb interventions" have been modified from the work of Jerome Price (1990) and have been successfully used not only with adolescents who run away, but with those who resort to other "aces" as well. These interventions include the following:

1. Selling, pawning or removing the teenager's prized material possessions (e.g., stereo equipment, makeup, compact disc [CD] collection, or telephone) if the adolescent runs away.
2. Instituting a 24-hour watch, or having a parent, neighbor, or security guard accompany the teenager everywhere he or she goes until the risk of further running away has subsided; this entails being at school, sitting in during class, and escorting the teenager between classes, so that the teen cannot run away as soon as he or she is out of the parents' sight.
3. Removing all clothing belonging to the teenager except for what the parents choose for the teenager to wear (running away will be more difficult if the teen only has a few items of clothing).

These interventions can work effectively for two reasons. First, today's teenagers are extremely materialistic and do not like the thought of having their material possessions removed or sold without their consent. Second, teenagers want authority figures "off their case." Therefore, teenagers will not like the idea of having one or both parents in school with them or having the parents pick out their clothes. Again, if the consequence is more difficult for the teenager than continuing to run away, the behavior can be stopped immediately. Each of the atom bomb interventions is outlined in detail below.

Selling, Pawning, or Removing the Teenager's Prized Possessions

Before the teenager returns home from running away, parents are instructed to confiscate the teenager's possessions (e.g., stereo equipment, makeup, CD collection, telephone). They are asked to take these items either to their offices or to a friend's house so that the teenager cannot get them. When the teenager returns, parents are instructed to give the teen a pawn ticket and have him or her read it. Parents must then walk away calmly and without giving the standard lecture or sermon. The pawn ticket will state the following information:

> Good for one [fill in item or items]. We have secured these items in a safe place, and you may have them back unharmed if you do not leave the house again without permission for 7 days, starting today. If you do leave without permission in the next 7 days, these items will be pawned or sold. If they are sold, they will not be replaced. [If the teenager is in competition with a brother or sister, the sibling can receive the money for items sold. The teenager is told this in writing on the pawn ticket.]

A 7-day period is used because it is enough time to make an impact, but not so long that the teenager will feel that he or she has nothing to lose and stop trying. However, if running away continues, parents have the option of extending the time limit. The parents can also use a shorter time period if they know that a 1- or 2-day removal of prized possessions would stop this behavior.

Items pawned should be things the teenager cares about, but not everything the teen owns. The first offense should only result in a warning. If the behavior continues, more and more items can be placed in storage for longer and longer periods of time. The teenager should be told ahead of time that if he or she steals other items from the home in retaliation, his or her own items will immediately be sold to the pawn shop.

The teen may argue that he or she bought some of these items and therefore they cannot be touched. The parents can reply that possessions are taken all the time to pay off debts. They can also remind the teenager that he or she is receiving free room and board in the parents' house. If this explanation is still not good enough, parents are instructed to refrain from further explanation. At this point, no reason will ever be good enough; further rationales only run the risk of making the confrontation more volatile.

Instituting a 24-Hour Watch

A 24-hour watch can be used if the first intervention does not work, if the problem is chronic, or if the teenager doesn't value material possessions. Parents must be told that it will be more economical to stop the problem of the short term, even if they have to pay someone to watch their teenager during the times that the parents cannot watch him or her, than it will be to spend hundreds of dollars on hospitalization or institutionalization. Moreover, the teenager could be killed in the streets if he or she continues to run away.

Parents are reassured that it will only take 1 to 2 weeks out of their entire lives to make the consequence of running away so noxious that the teenager will be reluctant to try it again. It is best to try to get a parent or a close friend to do this job before going outside the family for assistance. If the parents have to go outside the family and ask church members, neighbors, or a security guard, the parents must interview each one personally until they find the right person. They must instruct the church member or security guard not to touch the teenager physically. If the teenager starts to run, they should follow him or her and contact the police and parents to give them the exact location.

At night, one parent must sleep in the room with the teenager (or, if this is not possible, lock him or her in a room without windows) so that the teen cannot sneak out at night. During this time, all privileges are suspended; these include using the phone, seeing friends, playing video games, and watching television. When the teenager is home, he or she will be with the parents at all times. The 24-hour watch is not stopped until the counselor is consulted and it is determined that the teenager wishes to be given another chance.

A version of this strategy consists of the establishment of a consequence in which the teenager is only under watch for the actual length of time he or she was away (or double that time, depending on the particular teenager). This amount of time may be enough to stop the extreme behavior and can be tried as an initial step before proceeding to the "big gun" of a 24-hour watch. Parents may also be more willing to try this as a first step because it is more convenient for them.

Removing All Clothes

Removing the teenager's clothes is similar to removing his or her material possessions. As with material possessions, the clothes are taken before the teenager returns home. The pawn ticket will state the following information:

> This ticket is a voucher for your clothes. We have secured these items in a safe place, and you may have them back unharmed if you do not leave home again without permission for the next 7 days, starting today. If you do leave home without permission in the next 7 days, these items will be sold. If they are sold, they will not be replaced. [If the teenager is in competition with a brother or sister, the sibling can receive the money for items sold.]

The teenager is responsible for washing the one outfit he or she is allowed to wear while the other clothes are in storage. If this one outfit starts to smell, the teenager has the choice of either washing the outfit or adding 1 more day to the pawn ticket.

Implementation. First, in front of the teenager, the parents concretely define what constitutes "running away." Is it leaving the house at any time without permission? Leaving home for more than 24 hours? Or leaving to cool down after a heated argument? The teenager is then asked to repeat what was stated, to ensure that he or she understands how "running away" is defined. The definition of the behavior is then written down as part of the contract.

The teenager is told that since other punishments have not worked, the next punishment if he or she runs away again will be extremely severe. The teenager will immediately want to know what the punishment is, but the parents should not reveal the consequence until they have to enforce it. This secrecy is important, because in the past the teenager has gotten an explanation for every parental action; the teenager has then used his or her enhanced social perception to sabotage the consequence. The secrecy of the consequence symbolically places power back in the parents' hands and keeps the teenager off balance.

Second, after this message is delivered, the teenager is asked to leave the room as the counselor and parents customize which atom bomb intervention they want to use. What may work for one teenager may have no effect on another. For example, some teenagers may not care at all if their personal items are sold, but would not like to have adults attend school with them. As stated earlier, a good rule of thumb is to use a less extreme strategy first (selling, pawning, or removing the teenager's prized material possessions) and only go the "big guns" (24-hour watch, removing all the teen's clothes) if the running away continues or is already chronic. It is good to punish less severely when possible, to avoid the resentment that can accompany harsh consequences. In addition, the parents should not use all of their ammunition during a first strike. It is always good to have reserve interventions on hand if needed in the future.

It is important to note that even though the teenager should not know the atom bomb consequence beforehand, the parents must know what it will be and how they are going to implement it. The better thought out and more precise the plan is, the more successful the parents will be in implementing it. The plan should be written down in detail before the parents leave the counselor's office. If the counselor is running out of time, it is better to tell the parents to hold off on implementing the plan until the next meeting when it can be fully outlined, rather than run the risk of failure.

Third, without the teenager present, the counselor and parents must troubleshoot and map out solutions for each "what if" scenario. For example, what will the parents do if their son refuses to let them pawn his possessions or their daughter hides her clothes? These potential problems must be worked through beforehand, using a troubleshooting process similar to that outlined in Chapter 4. The counselor should also outline the following procedures the parents should follow if the teenager runs away in the future.

1. The parents should call the police and, if more than 24 hours pass, file a missing person's report.

2. After 24 hours pass, the parents should find a picture of the teenager and print up flyers to be posted all around school and the places he or she frequents. A small reward should be offered for information on the teenager's whereabouts. Parents will be surprised at how many friends and parents will blow the whistle for a small reward, and/or at how the embarrassment of flyers can make running away less enticing.

3. The parents should enforce the atom bomb consequence when the teenager returns without guilt trips, sermons, criticism, or lectures. Parents must be told that their silence alone is the best medicine. The teenager will not be expecting this treatment. At the same time, parents must be told not to give their teenager the "cold shoulder," but to attempt to restore good feelings as quickly as possible. For example, one mother thought this idea was absurd, but agreed to try it because she had a great rapport with the counselor. When the mother tried it, she could not believe the difference. The daughter showed remorse and even apologized later. The daughter reported that this one act of kindness without any lecture was one of the biggest reasons why she stopped running away.

4. The parents and counselor together should try to discover the destructive issues in the home and work to solve them. For example, in one family the issue was extreme marital conflict, which emerged only after the parents stopped being in a constant state of crisis. Once the teenager's behavior was stable, the counselor was able to help the parents see how the marital problems contributed to the running away. On this basis, the parents were willing to engage in marital therapy with the counselor.

Strategy 2: The Bathroom Strategy

The bathroom strategy is an effective intervention to eliminate not only running away, but disrespect and threats or acts of violence. It is typically used as a last resort when running away persists and when other strategies have failed. This strategy should be used only by a seasoned counselor. I define "seasoned" as someone who has seen at least 100 difficult adolescent cases. Beginning counselors or interns should not attempt this strategy.

In essence, the length of time the teenager is away from home without permission is the length of time the teenager will be required to spend as punishment in the bathroom. For example, if the teenager is gone 5 hours, the teenager will spend 5 hours in the bathroom upon returning home, and so on up to 24 hours. If the teenager is gone 24 hours or longer, the first offense will result in a sentence of 24 hours. Each 24-hour period thereafter will result in the addition of 6 more hours to the sentence. If immediate punishment is not possible because of the parents' work schedule, they can wait to enforce the consequence on a day off or on the weekend; however, the parents should not tell their teenager about this ahead of time, to keep him or her off balance. In case of emergency, at least one parent must be in the home the entire time the teenager is in the bathroom. The parent must provide food and water to be eaten in the bathroom. However, no books, television, music, or other items are allowed, except for a pillow and blanket.

Parents use the bathroom instead of the bedroom as the time-out facility because it is usually the most boring room in the house and the most difficult to escape from. The teenager can also use the facilities in the bathroom. In addition, the adolescent's bedroom has too many entertainment items (television, radio, stereo equipment, etc.) and should be seen as a place of sanctuary rather than a place of punishment. The teenager is told about this plan of action beforehand and is warned that it will happen if he or she runs away in the future.

Parents are given the following rationale for the use of this strategy. First, teenagers value their freedom above all else; therefore, this strategy can sour the idea of running away very quickly, because it represents a loss of freedom. Second, this strategy mirrors what would take place if the adolescent were institutionalized. The only difference is that the parents would be paying thousands of dollars to have the institution babysit the teenager. When the adolescent returned home, the behavior would start all over again, because outside forces rather than the parents would have brought about any changes. Hence, the teenager would have no reason to respect the parents' authority and would believe that he or she was capable of stopping the behavior unassisted. Finally, other consequences have not worked, so something different and extreme needs to be tried. If not, the behavior will continue to worsen, and the teenager will be at greater risk of getting hurt or killed in the streets. This rationale must be fully described by the counselor and accepted by the parents; otherwise, they will be unwilling and unable to follow through with this consequence.

Implementation. Before this intervention is initiated, the bathroom is totally stripped. All toiletries and glass shower doors are removed, if possible. The door handle should be turned around so that the door can be locked from the outside. Additional restraints are placed on the outside of the door as needed. If the teenager is strong or extremely violent, a metal door can be purchased and installed. If the teenager becomes violent or starts destroying property, he or she is told to stop, or else a takedown procedure will be initiated immediately.

A "takedown" is a nonviolent method frequently used by hospital staff to stop extreme behavior and prevent patients from injuring themselves. In a takedown, the adolescent is put on the ground and rolled onto his or her stomach. The parent then sits on the adolescent's buttocks and leans his or her body weight forward to grab the teenager's wrists and securely hold them down. In this way, the adolescent is immobilized and unable to bite, spit, or kick the parent. The parents can use role playing to practice how they will initiate and complete a successful takedown. (The adolescent, of course, should not be present.)

Parents are also shown how to be nonreactive if the adolescent tries to escape from a takedown position. It is emphasized that for this strategy to be effective and nonabusive, the parents must remain calm at all times. To ensure that this goal is met, the counselor goes through a dry run of the takedown procedure, in which he or she role-plays the adolescent and tries to push every parental button possible. The counselor may even ask the parents to physically go down on the ground in a takedown position, to make the role play as real as possible. If there is a problem, the counselor freezes the role play and highlights how the parents could correct their reactions.

Parents are also shown how to recognize when their teenager's muscles begin to relax in a takedown. They are instructed to ask the teenager whether he or she is ready to get up to start a time out and voluntarily go into the bathroom. The teenager must be able to verbalize in a clear, calm voice why he or she had to be taken down. This procedure is initiated to prevent a "false calm," in which the teenager is pretending to be calm when in fact he or she is not. A teenager who cannot tell the parents why he or she was taken down in a calm voice is not ready to be let out of a takedown position. Parents are forewarned that initially several takedowns may have to occur within the space of an hour or so before they are successful. This same procedure is followed over and over until the adolescent can sit calmly in the bathroom for the required time.

The parents and teenager are told beforehand that if the teenager hits the parents when they try to restrain him or her, or if the teenager does major property damage, the police will be called and physical assault or property damage charges will be filed. This mirrors the real world and what would happen if the teen were an adult. If the teenager claims abuse when the police arrive, the parents are told to let the officer in calmly.

CLINICAL EXAMPLE

When the police arrived in the case of 16-year-old Greg, the father tried to prevent the police from entering until the counselor could be reached. This only agitated the police officers, and they arrested the father for obstruction of justice. The police felt that the father had something to hide. The police told the counselor that if they had been let in immediately and given a document describing this intervention, there would have been no problems.

Parents must be forewarned that adolescents will frequently attempt to triangulate outside forces like the police or child protective services workers, in order to disempower the parents and get them off their backs. Many parents can relate horror stories of this happening and are understandably reluctant to implement this strategy.

If this happens, the counselor tells the parents that things will be different this time, for three important reasons. First, they will be given a handout (Figure 6.1) describing the bathroom strategy and stating that it has been cleared by child protective services. (The counselor can copy this handout and give it to the local child protective services supervisor for clearance.) A letter will also be provided by the counselor stating that the teenager is under his or her care and giving a phone number so that the counselor can be contacted if necessary. (Figure 8.5 in Chapter 8 is an example of such a letter.) The parents will calmly hand the letter and the handout to the police officer or child protective services worker when he or she arrived. Second, the counselor will be on call 24 hours a day, 7 days a week. Parents are instructed to call immediately if there are any unanticipated problems or if the police or child protective services are called. The counselor assures the parents that he or she will be their advocate and defend them if these problems occur. Third, the counselor will make home visits if requested to help the parents with this strategy and will come to the house if the police or child protective services are called. This kind of commitment is necessary if this strategy and others are to be effective. It empowers the parents and gives them the confidence and energy they need to take back control of their own household. This strategy is not for those counselors who prefer 1 hour of office therapy per week. However, the rewards are great, because this strategy can work very quickly to stop the behavior within just days or weeks of its implementation.

The purpose of this handout is to explain the rationale, purpose, and benefits of the bathroom intervention. After reading this handout, if you have any questions or concerns *please do not hesitate* to contact me immediately regardless of the day or time. I can be reached 24 hours a day at [place number here]. I will return your call as quickly as I can. This intervention has been cleared by child protective services (CPS), as indicated by the signature of the CPS supervisor.

This intervention has been used with many other teenagers who chronically leave home without permission. It is used only as a last resort and after all other consequences have been tried and have failed.

In this intervention, the length of time the teenager is away from home without permission is the length of time the teenager will be required to spend as punishment in the bathroom. For example, if the teenager is gone 5 hours, the teenager will spend 5 hours in the bathroom upon returning home, and so on up to 24 hours. The bathroom is used instead of the bedroom as a time-out facility because it is usually the most boring room in the house and the most difficult to escape from. Otherwise, the teenager will run out the door when the parent's back is turned or climb out the bedroom window. In addition, the teenager's bedroom has too many entertainment items (television, radio, stereo equipment, etc.) and should be seen as a place of sanctuary rather than a place of punishment.

Adhering to state laws on abuse and neglect, in case of emergency or fire, the parent or another adult is in the home and awake the entire time the teenager is in the bathroom. Parents provide food and water to be eaten in the bathroom. No books, television, music, or other items are allowed, except for a pillow and blanket, in order that this not be an enjoyable experience. Before this intervention is initiated, the bathroom is totally stripped. All toiletries and glass shower doors are removed, if possible. The door handle should be turned around so that the door can be locked from the outside. Additional restraints are placed on the outside of the door as needed. If the teenager is strong or extremely violent, a metal door is purchased and installed.

If the teenager tries to destroy property in the bathroom, the police are called and charges are immediately filed, or a "takedown" procedure is initiated. A takedown is a nonviolent method frequently used by hospital staff to stop extreme behavior and prevent patients from injuring themselves. The police are called in only if the teenager is physically stronger and bigger than the parent in charge. If this happens, the parent will wait for the other parent to come home or (in the case of a single parent) for the person in the community who has been designated to help the parent to arrive. The teenager is told ahead of time that he or she will be placed in the bathroom for however long it takes the other parent or community member to get to the house, because of the inconvenience.

In a takedown, the teenager is put on the ground and rolled onto his or her stomach. The parent then sits on the teenager's buttocks and leans his or her body weight forward to grab the teenager's wrists and securely hold them down. In this way, the teenager is immobilized and unable to bite, spit, or kick the parent. The parents use role playing to practice how they will initiate and complete a successful takedown in a nonreactive fashion.

The rationale for this intervention is that the teenager values his or her freedom above all else. Therefore, this intervention can sour the idea of running away very quickly, because it represents a loss of freedom. Without this secured facility, the teenager will leave whenever he or she feels like it and be at a greater risk of getting hurt or killed in the streets. When this intervention is working, the teenager will sometimes call the police and/or CPS, or get another parent or peer to call and claim abuse, when there is no evidence of abuse. The teenager does this simply to create a crisis and get the parents to back off.

I [name of CPS worker] have read this handout and have cleared this strategy for use.

Signed,

CPS Worker

FIGURE 6.1. Parent handout: Description of the bathroom strategy. This handout can be modified to use with disrespect and threats or acts of violence. From *Treating the Tough Adolescent* by Scott P. Sells. Copyright 1998 by The Guilford Press. Permission to photocopy this handout is granted to purchasers of *Treating the Tough Adolescent* for personal use only (see copyright page for details).

CLINICAL EXAMPLE

Fifteen-year-old Lynette left the house whenever she did not get her way or was grounded. She told the counselor in the first session that no one could stop her. The police had been called and did nothing. Her single mother was small in stature and admittedly afraid of Lynette.

With the mother's permission, the counselor contacted two neighbors, a best friend and minister. At the next meeting, each person was asked "what if" questions and went through a dry run of how he or she would implement the bathroom strategy. The counselor role-played the part of Lynette and tried to push each person's buttons to make them lose control of their emotions.

The mother was instructed to look at her watch as soon as Lynette left the house without permission and to calculate how long she was gone. All the doors to the house would then be locked. When Lynette came back home, the mother would refuse entrance until the counselor was called and at least one of the mother's friends could come to the house. After the counselor and one or more friends arrived, the mother would tell Lynette that she had until the count of three to go to the bathroom and serve her time quietly. The mother's friends were instructed to stand behind the mother but not say and do anything. The counselor was also in the background to choreograph the intervention and keep everyone on track. After the count of three, the mother would gently take Lynette by the arm and guide her to the bathroom. If she grew violent or refused to move, the mother would initiate a takedown. Friends would grab Lynette's legs, while the mother held her down by the shoulders. These takedown procedures were practiced beforehand in the office, with one of the neighbors playing the part of Lynette.

Because of this preparation, the intervention was a success. The following week, when Lynette ran away for 3 hours, everyone played his or her role as instructed. While everyone stood physically behind the mother to show support, Lynette quietly went into the bathroom. When she started destroying property in the bathroom during her second hour, the neighbor was there as planned to help the mother open the door and perform a takedown. This intervention occurred only twice before Lynette decided to give up running away. She later told the counselor that she was "sick of the bathroom" and would rather stop running away than have to lose her freedom.

Exceptions to the use of this procedure include the following:

1. If the adolescent is physically stronger and bigger than one parent, that parent should not use a takedown procedure. Instead, the parent should wait for the other parent to come home or (in the case of a single parent) for a person in the community who has been designated to help the parent to arrive. The adolescent should be told ahead of time that he or she will be placed in the bathroom for however long it takes the other parent or community member to get to the house, because of the inconvenience.

2. If the parent cannot physically initiate a takedown and the adolescent

commits acts of violence or destruction of property before the other parent returns or the community member arrives, the police are immediately called and charges are filed.

3. The procedure becomes less and less effective as a teenager gets older and physically stronger. It is most effective for adolescents between the ages of 12 and 15. However, this procedure has been used effectively with adolescents as old as 17, and its use should be determined on a case-by-case basis.

4. This procedure should not be used if one or both of the parents react to the teenager in a hot-tempered manner or are prone to physical abuse. However, as stated earlier, many parents are physically or emotionally abusive because they feel out of control and do not have a better set of tools to be in charge. Once this strategy is initiated, the parents have the tools to be in charge without being abusive. Hence, again, the use of this procedure should be determined on a case-by-case basis.

5. This procedure should not be used if an adolescent is physically stronger than a single mother and she has no support system. In some cases, a counselor can help the mother locate someone through the church or the neighborhood to help the mother temporarily, as noted above. In this case, the counselor goes over these procedures with both the mother and the neighbor before the plan is initiated.

Strategy 3: The Gandhi Strategy

The Gandhi strategy was developed by Neil Schiff (Schiff & Belson, 1988) and has been successfully used for adolescents who run away, are truant, or threaten or commit acts of violence. This strategy was named after the Indian leader Mohandas K. Gandhi, a noted advocate of nonviolent protest, because the parents commit themselves to an all-day nonviolent sit-in with their teenager.

Parents must be told that their teenager will be so miserable the first time this strategy is implemented that they will probably not have to resort to it a second time. Parents who understand this rationale are usually willing to go to this extreme, once it is clear that the strategy is time-limited. This strategy is very effective because teenagers would rather stop their problematic behavior than face an entire day staring at their parents.

Implementation. The parents take the day off from work and sit in the living room all day with their teenager. No television or phone calls are allowed. Instead, each party is required to sit and stare at the others without saying a word. No one is allowed to leave the room.

This strategy should be implemented the next time the adolescent returns home from running away. The adolescent and/or parents are likely to recoil at the idea of spending an entire day in this manner. This recoil is sometimes sufficient to stop the adolescent from continuing the behavior. However, for this intervention to work, the adolescent must be convinced that one or both parents will participate in an all-day sit-in if necessary.

CLINICAL EXAMPLE

Sixteen-year-old Miko was referred because of running away. When the parents attempted to stop her from leaving the house to see her boyfriend without permission, Miko would become hysterical and run away. The police would then be called, and Miko would be taken to the hospital for observation.

At their first meeting, the counselor recommended the Gandhi strategy the next time Miko ran away. Miko immediately recoiled at the idea that she might have to sit in the living room with her parents an entire day without talking. The father also reported that he would be unable to take off work to spend all day with his daughter. However, the counselor was able to convince the father that nothing else to this point had worked and that this strategy was worth a try. In addition, the counselor made the father and mother aware of the fact that Miko had recoiled at the idea. This alone was a good sign that the consequence would be effective. The father was instructed to sit in front of the door to block the daughter from running away. The parents were also shown ways to be nonreactive to Miko if she started to scream or throw a temper tantrum. Two days after this meeting, Miko tested this consequence by running away. The next day the father took off work as promised, and the parents and daughter had an all-day sit-in. Miko hated this intervention to such a degree that she never ran away again.

Strategy 4: Poisoning the Adolescent's Safe Houses

One reason a teenager can run away from home is often that he or she has one or more "safe houses" to go to. Many times, the parents at these safe houses do not know that the teenager is there or think that the teenager has permission to sleep over. In other cases, a teenager may have been able to convince these parents through lies or half-truths that he or she is being abused. With only one side of the story, these parents may believe the teenager and feel that they are protecting him or her from further abuse by letting the teen stay in their home.

To counter these problems, the parents must do everything in their power to find these safe houses and "poison" them by making the teenager no longer welcome. To accomplish this goal, the parents have several options.

Implementation. First, parents can begin calling their teenager's friends to locate where he or she might be staying. Parents must be persistent because friends will often protect the teen and may not initially reveal any information. If this happens, the parents can talk to the parents of their teenager's friends. They can ask the parents to put pressure on their sons or daughters to reveal the runaway teenager's whereabouts. Pressure from both sets of parents may be enough to force or convince a friend to give the correct information. In addition, as noted earlier, parents can find a picture of the teenager and print up flyers to be posted around the school or at the places he or she frequents, with a small reward offered for information on the teen's whereabouts.

Second, once the parents find a safe house, they should first approach the situation with the assumption that the parents either are unaware of the teenager's presence or have been given misinformation. Given this assumption, the parents should go directly to the safe house during the evening after work on a surprise visit to talk to the parents at that house. The parents should first try to reason with the safe house parents to clear up any misinformation. Many parents will be receptive to this approach and gladly turn over the teenager. The parents then tell the safe house parents in front of their teenager that if the teen should run away again, they will immediately give the safe house parents a call. The two sets of parents then exchange phone numbers. This collaboration between parents is important for the runaway teenager to see and will increase the likelihood that this safe house is now poisoned.

Finally, if the safe house parents are uncooperative, parents should initiate Plan B by telling the safe house parents that they are harboring the teenager illegally. If this continues, the teen's parents will contact the police. One parent even picketed on the lawn of a stubborn parent with a sign saying that the parents in this house were housing her daughter illegally. This embarrassed the safe house parents so much that they soon gave up the daughter. In addition, the parents can send the safe house parents a certified letter stating that they have now been officially informed that they are harboring their son or daughter illegally. The letter should also state that if the safe house parents do not immediately release the teenager, a copy of the letter will be delivered to the police. Most families will give up the teenager at this point, because they do not want any trouble with the law.

The more safe houses the parents poison, the more difficult it will become for the teenager to run away. In addition, word will spread that the parents will harass anyone who harbors their teenager in the future. Consequently, other parents will be less likely to provide a safe house to this runaway teenager. To ensure further that this objective is met, the parents can tell the teenager that they will have to meet all of the teen's friends. Each friend they meet has to provide his or her parents' names and phone numbers. The parents are then called to confirm that the number is valid. All information is written down on a list to establish a phone tree. This list can then be used if the teenager runs again. The more preventive measures that are taken, the more likely it will be that these safe houses will be contaminated and make it more and more difficult for the teenager to run away in the future.

Strategy 5: Using Positive Reinforcers

As soon as the running away stops or lessens, it is important for the parents to find positive ways to let the teenager know that they appreciate the teen's efforts to improve his or her behavior. Often the teenager is exposed only to criticism or other negative reinforcers even when he or she attempts to do better. When this happens, the home environment becomes toxic and the teenager stops trying. A vicious cycle is created, with the teenager failing to improve and the parents being highly critical. It is extremely important that the counselor make the parents aware of this cycle and show specifically how it contributes to running away.

CLINICAL EXAMPLE

Thirteen-year-old Paul's father constantly criticized him. Even when Paul initially stopped running away, it was never good enough for the father. Instead of praising Paul for not running away, the father moved immediately to criticize another problem area. During the session, the teenager's slumped body language suggested defeat. Paul ran away the next day; the father's reaction was to shout "Here we go again!" and throw his hands in the air. Paul later reported that he stopped trying because he felt that nothing he did would ever be good enough.

The counselor had a good rapport with the father and asked him to experiment with eliminating all criticism for 2 weeks. Each time the father criticized, his wife would fine him. By the end of the first week, he had paid over $30, which she spent on needless luxury items. The father did not like to part with or waste money. The next week the father reported that until he tried to stop criticizing, he had not realized how much he did it without thinking. At this point, there was a dramatic shift in the father's thought processes, and he began to praise and acknowledge Paul's efforts in a very sincere and caring manner. Paul later reported that the main reason he stopped running away was the effort his father had made to stop criticizing him.

Strategy 6: Trust Building, When Possible

The counselor must teach parents the importance of giving the teenager the means by which he or she can begin to build trust. Trust is the cornerstone of all relationships. Therefore, if the teenager feels that there are no opportunities to trust, he or she will begin to lose hope that things will ever improve;

consequently, the teen will stop making any effort to change. However, trust may have become an extremely difficult concept for the parents to understand or commit themselves to, because they have been "burned" so many times in the past that they hesitate to let their guard down and try again.

Implementation. If this happens, the counselor must take charge and convince the parents to find ways to let their teenager build trust. This is a difficult challenge but can be accomplished through two different avenues. First, the counselor may need to stop the extreme behavior by helping the parents implement one or more of the consequences above. This can bring the family a temporary sense of peace, and can help the parents to develop trust in the counselor as an expert. Second, the counselor assures them that the plan to rebuild trust will be a slow, step-by-step process. If the teenager breaks the rule and runs away or does not come back at curfew, there are predetermined consequences that will be reinforced. The only difference from before is that the teenager and family will get back on track as quickly as possible, in order to provide means by which the teenager can continue to try to rebuild trust.

CLINICAL EXAMPLE

Fourteen-year-old Barbara would run away from home as soon as her parents enforced any rules she did not like. Over time, the mother felt so burned out and betrayed by Barbara that she refused ever to trust the daughter again. She insisted that Barbara had to be placed under constant surveillance. Barbara resented the mother for this and stated that she would no longer try if her mother continued to expect the worst. When the counselor tried to bring up the concept of trust, the mother immediately yelled at him for taking the daughter's side. However, after the counselor succeeded in helping the parents to apply the bathroom strategy to stop the running away, the mother was willing to take a second look at the trust issue, because the counselor had been able to accomplish a miracle in her eyes.

Armed with this success, the counselor set about the task of convincing the mother that she had his 24-hour support if her daughter relapsed and ran away again. Trust could be earned in the following manner: (1) For each day Barbara came home on time, she would receive 1 hour added to her curfew time; (2) Barbara could keep that hour as long as she continued to come home on time; (3) if Barbara was more than 10 minutes late for curfew, she would lose that extra hour and be grounded the next day. After the consequence was administered and served, Barbara would immediately have the opportunity to regain her hour back and earn trust if she came home on time the next day. In this way, the daughter continually received opportunities to build trust, while still receiving consequences if she was late for curfew.

A "regaining trust" contract should be written after the teenager's behavior starts to improve; otherwise, the changes may be only temporary. Often the best beginning is to ask the teenager directly what he or she thinks are reasonable steps to move toward regaining trust. Most teenagers want their freedom. Consequently, the parents can give or take away hours of freedom, based on coming home on time and checking in at predetermined time intervals.

One parent got very creative and designed 1-hour coupons that could be used for more phone time (up to 2 extra hours per night) or up to 1 extra hour of curfew on weekends, as long as the teenager was not grounded and obeyed curfew. The teenager later reported that this symbolized trust because he had an opportunity to earn back his freedom even if he relapsed. In the past, he would have been grounded for 2 months with no chance of regaining his freedom.

Strategy 7: Predicting Relapse

Predicting relapse is one of the most important strategies to consider when dealing with running away and other extreme behaviors. However, many counselors and parents fail to recognize that relapse is normal and should be expected. Consequently, when teenagers relapse, parents and counselors alike feel betrayed and angry that they put in so much time and effort. They may also feel that they are "back to square one" and that things will never change. At this point, many parents drop out of counseling because they feel defeated and take the relapse very personally.

CLINICAL EXAMPLE

Sixteen-year-old Alicia had stopped running away for 3 weeks, had gotten a job, and was behaving more respectfully to her parents. The session ended with everyone thinking that counseling was over and with Alicia promising that this time things would be different. The parents even went out for a special dinner to celebrate. However, the next weekend was the 4th of July, and Alicia stayed out all night. The parents felt so betrayed and hurt that they almost quit counseling. Without any preparation for a relapse, the parents were completely caught off guard and saw the relapse as a personal slap in the face, rather than as a normal part of the change process.

Implementation. To prepare the family for relapse, it is critical for the counselor to do two things. First, the counselor must tell the parents that relapse is a normal part of the change process. As with any change, there will be ups and downs. Therefore, the goal of treatment is not to expect the behavior to stop forever instantaneously, but rather to space the relapses further and further apart until they no longer occur. This normalization helps reduce blame and increase the understanding that a relapse is to be expected. When the parents accept this fact, they are less likely to give up all efforts when one occurs.

Second, the counselor must instruct the family that the time to plan for and anticipate a relapse is, ironically, when things are going well. Both the parents and the teenager may vehemently disagree with this statement. They may say that the counselor does not know what he or she is talking about, because things have never been better. The counselor must tell the family that the planning is only a precaution. This type of paradoxical intervention often succeeds because the family's instinct is to resist the counselor's prediction by doing their best to prove him or her wrong. This supports the teenager in battling the urge to relapse. Even if the teenager does relapse, the parents and counselor have devised strategies and consequences to handle such a contingency. This creates a win–win scenario for both the family and the counselor. If the teenager does not relapse, the family feels empowered and proud for proving the counselor wrong. If the teen does relapse, the family is not caught off guard and can perform damage control by immediately getting back on track.

CLINICAL EXAMPLE

Fourteen-year-old Peter continued to relapse after each week of perfect behavior. The parents would immediately state that they were "back to square one" and redouble their efforts by becoming overly strict. After consultation, the counselor decided to use a paradoxical intervention and normalize relapses. He had a good relationship with Peter and playfully suggested that Peter was about due for another relapse because things were going too well. The counselor told Peter and his parents that relapses were normal and should be expected. He suggested that peter intentionally sabotaged his behavior improvement because he was afraid of success. Both the parents and Peter vehemently disagreed and were reluctant to talk about the possibility further.

The counselor stood by his assessment and put a $5 bill on the table. He told Peter that he would bet him $5 that he would relapse. Smiling, Peter replied that he would take that bet and that he was not scared of success. The counselor then prepared the parents with "what if" scenarios in case Peter relapsed. The parents decided that if Peter relapsed they would not get angry, but simply place him in the bathroom for as long as he was gone without permission. After this integral session, the weekly relapses immediately halted, proving the paradoxical intervention a success.

The counselor must continue to predict and plan for relapses throughout treatment. This is especially true when things seem to be going well. If the teenager is challenged to maintain the positive behavior and prove the counselor wrong, the relapse may not occur. In many cases, it seems as if normalization is the immunization needed to stop relapses.

ACE 2: TRUANCY AND POOR SCHOOL PERFORMANCE

Truancy and poor school performance are combined into one "ace" for two reasons. First, they both involve the school system on some level. Second, both behaviors have the desired effect of neutralizing the parents' authority. A teen's missing school makes parents anxious and fearful because the teenager is unsupervised during these times. Moreover, many parents value education, and if a teenager is failing in school because of fighting or lack of effort, parents can get just as anxious and frustrated as they can over truancy. In fact, poor school performance can contribute to making the parents so angry that they are ineffective, and thus it can have the same effect as truancy often does.

Truancy and poor school performance can be stopped, but, to do so, the parents must have a concrete plan of action and must work in close collaboration with school personnel. However, when parents contact teachers, guidance counselors, or other school staff members, the school personnel may blame the parents (either aloud or silently) for the teenager's problems and lack of communication. This removes the accountability from the teenager and strengthens the friction between the two systems, making collaborative efforts difficult without outside assistance.

This outside assistance comes in the form of the counselor, who coaches parents on how to collaborate with school personnel to increase cooperation. The parents are then better prepared and better able to enlist the school's support of the behavior contract. Mutually directed blame is suddenly replaced with cooperation when the teenager is held responsible for his or her actions by both school personnel and the parents.

CLINICAL EXAMPLE

Sixteen-year-old Elena continually skipped school. After 3 months, her teachers gave up trying to contact the parents and blamed them for Elena's problems. The parents, in turn, attributed Elena's truancy to the incompetence of the school personnel. The counselor helped the parents develop a plan of action that included the consequences of grounding Elena and having her father go to school with her the next day and sit in on each class. The parents met with each teacher to discuss the contract while Elena waited outside in the lobby. The counselor also attended to keep the discussion on track while the parents took charge and told the teachers that, although it was not their job to babysit Elena, they would appreciate the support of the teachers in monitoring rules and enforcing consequences. After working out the details with each teacher and troubleshooting future problems, the parents brought Elena into the meeting and presented the contract. The teachers, the counselor, and the parents were thus able to present a united front.

The following strategies have been used to develop successful contracts with the school and effective consequences at home to stop truancy and poor school performance: (1) working collaboratively with the school system; (2) attending school with the teenager; (3) having the teen come to work with a parent or dress like a "nerd"; (4) implementing in-home consequences; and (5) home schooling or switching schools. In addition to these strategies, the counselor must employ some of the strategies described above in connection with running away: using positive reinforcers, building trust, and predicting relapses.

Strategy 1: Working Collaboratively with the School System

When the parents meet with the school personnel, the teenager should wait outside while the parents give a written plan to each teacher or guidance counselor present. Witnessing any disagreements between parents and school personnel would only provide the teenager with more ammunition to defeat the parents. After the details have been worked out, the teenager is asked to come back into the room. The parents read the contract to the teenager, explain everyone's role, and outline how the teen's behavior will be monitored. The meeting is then quickly concluded so that the teenager does not have an opportunity to unravel the plan. The counselor should be present at the school to advocate for the parents and to mediate when necessary by keeping all parties on track. The actual letter written by the father of 13-year-old Jay is reproduced in Figure 6.2 to serve as a model for implementing this strategy successfully. It illustrates two essential principles: keeping solutions problem-focused, and promoting open communication and accountability.

Keeping Solutions Problem-Focused

Most parent–teacher conferences are nonproductive. Teachers will often comment on how bad the teenager is, with body language and tones of voice that communicate hopelessness. The teachers and parents then lecture the teenager on how he or she has to improve, without taking any steps to map out exactly how this will be done. This pattern of futility repeats itself in future parent–teacher conferences, and progress is never made.

However, note in Figure 6.2 that Mr. Smith took charge by setting the tone of the meeting as one of solutions, not problems. Mr. Smith did this by clearly defining everyone's role and outlining how he and the teachers could work together as a team. The positive direction and concrete plan of action encouraged teachers who had previously been negative to become cooperative and helpful. The purpose and problem-solving tone of the meeting are

Kevin M. Smith
A-1 Group
123 Darby Lane

Office Number: 555-5555
Home Number: 444-4444

January 9, 1997

Track 4 Teachers of Jay Smith:
Ms. Watkins
Ms. Gordon

Ms. Bixler
Ms. Fargason

Dear Teachers,

Jay, his mother, Dr. Scott Sells, and I have had considerable discussions over the Christmas break about what Jay needs to do to turn around his behavior and performance in school. **The purpose of today's meeting is to coordinate our actions and set up guidelines for Jay.** Jay's mother has been kind enough to allow Jay to live with me during this trimester, so I can concentrate my full attention on helping him improve at school.

I will not tolerate Jay's being disruptive in any of your classes, nor will I tolerate his not turning in assignments. I am therefore requesting your help as follows:

1. I am giving each of you two postcards with my return address. If you have any problems with Jay or if he misses any assignments, please drop off these cards in the mail, and I will respond immediately.

2. Place any comments about Jay's behavior, lack of attentiveness, or missed assignments in his daily planner. I will review this planner with him on a daily basis. This planner will serve as a way for us (you four teachers and myself) to communicate with one another.

3. Call me at either of the numbers listed above, and I will immediately come to school. I am about 5 to 10 minutes away from the school. I will sit with Jay in class to assure that he pays attention and does not disrupt your teaching.

Jay knows ahead of time that there will be consequences at home for any negative comments in his planner or any postcards. I have asked Jay to continue to have each of you initial his planner every day to assure that he writes down the assignments correctly and allow you to make any comments to him or me about his behavior and performance in the classroom.

I thank you for your extra efforts. Jay knows that this will be an exceptionally important trimester for him and that he is now making a fresh start. I want to work collaboratively with all of you to make this Jay's most productive trimester. I would like to meet again in a month to discuss his progress and review this plan.

Very truly yours,

Kevin M. Smith

FIGURE 6.2. Parent handout: Example of a letter written by a parent to school personnel. From *Treating the Tough Adolescent* by Scott P. Sells. Copyright 1998 by The Guilford Press. Permission to photocopy this handout is granted to purchasers of *Treating the Tough Adolescent* for personal use only (see copyright page for details).

clearly stated in the first paragraph of the letter: "The purpose of today's meeting is to coordinate our actions and set up guidelines for Jay." The counselor helped Mr. Smith draft this letter a week before the scheduled meeting. The counselor was a vital part of the plan, but the father conducted the meeting himself. The counselor acted as a mediator to keep the discussions focused and on track.

Promoting Open Communication and Accountability

A major reason why teenagers are truant or perform poorly in school is the parents' inability to "nip the problem in the bud." Problems may happen throughout the week, but the parents often have no knowledge of these problems until days or weeks later, or only learn about them when they receive a report card or a letter or phone call to schedule a required parent conference (RPC). Even this communication can fail if the teenager gets to the mailbox before the parents to prevent them from getting a report card or an RPC notice. The teenager believes that this will stop the school and the parents from working together. The teenager also realizes that he or she will not be held accountable if the school and his parents are at odds or fail to communicate.

To counter this possibility, the counselor must teach the parents to be proactive in establishing good communication with their teenager's school. The counselor can help the parents understand that since the school has so many students, it is impossible for teachers to call or communicate with each and every parent. It is up to the parents to make it easier on the teachers to communicate with them, just as Mr. Smith did with just three simple yet effective actions, as described in Figure 6.2:

1. The father gave each teacher two stamped self-addressed postcards. If the teachers did not have time to call, they could quickly list any problems, absences, tardies, or missed homework assignments on a postcard and drop it in the mail to Jay's father. Consequences at home could then be swift and immediate to stop the behavior before it worsened.

2. The father provided Jay with a daily, not weekly, logbook in which Jay's teachers were asked to complete a daily progress report. The report (not described in Figure 6.2) was divided into three columns. The first contained the class period; the second listed the homework assignment for that particular class and/or any behaviors the father should be aware of; and the third held the teacher's signature to verify Jay's attendance and his completion of the homework assignment. Jay was required to bring his logbook home to his father each day. If he did not, there would be severe consequences at home. Jay also bore the responsibility of getting all of the teacher's signatures and filling out the homework assignment each day. This logbook system provided

Jay's father with constant communication with the teachers and immediate feedback on Jay's progress and daily attendance.

3. The father encouraged the teachers to use him as a disciplinary resource if Jay broke any rules at school. He did this by giving the teachers phone numbers where he could be reached if there was a problem, and offering to come to the school immediately if he was called.

With this well-organized plan, Jay suddenly became accountable for his actions on a day-to-day basis. Problems could now be identified and addressed before they became chronic or resulted in Jay's suspension or expulsion.

Strategy 2: Attending School with the Teenager

A very effective strategy if done correctly is one in which a parent attends school with the teenager. In this developmental stage of their lives, teenagers are very self-conscious and want to look "cool" in front of their friends. They will definitely not like Mom or Dad following them to each class and sitting right beside them—especially if Mom comes to school in fuzzy slippers with rollers in her hair, or Dad wears loud, colorful plaid pants and a pocket protector. This intervention is one of the parents' "big guns" and should be used only if other strategies are ineffective or the problem is chronic.

Implementation. Before a parent escorts the teenager to school, the principal and teachers must be notified ahead of time and must grant their permission. Sometimes the counselor must intervene and speak with the principal to emphasize the plan's benefits before permission is granted.

Once the approval of school personnel has been obtained, the counselor must prepare the parents in private and must troubleshoot possible outcomes. First, the counselor must stress with the parents that it usually takes one to three visits to the school before this strategy works. The parents may object, saying that it is too costly to take off work for so many days. In response, the counselor should point out that the parents will be forced to miss many more hours of work in the future if the problem behavior continues or worsens. Without strong interventions, the financial and emotional costs to the family will only increase.

When all parental concerns have been dealt with, the counselor explains each procedural step as follows:

1. The teacher notifies the parents when the teenager is truant, absent, or tardy, or the parents proactively contact the school attendance officer to find out the information each day. A parent then accompanies the teenager

to class the next day or the first day the parent can get time off from work. The penalty for the first offense can be a "warning shot," with the parent only attending a few classes. However, if it happens a second time, the parent should go for the entire day. This includes eating lunch with the teenager in front of his or her friends. This procedure works best when both parents are able to miss work and go together the first time as a symbol of a united front.

2. If the teenager has severe behavioral problems (hitting other kids, destruction of property, swearing at teachers), these should be defined ahead of time. If any of these behaviors occur at school, the parents ask the teachers to call them or note it in the daily progress report. The parents will then make arrangements to come to school the next day possible to support the teacher and make sure the teenager behaves properly.

3. If the teenager refuses to do homework, one or both parents can also go to school the next day or the first day they can get off work. Not only does this communicate to the teenager how serious this behavior is, but it shows that the parents will do everything in their power to see that the teenager puts forth his or her best efforts in school.

Strategy 3: Having the Teen Come to Work with a Parent or Dress Like a "Nerd"

If neither parent can take time off from work to accompany the teenager to school, a parent can instead modify the strategy by taking the teenager to work or dressing him or her like a "nerd" (i.e., a shirt, tie, and suit for a boy, or a blazer and skirt for a girl). If the teenager goes to work, he or she is required to simply sit all day doing nothing. This can be done on a daily basis until the teenager decides that he or she would rather go to school than "die of boredom." In addition, one parent made his son dress in a shirt and tie for every day he missed school. The teenager was so self-conscious about his looks that he decided he would rather go to school than suffer the embarrassment of being labeled as a "nerd."

CLINICAL EXAMPLE

Thirteen-year-old Jon refused to go to school and preferred to stay home and watch cable television with his friends who came over. The father was a single parent who was unable to take time off from his construction job to go to school with Jon. Therefore, Jon was required to go with his father to work and sit on a woodpile all day in the hot sun doing nothing. When he got home from his father's workplace, Jon was required to sit in the bathroom the rest of the day with no television, music, or books. This intervention only lasted 2 days before Jon was begging his father to let him go to school.

Strategy 4: Implementing In-Home Consequences

In-home consequences can be implemented for the following behaviors: (1) truancy; (2) missing or incomplete daily progress reports; (3) missed homework; or (4) behavior problems at school. Each of these behaviors is fully defined within a written contract, and consequences are predetermined.

Grounding

Grounding is most effective when it is implemented on a 1:1 ratio (1 day of grounding for each violation). The 1:1 ratio is suggested because many parents take away privileges for weeks on end. If the grounding goes on for a long time, it is actually harder on the parents than on the teenager, as the parents are responsible for closely monitoring the teenager's behavior to enforce the consequence. In addition, a teenager who is grounded for too long may feel that he or she has nothing more to lose by skipping school to visit with friends.

Grounding should take place on the days when it is the most meaningful to the teenager. For most teenagers, these days are usually Friday, Saturday, and Sunday. If grounding takes place during the week, it may have little impact. Therefore, for each violation the teenager is grounded for one weekend day and night, beginning Friday. For example, a teenager who violates a school rule on Monday is grounded on Friday. If second and third violations occur that same week, the teen will be grounded Friday, Saturday, and Sunday. If subsequent violations take place in the same week, the parents postpone the grounding until the next Friday, Saturday, and so on. Teenagers are told beforehand how their parents define grounding. Most often it means no television, no phone, no car, no stereo, and no friends, but it is up to the parents to decide. Troubleshooting is also initiated, with the teenager being informed of the consequences that will occur if he or she retaliates in any way.

Going to the Bathroom or Going to School

If the teenager refuses to go to school, the teen is told that he or she has just chosen "Plan B," which is to go straight to the bathroom and sit there until the next school day. The next day the teenager will be required to go to school again, and the parent will accompany him or her and sit in class. If the teenager still refuses, he or she will stay in the bathroom another day. Unless the teenager is extremely stubborn, this procedure will only need to be initiated 1 or 2 days. If the behavior continues and the parents cannot take the day off, they can have a trusted friend watch the teenager in the bathroom. If there are any problems or property damage, the friend calls the parents immediately. Property damages result in charges being filed with the police.

The friend is asked simply to monitor the teenager and not to take any physical action.

Using Positive Reinforcers

It is important to use positive reinforcers whenever possible. Each week that the teenager has documented perfect school attendance, all progress reports signed, all homework completed, and no extreme behavior problems, something positive should take place and continue until school problems resurface. This can include the privilege of riding a bike to school, an extra hour of curfew on the weekends, extended phone time, or special outings. It is important to choose the reward that best motivates the particular teenager. The teenager should be told that these privileges are not permanent and will be taken away if the problem behavior resumes.

If possible, the reinforcer should immediately follow a day of perfect attendance or good school performance. For example, one teenager received a coupon for an extra hour of freedom on the weekend for each day of perfect attendance, while another teenager received a coupon for one extra hour of phone time. The parent of a third teen got creative and grounded the teenager for a week, but reduced the grounding time by 1 day for every day the daily progress report was completed and the daughter was not truant. As noted earlier, it is important for the counselor to help parents to remove themselves from a strictly punitive stance by incorporating both positive and negative consequences.

Strategy 5: Home Schooling or Switching Schools–
A Last Resort

When given the chance, the teenager will opt for home schooling and make "pie in the sky" promises to entice the parents to try this option. The problem is that a teenager who is unable to change his or her behavior in a regular school setting will generally not miraculously change it within a home school setting. After an initial honeymoon period, teenagers may actually exhibit worse behaviors, because they have too much time on their hands and are often left unsupervised. Once the taste of freedom sets in, it can be nearly impossible to get such teenagers back into public school.

If home schooling is not the issue, switching schools often is. Teenagers may think that switching to a new school can magically solve their problems. However, the problem behaviors will follow the teenagers no matter what school they attend. Switching schools should only be considered an option when it can be determined that a teenager is in danger of being physically hurt, and school officials are unable or unwilling to get involved.

The counselor should instruct parents to consider home schooling or switching schools only under the following conditions:

1. All the strategies described above have been tried and have failed on a consistent basis.

2. The teenager maintains a part-time or full-time job and pays the parent the equivalent of one semester's charges before home schooling begins. The teenager is not allowed to pay after the fact or as he or she goes unless an automatic paycheck deduction can be set up through the teen's employer. Parents can find out the costs by contacting the school. Often schools provide these home services at little or no charge; in that case, the money the teenager pays the parents can go into a savings account and be used as a future reward or punishment. For example, if the teenager achieves a grade of C+ or better in every subject, the teenager will get the money back as a reward. If not, the parents get the money.

3. If no schooling option is working out and the adolescent is 16 to 18 years old, the teenager must obtain and maintain a full-time job before he or she is allowed to drop out. The teen must also pay for and pass a high school equivalency examination and obtain a general education diploma (GED).

ACE 3: SUICIDAL THREATS OR BEHAVIORS

Whether or not to hospitalize a teenager who threatens or attempts suicide is a difficult decision for anyone to make. It should depend on the seriousness of the threat or attempt, any previous threats or attempts (and their seriousness), the parents' commitment to keeping their son or daughter alive, and the parents' ability to work together as a team to prevent suicide. Even if suicidal threats are determined to be a form of manipulation, the teenager may still be successful in accidentally killing himself or herself. Therefore, all threats and behaviors must be taken seriously, and the counselor must carefully assess each of these factors.

The 24-Hour Watch Strategy

The 24-hour watch as a strategy for dealing with suicidal threats or behaviors was developed by Jay Haley (1980) and has been used successfully with suicidal adolescents. (It has been described earlier as one of the "atom bomb interventions" for running away.) When parents institute a 24-hour watch, they continuously observe their teenager and are careful never to leave him or her alone until the risk of suicide (or running away) has passed. This means going to school with the teen, going out with the teen and his or her peers, and sleeping in the same room if possible. This will test the patience of the parents, but helps them take a firmer position in demanding normal behavior from the youth. This technique also mirrors what would take place in a hospital setting. In a hospital, if the adolescent was deemed at risk for suicide or flight, he or she would be placed in a locked unit and closely monitored at all times. However, if the youth is hospitalized, outside experts are the ones changing the behavior, not the parents. Thus, as noted earlier, the youth is likely to use these same extreme behaviors again when he or she returns home and is faced with tough rules or consequences. If this happens, the cycle of being in and out of institutions may never end. A case example illustrates how the 24-hour watch can be implemented for suicidal behaviors.

CLINICAL EXAMPLE

Fifteen-year-old Carrie was referred to counseling for running away and chronic truancy. During the course of treatment, the parents began to put aside their differences temporarily and enforce the rules of curfew and going to school. As a result of these changes, Carrie threatened suicide by holding a razor blade to her wrist if the parents tried to prevent her from leaving the house late at night. When this happened, both parents were ready to hospitalize Carrie and frame her behavior as a mental illness.

The counselor immediately took charge and reframed her behavior as manipulative and childish. He pointed to the fact that there had been no previous suicide threats until the parents began to exert their joint authority. Furthermore, if they hospitalized Carrie, they would have to pay thousands of dollars to have someone do exactly what they could do at home. In addition, she would get the message that she was not responsible for her behavior and that she could get authority figures to back off if her behaviors were extreme enough.

Because Carrie had no previous history of suicidal behavior, and the parents were invested and motivated, the counselor was able to initiate the 24-hour watch strategy. First, both parents had to agree that, for safety reasons, they could not end the watch on their own. The final approval to terminate the watch had to come from the counselor in collaboration with the parents. Second, they had to remove all razors, sharp objects, and chemicals from the bathroom and the rest of the house immediately upon returning home. The parents then had to call the counselor by phone to verify that this had been accomplished. Third, they would have to arrange their work schedules so that one parent would be able to watch Carrie at all times. Fourth, the parents had to get permission from Carrie's school to be on campus. The counselor would also call the school to advocate for the parents. However, if there were any problems with the school or Carrie refused to go, she would stay confined to her room all day; until the crisis was over, all privileges (phone, car, etc.) would be suspended. Fifth, since Carrie was prone to run away at night and the parents had to get some sleep, Carrie would be confined to a bathroom with no windows and given only a sleeping bag and pillow. The bathroom would be stripped down and made suicide-proof. Sixth, since Carrie was in danger of hurting herself, she could not see her friends or leave the house except to go to school, in which case her parents must accompany her at all times. This would continue until the risk of suicide and running away had passed. Finally, the counselor would be on call 24 hours a day and available if any problems occurred.

By the second day of the watch, the daughter was so unhappy about losing all her freedom and being treated like a "mental patient" that the symptoms of suicide immediately stopped and never returned again. In addition, the parents became firmer and began to expect normal behavior from Carrie. In this way, the consequence of the 24-hour watch made it more difficult for Carrie to maintain suicidal behaviors and running away than to give up her freedom and independence.

In sum, suicidal threats or acts should never be taken lightly. The counselor has to be available 24 hours a day, 7 days a week, and must be ready on a moment's notice to conduct home visits. If the parents do not have the time, energy, or commitment, the counselor should initiate hospitalization rather than place the teenager at risk.

ACE 4: THREATS OR ACTS OF VIOLENCE

Threats of violence must be separated from acts of violence. Both must be dealt with quickly, but in a slightly different manner. When threats of violence take place, the counselor must teach the parents how to stop such threats from advancing into action. If real violence does ensue, it is a time for action, not more talk. This action includes the use of physical restraints (i.e., takedowns) and/or getting the police involved. As with the other "aces," relapse prevention should be conducted whenever things seem to be going well.

As stated earlier, threats of suicide and acts or threats of violence fall into a special category. These behaviors are potentially lethal and therefore must be dealt with immediately. The strategies outlined below should be predetermined, clearly written into a contract format, and signed by all parties. Less seasoned counselors should seek the direct supervision of more experienced counselors before attempting to intervene in this area.

Threats of Violence

"Threats of violence" are defined as threats to kill or injure siblings, parents, or animals or to destroy property. Teenagers usually have no intention or desire to commit these acts, but many times they use threats to do so as a last resort to get the parents to back off or to scare them away. In the past, this has worked because parents will lose control of their emotions or take the threats personally.

At this point, the temptation is high for the parents to become aggressive or lecture in response. However, now is the time to stay calm. If not, threats can easily escalate into violence. To combat this ace, parents are taught the following two strategies:

Strategy 1: Exiting and Waiting/Staying Short and to the Point

As described in Chapter 5, parents are taught to tell the teenager that threats of violence are not acceptable (i.e., to stay short and to the point), and then to exit from the situation immediately and wait. Consequences can be administered after the teenager has calmed down. If the teenager starts to follow the parent in anger, the parent may have to go to the next strategy and place the teenager in time out.

Strategy 2: The Bathroom Strategy

The bathroom strategy is used *only* if the first strategy is not working. Otherwise, the parent risks unnecessary escalation and feelings of bitterness and resentment.

Parents are instructed to follow the same procedures as outlined for the bathroom strategy when a teenager runs away, with the following modifications:

1. The parents must tell their teenager ahead of time that he or she will be given one warning to stop the threats of violence. Parents can also give the teenager a count of 3 as a warning.

2. If the teenager still does not stop, he or she is immediately escorted to the bathroom for an initial 15 minutes of cool-down time. Time out does not start until the teenager is quiet. If the teenager will not go to the bathroom or becomes violent, the parent will use the takedown procedure and call the police if the parent is physically hurt.

3. Each time the teenager threatens violence again that same day another 15 minutes is added. The teenager starts fresh the next day. Below is a summary of a hierarchy of consequences:

> *First offense*: 15 minutes
> *Second offense*: 30 minutes
> *Third offense*: 45 minutes (and so on)

These times can be modified, depending on the particular teenager. A teenager who is particularly stubborn may need to begin at a longer starting time (e.g., first offense, 30 minutes; second offense, 1 hour; etc.). Some teenagers can negotiate going to the bedroom for a first offense as an acceptable compromise. Positive reinforcement can be used in the following manner: The teenager is told up front that he or she can cut time out in half by going to the time-out area calmly and without an escort. For example, if the first offense is 15 minutes, it can be cut to 7 minutes; if the second offense is 30 minutes, it can be cut to 15 minutes; and so on.

Acts of Violence

"Acts of violence" are defined as property damage, hurting oneself, or physically assaulting another person (the third behavior is also known as "battery"). If the teen's behavior gets this far, the parents cannot exit and wait, but must use one of the following strategies to take action.

Strategy 1: Filing Assault Charges

If the teenager commits an act of violence against another person, a parent or sibling must be instructed beforehand to exit as quickly as possible, dial 911, and tell the operator that someone has been physically assaulted. This makes the call a high priority and may get the police to the household quicker; otherwise, the police may drag their heels while the teenager becomes more violent. Once the police arrive, the parents must file assault charges and request that the teenager be booked.

Police officers will tell the parents that once the teenager is booked, the station will try to contact the parents immediately to come and get the teen. However, if the parents do not answer the phone and pretend that they are not home, the police have to hold the teenager overnight. This can send a powerful message and make the teenager think twice before committing another act of violence.

Many parents will say that they cannot bring themselves to have their son or daughter arrested. In addition, the parents are afraid that it will make their son or daughter angrier when the teen is released. However, in the real world, people do get arrested for assault. Therefore, the counselor must somehow convince the parents that they must mirror the real world, instead of waiting until it is too late and their teenager is bigger, stronger, and unreachable. Otherwise, the teenager may physically assault the parents, a future spouse or partner, or someone outside the family in the future. Most parents can understand this rationale.

In addition, parents must be informed that although their son or daughter may be upset upon returning home, they are less likely to commit violence when they know the police will be called again. Even if the teenager only gets a slap on the wrist, more serious penalties may be imposed in the future. The parents must have a documented history of these offenses to get the police and the courts to take more serious action.

CLINICAL EXAMPLE

Fifteen-year-old Peggy was referred to counseling by the foster care agency because she hit and pushed anyone who tried to enforce consequences. To combat this problem, the counselor spent an inordinate amount of preparation time with each of the outside parties. The foster parents, foster care workers, and probation officer met with the counselor for over 3 hours to formulate a no-violence contract and to clarify roles.

Every possible scenario was discussed beforehand and troubleshooting was conducted. Each person was asked "what if" questions and went through a dry run of what to do and how to react in each situation. The counselor role-played the part of Peggy and tried to push the buttons of each party. The course of action was then written down in a contract format. Each person was asked to repeat his or her understanding of the contract and the role he or she would play if there were any future threats or acts of violence. Any misunderstandings were clarified. The counselor committed himself to be available on a 24-hour basis, to conduct home visits if necessary, and to wear his pager at all times. Peggy was then asked back into the room.

Peggy was told that there would be zero tolerance for any future threats or acts of violence. "Threats or acts of violence" were then defined in concrete terms. The plan was that if this rule were violated, the foster parents would exit from the situation and immediately call the police and the counselor. The counselor would then call the foster care worker and probation officer at work or at home, depending on the day and hour. Peggy would be placed in detention immediately and assault or battery charges would be filed. Peggy was told that her contract mirrored the real world. People were going to start treating her as a normal teenager who was accountable for her actions. Everyone then signed the contract.

Peggy tested this contract the next week by picking up a hot curling iron and throwing it into her foster mother's back. The foster mother was prepared, however, and executed the plan flawlessly. Peggy was placed in detention and assault charges were filed. Each of the parties went to the detention center for a counseling session. During this session, Peggy was held accountable for her behavior. Each person in the room had a chance to tell Peggy how her actions affected him or her. Peggy then apologized, on her knees, to each person. This intervention had a dramatic impact on Peggy. After being released from detention, the violent behavior stopped.

This case was successful because of the amount of preparation beforehand. The roles of the foster parents and outsiders (i.e., probation officer, foster care worker) were clarified until everyone was "on the same page." This type of coordination is critical to stop acts or threats of violence. (The art of working with outsiders is outlined in Chapter 8.)

Strategy 2: Filing Property Damage Charges

When a teen commits property damage, parents are instructed to follow the same procedures as they would with assault charges. However, there is an important difference: Many police will tell the parents that property damage is their problem and will refuse to get involved. At this point, parents should ask to speak to the desk sergeant and keep going up the line until the police finally book the teenager. When possible, parents should handle this problem themselves by making the teenager work off the damage through hard labor or through a paying job (see Strategy 4, below). This mirrors the real world and is more effective than police involvement, which is often unpredictable.

Strategy 3: Doing a Takedown

If the teenager can be handled physically by one parent and the parent can stay calm under stress, that parent should do a takedown until the teenager is calm and then place him or her in a locked bathroom. The procedure has been described earlier in the section on use of the bathroom strategy when a teen runs away.

Strategy 4: Reparation for Property Damage

A teenager who damages or destroys any property (e.g., who kicks a hole in a wall) must repair the damage himself or herself under the parents' supervision and within a specific time period (e.g., 20 days). If repairing the damage personally is not an option, the teenager must give the parents money to pay for the damage (sometimes in equal monthly installments) or work it off through hard labor (e.g., extra chores, cleaning the garage, feeding the homeless, helping out at a nursing home, etc.). This strategy makes the teenager responsible for his or her own actions, thereby decreasing the probability that this same behavior will happen again.

To implement this strategy, parents must first find out what the damage is and how much repair or replacement will cost. Second, depending on the cost, the parents work out a payment plan of weekly or monthly installments. Third, the parents then go to the teenager with the total amount owed and the payment plan. Fourth, the parents take collateral in the form of personal items whose value is approximately equal to the total amount owed. Several items (stereo, CDs, clothes, makeup) that together come close to the total amount may have to be collected. Parents must not wait to take these personal items; otherwise, the teenager may try to hide these items, and the parents will lose any leverage. Parents then make up a pawn ticket like the one below to give to the teenager.

Good for one [fill in item or items]. We have secured these items in a safe place, and you may have them back untouched and unharmed if you pay us the amount owed by this date [or this amount by the first day of every month]. If payment is not received by this date, these items will be sold to cover this payment. Once sold, these items will not be replaced.

ACE 5: DISRESPECT

"Disrespect" can mean different things to different parents, and the definition must be custom-fit to the particular household. For most households, the following disrespectful behaviors can be listed on the written contract:

1. Swearing, yelling, or using gestures (e.g., giving the finger, rolling the eyes).
2. Not following directions, or refusing to comply when asked to do something (homework, chores, etc.), even after one warning is given.
3. Mimicking or imitating the parents in an unflattering manner.
4. Following the parents all over the house and nagging them or screaming at them.
5. Lying that can be proven by the parents.

The counselor must ask parents the following question: "What does your teenager do or say that is disrespectful or displays a bad attitude?" Once disrespect is operationalized into concrete behaviors, the parents are ready to apply the necessary consequences.

It is important to note that disrespect was not originally included in my formulation of the "aces" that need to be neutralized. However, this is a good example of how research findings can refine and inform clinical practice (see Chapter 12 for a full discussion). In this case, qualitative focus group interviews and quantitative outcome research with over 82 families informed me that disrespect can be every bit as poisonous as the other four "aces." Many parents ($n = 31$) reported that disrespect pushed their "buttons" to a greater degree than all the other aces combined. In turn, this caused the parents to lose their tempers and their capacity for rational thought. Instead, parents reacted out of emotion and were unable to maintain consistency or follow through on predetermined rules and consequences.

Strategy 1: Exiting and Waiting/Staying Short and to the Point

Parents are coached to recognize when their teenager is being disrespectful or metaphorically "throwing up" on them by yelling, swearing, screaming, or talking to them like dirt. As stated earlier, parents can then quickly tell their teenager that this is not acceptable and exit from the conversation immediately. Parents are taught that a teenager needs an audience to be disrespectful. If the audience is gone, the teenager must find new ways of getting his or her point across in a more respectful manner. The counselor must also reiterate that the parents do not owe their teenager an explanation and must be short and to the point. The longer a parent is engaged in a confrontation or explanation, the greater the opportunity for the teenager to be disrespectful and defeat the parent.

CLINICAL EXAMPLE

Seventeen-year-old Jessica would constantly use the "ace" of disrespect by swearing and screaming to push her father's buttons. The father would then back off, and his consequences were ineffective. However, after being shown how to exit and wait and how to stay short and to the point, the father began to exit any time his daughter started becoming disrespectful. At first, Jessica escalated more often when she lost her audience and felt ignored. However, when this happened, the father immediately placed the daughter in the bathroom (for a half-hour the first time and an hour the second time). Jessica hated to be ignored and placed in isolation. As a result, the disrespectful behavior quickly ended, and Jessica learned how to talk to her father in a calm and respectful manner.

Strategy 2: The Bathroom Strategy

The same procedures are used that were outlined in the section on the bathroom strategy for running away, with the following modifications:

1. The teenager is told ahead of time that he or she will be given one warning to stop being disrespectful. A count of 3 can be given to represent a warning. The parent defines these disrespectful behaviors ahead of time in a written contract.

2. The teenager is told beforehand that if a disrespectful behavior does not stop after the warning, the teen will be escorted to the bathroom for a 15-minute cool-down period. Time out will not start until the teenager is quiet. Each time the teen is disrespectful again during the same day, another 15 minutes will be added. The teenager will start back at a 15-minute baseline the next day. If the teenager goes immediately and is quiet, he or she can be rewarded by serving only half of the original time.

3. The teenager is also told beforehand that if he or she becomes violent, a takedown will be immediately initiated, and the police will be called if parents are physically assaulted.

Parents can use the first strategy in conjunction with the bathroom strategy. That is, parents can be brief, exit, and wait, but if the disrespectful behavior continues the teenager can be placed in time out until the behavior stops. In either case, the parents how have the tools to control the mood and direction of the argument, without the need for violence that often accompanies disrespectful behavior.

Strategy 3: Grounding, Fines, or Loss of Transportation

Depending on the particular teenager, grounding, fines, or loss of transportation can be very effective. These can be especially effective if the teenager is caught in a lie. A lie is a behavior or action rather than a temporary mood. Therefore, a loss of freedom may have a longer and bigger impact on lying than a short period of time in isolation may have. The following predetermined consequences are suggested for lying or for a disrespectful attitude that continues over a long period of time:

> *First offense*: Grounding the next weekend day (no phone, TV, friends).
> *Second offense*: Grounding another weekend day (no phone, TV, friends), fine, or loss of car or any transportation for next day or weekend day, depending on what has the greatest impact.
> *Third offense*: Fine or loss of car or any transportation for next day or weekend day, depending on what has the greater impact.

The teenager is told ahead of time that for every complete day of respectful behavior and following directions, he or she can have a 1-day reduction of grounding, fines, or loss of transportation. For example, a teen who was grounded for being disrespectful the day before can gain that day back for being respectful the next day. This is done to incorporate both positive and negative consequences. (See also Strategy 4, below.)

In regard to loss of transportation and fines, it is important to note that often parents will still give a teenager money and transportation even after the teen is extremely disrespectful; this sends a bad message to the teenager. Instead, a teen can be fined a predetermined amount of money for each disrespectful behavior. In addition, loss of transportation for a weekend day and evening can be implemented for any disrespectful behavior. With the counselor's help, parents can get very creative and find the consequence or combination of consequences that will stop the extreme behavior.

CLINICAL EXAMPLE

Thirteen-year-old Max was extremely materialistic and hated the idea of giving up a percentage of his allowance, which was the consequence his parents imposed for disrespectful behavior. In addition, the money would go to his twin brother, with whom Max was in fierce competition. When this consequence was implemented, disrespect stopped immediately. Max did not want his twin brother to receive any of his allowance.

Strategy 4: Using Positive Reinforcers

The counselor should coach parents to balance "tagging" the disrespectful behavior with reinforcing times when the teenager is respectful. Parents are informed that this new approach will at first seem contrived or mechanical, but they are asked to keep trying until it becomes second nature. Parents are taught how to focus on behaviors that are not disrespectful, using comments such as the following: "Jack, I really appreciate the fact that you did not swear, yell, or lie today," "I want to tell you that I see you trying, even though it might not be easy for you," "Ted, I saw that you almost lied, but then held it together and told me the truth," or "I really appreciate you not swearing." Parents are taught to focus on the specific respectful behaviors, rather than to make generalized comments such as "Thanks for doing a good job or being respectful."

In addition to praise, parents can get creative and come up with coupons that they can give to their son or daughter if the teen exhibits respectful behavior or a good attitude on a daily or weekly basis. Some of these creative ideas include the following: (1) A "Get out of jail free" card (a teenager who is grounded can use this card to reduce grounding by 1 day); (2) a phone card, good for 1 hour of extra phone time; (3) a money card, good for a specified amount of money; or (4) a special outing card, good for movie, lunch, or dinner with Mom or Dad.

SUMMARY

Treatment will fail when a counselor cannot give parents or authority figures a menu of effective consequences to stop extreme behaviors. Therefore, this chapter is intended to give the counselor a road map or set of procedures for helping parents to stop these extreme behaviors and create the opportunity for permanent change.

It is important to note that consequences to stop extreme behaviors will be severely hindered or ineffective if other key areas within the home are not addressed and changed. (Although these points are made in the text in regard to running away, they often apply to the other four "aces" as well.) These areas include the following:

- One or both parents are overly strict, harsh, punitive, or focused on the negative.

- One or both parents constantly push the teenager's buttons.
- At least one parent has an addiction of some type.
- Undisclosed sexual abuse has occurred or is occurring in the home.
- There is physical violence in the home.
- Marital conflict and/or parental depression exists.
- A boyfriend, girlfriend, or peer group is pulling the teen away from the family.

Counselors must therefore integrate the principles of earlier chapters with the consequences in this chapter to stop both the identified "aces" and these other key problem areas. One problem or set of problems cannot be worked on in isolation from the other.

The following is a summary of the major points contained within this chapter:

1. Procedures have to be extremely concrete and written in a contract format before the parents go into battle and implement these strategies. In the heat of battle, the parents must have this contract to refer to and consult.

2. A consequence must be severe enough that a difficult adolescent would rather give up an "ace" than continue to suffer the punishment. Otherwise, there is no reason to give up the extreme behavior.

3. These methods are not for counselors who do not like this type of intensity or possess the willingness to commit themselves to 24-hour-a-day, 7-day-a-week availability. When these methods are put into place, an adolescent will have an initial intense and negative reaction. The process can be like stirring up a sleeping rattlesnake. Hence, the parents will need a great deal of support and hand holding until the initial crisis is past and they get stronger.

4. Counselors must also possess an innate ability to "think on their feet" and change tactics midstream if an intervention appears not to be working. Families of difficult adolescents can rapidly lose hope and experience burnout. Therefore, counselors only have a small window of opportunity to make an impact before they lose clients.

5. The counselor must troubleshoot with the parents and help them anticipate everything that could go wrong before it happens. Otherwise, the consequence will fail on impact. Adolescents have enhanced social perception abilities and will work overtime to "outthink" parents and defeat all attempts to neutralize the "aces."

6. Counselors must normalize, predict, and anticipate relapse. One of the biggest reasons why counseling fails is a lack of attention to this relapse process. When things are going well, it is not the time to rest, but the time to prepare for possible hurricane winds ahead. Consequently, a counselor must predict relapse and design strategies and a concrete plan of action if the extreme behavior should resurface.

CHAPTER 7

Restoring Nurturance and Tenderness

Parents and counselors may successfully design interventions to stop the "five aces," but still may fail to achieve permanent change. Parents must maintain their authority by balancing a "hard" and a "soft" approach with their teenagers. On the hard side, they must be tough by effectively and consistently enforcing rules and consequences, neutralizing the "five aces," and determining the mood and direction of confrontations. However, parents must also show empathy and consideration for each other and their teenager, help the teenager feel loved, and provide special times together to promote positive parent–child interaction. An imbalance of these two types of approaches can lead to serious emotional or behavioral problems in the teenager.

The aim of this chapter is to demonstrate how to restore the nurturance that has been buried under months or even years of extreme conflict. First, counselors are shown when to introduce the topic of nurturance and what factors within a family influence this decision. For example, should a counselor address the establishment of goodwill before strict discipline, or should he or she approach both areas at once with the parents? Next, seven strategies for successfully reviving tenderness within the family are described. Two further sections explain (1) how to help the parents use soothing sequences of communication to cultivate discussions that are positive rather than destructive, and (2) how to help the parents implement the seven strategies and overcome potential obstacles to doing so.

WHERE TO BEGIN

The counselor must first decide when to introduce the topic of nurturance to the parents and teenager. One choice is to initiate feelings of goodwill before behavior problems are addressed. In some cases, the behavior problems are so minimal that the soft side of nurturance is the only area that needs to be addressed. However, with difficult adolescents this is the exception rather than the rule. A second choice is to address the hard and soft sides concurrently. This is possible when behavior problems are less extreme or when problems first emerge; in both instances, family members are not burned out, and the negative interactions have not yet had a serious impact on the family's closeness. A third choice is to stop extreme behaviors through hard-side interventions (i.e., to neutralize the "five aces") before proceeding to the soft side. When treating difficult teenagers with severe behavior problems, the counselor will be most successful with this third approach. Years of conflict have taken their toll on the parent–child relationship. The parents feel out of control, helpless, and disempowered. Consequently, nurturance cannot be addressed until the teenager's "aces" have been neutralized and the parents' position of authority has been upheld. Only then will the parents have the peace of mind and energy necessary to bring tenderness back into the relationship. Each of these three choices is explained in detail below, with case examples to highlight major points of discussion.

Addressing the Soft Side before the Hard Side

Addressing the soft side first is most appropriate for families with adolescents who have not yet developed serious behavior problems. In such a family, the adolescent is still respectful and follows rules, but exhibits a change in temperament (e.g., becoming moody, depressed, or distant). The counselor determines which of the following three possibilities best correlates with this sudden change in mood: (1) a normal developmental need for autonomy that accompanies adolescence; (2) a negative reaction to an overprotective parent; or (3) a result of drug or alcohol use, negative peer relationships, or gang involvement.

If the counselor determines that the behavior simply reflects a developmental need for distance, the parents are educated about this need and shown how to strike a balance between autonomy and closeness. The counselor meets with each party separately to understand everyone's different needs and to seek possible areas of compromise. A new contract is then negotiated, with the counselor serving as a mediator between the parties.

CLINICAL EXAMPLE

Thirteen-year-old Jason's parents complained that although he did well in school and followed rules at home, he had suddenly become moody, angry, and uncommunicative. When Jason came home from school, he would go straight to his room and shut the door. Whenever either parent asked Jason about his day, he would reply, "I don't know" or "Fine." Jason also refused to go on trips with his parents and spent an excessive amount of time alone or with several close friends in the neighborhood.

When the counselor talked with Jason alone, he ruled out drugs or alcohol as the cause, and determined that the underlying problem was a developmental need for autonomy. Jason explained that his mother bombarded him with questions as soon as he walked into the door from school. He felt as if he were being interrogated, and stated that he needed his "space." The more his mother pressed, the more Jason shut down, and the more the mother insisted on a response. Jason began to head for his room as quickly as possible to avoid questions, which only made his mother more anxious. The mother than asked the father to go to Jason's room once a week to ask what the "real problem" was. Jason became so angry that he no longer wanted to participate in any family activities. This withdrawal led the parents to believe that Jason was using drugs. As a result, they refused to let him stay out late on weekends, even though he had returned home on time each week. Jason loved his parents but felt that they needed to "back off" and not "smother" him so much.

During this individual meeting with Jason, the counselor asked whether he would be interested in a solution that involved getting his mother and father to back off, while simultaneously enabling him to win back trust and lost freedoms. Jason was very interested. The counselor outlined the following plan of action to Jason:

1. The counselor would become a mediator by bringing all parties together and teaching them ways to communicate so that Jason did not feel interrogated and the mother felt satisfied that Jason was not shutting his parents out. This involved a customized signal designed by Jason to inform his parents when they were pressing too hard and that he needed time alone. The plan also involved Jason's expanding his answers beyond "I don't know" and "Fine."

2. The counselor reframed the problem as the parents' best way to show concern. If Jason told his parents basic information each day (e.g., happenings in school, moods, feelings), his parents would worry less and subsequently "back off."

3. Jason and his parents could plan times to do things together. The parents needed the closeness, even though Jason did not. However, this would be to Jason's advantage, since as his parents became less worried, they would be less suspicious and restore his freedoms.

4. The counselor would advocate for Jason that he get his curfew extended over time if he complied with the first three objectives. No promises could be made, but the counselor would try. Jason liked this plan and looked forward to meeting with his parents and forming this new contract.

The counselor then met with the parents alone. He framed Jason's behavior as part of his normal development as an adolescent, and gave concrete examples to support this rationale. The counselor then outlined the destructive communication cycle the parents had unknowingly created over the last year. This made sense to the mother; she had noticed that the more she pursued, the more distant Jason became. The counselor outlined the proposed plan of action and described how each problem area would be addressed. Then Jason returned to begin the mediation session.

During the mediation meeting, the counselor had Jason and the mother pretend that he was coming in the door from school and she was asking him questions. Jason gave his mother concrete suggestions on how to ask questions in a different way so that he would not feel smothered. The mother negotiated that Jason would eat dinner with the family again and that she would give him time in his room to "decompress" after school. Finally, the parents and Jason agreed to plan special outings together. Each time a different person would choose the activity, as long as it did not cost a great deal of money. The parents then agreed to let Jason resume his previous curfew time if he followed the plan on a week-by-week basis. Each of these points were then written down on paper for family members to refer to as needed, and the contract was signed by each party.

In this example, a balance was reached between Jason's developmental need for distance and the parents' need for closeness. Jason received autonomy while the parents achieved open communication on a day-to-day basis. The counselor was able to accomplish this goal by persuading each party to agree to areas of compromise, and by establishing a clear course of action.

If it is determined that a change in an adolescent's behavior is the result of enmeshment or overprotectiveness, the same basic principles apply, with some variations. The counselor must typically move at a much slower pace so as not to risk scaring the parents. The parents may already realize that they are overprotective, but to label the behavior as such is far too threatening. Therefore, the counselor must focus on establishing good rapport with the parents before addressing the enmeshment. Once the separation process begins, it should occur in conjunction with the promotion of nurturance.

Finally, a sudden change in mood may be brought on by a traumatic event, such as sexual abuse or induction into a gang or negative peer group. Drug or alcohol use is another common cause. In these cases, the counselor must immediately move to the third choice and solve these extreme behavior problems before issues of nurturance can be addressed. The parents will not have the time, energy, or desire to commit themselves to nurturance until these problems have been solved.

Addressing the Hard and Soft Sides Simultaneously

If the behavior problems are less severe or are just beginning to emerge, hard and soft approaches can be employed concurrently. For example, if the presenting problem is disrespect or not following rules, the counselor can establish clear rules and consequences to address the hard side, while addressing the soft side through the planning of special outings. With these relatively minor behavior problems, the parents and teenager have not yet developed a long history of negative interaction and unresolved bitterness.

CLINICAL EXAMPLE

Fourteen-year-old Brenda was brought to counseling because she refused to do chores and would have temper tantrums when she did not get her way. The father reported that Brenda had started withdrawing from the family and misbehaving about 5 months prior. As a result, the relationship between Brenda and her parents had become increasingly distant. Both parents agreed that the father had to be the "bad guy" and be tough with Brenda, because the mother was too scared of her temper tantrums. It had been a long time since the father and Brenda had gone out on any special outings or simply laughed and joked around together. The father loved Brenda very much and wanted to get back to the way things had been in the past.

Because the behaviors were relatively recent and the father wanted to restore affection, the counselor chose to address the hard and the soft sides simultaneously. The hour-long weekly sessions were subsequently divided into two parts. During the first half-hour, the counselor and parents met to design rules and consequences to stop Brenda's temper tantrums and refusal to complete chores or to comply with parental requests.

During the second half-hour, the counselor met with Brenda and her father. During these meetings, the counselor asked each to talk about times in the past when they were close. This shifted the mood in the room to one of softness rather than one of blame. The father recounted times when they had gone out to dinner together, and Brenda described times when her father used to hug her and not point out what she was doing wrong all the time. During these sessions, the counselor was able to persuade the father to plan special outings again and to look for positives on a day-to-day basis. These changes then influenced the daughter's behavior in a positive direction. She had fewer temper tantrums and increasingly began to comply with parental requests. The father then became even more loving as Brenda's behavior improved. Much later in treatment, Brenda reported that reconnecting with her father was the biggest reason why she stopped misbehaving.

In this case, the counselor was able to deal with the hard and soft sides together. The father was willing to confront the issue of restoring nurturance with his daughter, and her minor problem behaviors were stopped relatively easily, since she and her father did not have a long history of conflict.

Addressing the Hard Side First

In most difficult adolescent cases, the hard side needs to be addressed first. Parents with a difficult teenager often enter treatment after the problems have become severe and the parent–teenager relationship is already seriously damaged. When this happens, the parents enter the therapist's office burned out and angry with their teenager. Though they love the teenager, they often no longer like him or her. If the counselor introduces the concept of nurturance too early, it can end in disaster.

CLINICAL EXAMPLE

One father came to counseling because of 16-year-old Natasha's running away from home and alcohol use. Years of bitter confrontations over these issues had taken their toll on the father–daughter relationship; there was deep resentment on both sides. Instead of formulating strategies to solve these problems, the counselor focused on issues of nurturance that included forgiveness and planning special outings. The father was livid at such a suggestion and immediately walked out of the office in anger. He came back only after the counselor profusely apologized and promised he would help the father get Natasha to stop her destructive behaviors. After the father saw concrete changes in Natasha's behavior, he was more than willing to consider reconnecting with his daughter on an emotional level. He saw with his own eyes that his daughter was trying to change. This alleviated much of the father's past bitterness, and he was able to display forgiveness. This led to Natasha's also becoming more compassionate.

Counselors must understand the age-old principle of "starting where the client is." When a teen has an extreme set of behaviors and a long history of parent abuse, parents must see action before they will risk getting hurt emotionally. Both parents and teenager are afraid of taking the first step and reaching out on an emotional level. Each fears that the other will see any acts of kindness as a form of weakness and take advantage of it. Both parents and teenager also lack trust, so the counselor must move slowly. The first step is to address the hard side by helping the parents get the problem behaviors under control.

CLINICAL EXAMPLE

Steve was a 16-year-old boy who was required to come to counseling by the probation department. The parents told the counselor that they were only there because of the court's requirement. They had given up all hope and just wanted their son to be locked up. The last straw had come when Steve slapped and kicked his mother when she tried to ground him. After that incident, the father made Steve sleep in a tent in the backyard and refused to let him in the house. The mother then went on to say that Steve was no longer going to school and regularly used marijuana. These behaviors had been going on for years. The father said he had been fooled by Steve so many times and with so many lies that he now despised him.

After getting this background information, the counselor made a serious mistake. The counselor asked the father why he was so angry with the son and suggested that Steve needed forgiveness and love. The father became very agitated and told the counselor that he had tried to give his son a second chance over and over again, but each time felt as if he had been slapped in the face. The counselor did not recognize that the father was politely giving him feedback that he was going down the wrong road. Instead, the counselor continued to press the issued by trying to educate the parents on how nurturance needed to be brought back into the relationship. The body language of both parents communicated to the counselor that they were getting more and more angry. The parents missed the next session without calling to cancel or reschedule.

The counselor's supervisor heard what had happened and called the father to convince him to return. He told the father that he was an expert at solving the types of behavior problems Steve displayed, and he asked for just one session to prove it. The supervisor would work with the original counselor as a consultant. The father agreed to these terms. When the family returned, the counselor started off the session by apologizing to the parents for moving too quickly to a soft approach before first addressing the problems of violence, truancy, and drugs. The supervisor then stated that when these behaviors were solved, there would be time to reconnect bonds and heal old wounds. The father nodded and told the supervisor that this was what he had been trying to say all along, but that no one would listen. He loved his son, but until he could trust him again, he could not show his love and affection.

After the parents successfully implemented the bathroom strategy (see Chapter 6), the threats of violence quickly stopped. The father was then motivated to work with the school and even to go to school to stop the truancy. This worked, and the truancy stopped. After this problem was solved, the parents were motivated to tackle the drug problem by conducting random urinary analysis and not letting Steve out of the house until he tested "clean." Steve later said that he was happier because his dad was no longer calling him a "loser" and he was sleeping in his own bedroom again.

Since the father could see that Steve was trying to do better, it motivated him to try to get closer to his son on an emotional level. At this point, the supervisor introduced the idea of nurturance again, with a concrete plan to set up special outings between father and son. Even if Steve had a bad week, the father would use other strategies to stop the problem behavior but would still make time for special outings. The supervisor asked the father to separate the misbehavior from nurturance. The father agreed because he trusted the supervisor, who (in his opinion) was the only one who had helped turn Steve around. Before leaving the sessions, the father and son planned the date, time, and place for the first outing. The supervisor then engaged in troubleshooting to identify everything that could possibly prevent this outing from taking place.

After 2 successful weeks of special outings together, Steve was able to tell the father that he had always felt that his older brother was the "golden child" and he was nothing in his father's eyes. The father was able to tell Steve how he had wanted to be closer but couldn't because Steve was so close to his mother. As these issues were brought forth and worked through, father and son became closer. Steve's anger began to dissipate, and the threats and acts of violence ultimately stopped on a permanent basis.

In this example, the behavior problems took precedence and had to be addressed before nurturance was possible. When the counselor's efforts did not support this goal, the parents became agitated and did not return to the next session. However, once the counselor gained credibility, trust, and rapport by solving the original problems, the father was more than willing to look at issues of softness. As the family environment became less chaotic and the parents took charge, the day-to-day communication became less negative, and the parents felt more in control. In turn, this led to hope and positive interactions between parents and teenager.

STRATEGIES TO RESTORE NURTURANCE AND TENDERNESS

Once the counselor decides when to introduce the topic of nurturance, he or she must determine how it will be done. This is accomplished by using one or more of the following seven strategies:

1. *Education and normalization.* The parents and teenager are shown how they have reached a stage of emotional deprivation (or worse) over the years.

2. *Opportunities to build trust.* Teenagers reported in focus group interviews that when they lost the opportunity to build trust, they lost hope, and resentment soon set in. Parents are shown how to help their teenager regain trust while still holding the teenager accountable for future misbehaviors.

3. *A new approach to criticism.* Parents are shown new and better ways to criticize—ways that do not attack the teenager's personality or character, but merely comment on the current behavior.

4. *A new approach to praise.* A teen's self-worth is devoured by criticisms and enhanced by praise. Parents are shown how to praise their teenager in a way that will compliment behavior rather than evaluate it.

5. *Acceptance of underlying feelings.* Parents are shown the direct connection between how teenagers feel and how they behave. Teaching parents how to acknowledge their teenager's underlying feelings without condoning misbehavior can lead to a tremendous improvement in the relationship.

6. *Physical touch.* Parents are informed that normal physical touch and small signs of affection are extremely important to restoring tenderness with their teenager.

7. *Special outings.* When an adolescent has behavior problems, special outings often stop or become contingent upon good behavior. This only causes the relationship to become more distant and to lose much, if not all, of its caring quality. The parents and teenager are shown how to include special outings in their relationship again.

Strategy 1: Education and Normalization

No matter when the topic of tenderness is introduced, the counselor can show the parents and teenager how they have reached a stage of emotional deprivation (or worse). "Emotional deprivation" is defined as the parents' and teenager's inability to demonstrate acts of nurturance through physical signs of affection, conversations without criticism, or special outings together. It is the result of months or years of constant arguing and the failure of each party to make the first move to restore good feelings after confrontations. Education and normalization are used to reduce blame.

CLINICAL EXAMPLE

The father of 15-year-old Brittany was making the false assumption that his daughter refused hugs because she did not need or want them. Brittany pushed him away until he gave up. This perception changed only after the father was able to make the connection between the years of negative communication and subsequent emotional distance. Pushing away then became a normal reaction to years of bitter confrontations and a fear of rejection. With this new perception and understanding, the father continued to try to hug Brittany until an emotional connection was reestablished.

Both parents and teenagers are usually not aware of the big picture or of how they have reached their present situation; instead, each party blames the other. The counselor can reduce blame by giving both the parents and the teenager a handout (Figure 7.1) outlining the stages leading to and following emotional deprivation.

After the parents and teenager read this handout, the counselor asks them to select the stage they currently find themselves in. Many parents and teenagers are shocked to see how much their relationship has deteriorated and what the future holds if things do not change. On the positive side, many parents and teenagers begin to see how the problems have progressed over the years and how each party has played a role in the overall process. This realization can reduce blame and debunk the myth that one person has caused the total problem.

CLINICAL EXAMPLE

Fifteen-year-old Randy read the handout and told the counselor that his relationship with his father was currently at Stage 5. He stated that his peers had taken the place of his father. The father agreed but added that they were really in Stage 6, because the more Randy pulled away, the more he lectured, and the more Randy pulled away. Randy agreed and asked the counselor how to get unstuck.

The counselor told them that the answer was in front of them. To get un-

Stage 1: Behavior Problems	Stage 2: Negative Interaction	Stage 3: Conditional Love	Stage 4: Emotional Deprivation
A preadolescent or early adolescent becomes rebellious and has behavior problems.	The teen fails to comply with parental requests and lecturing, and negative interaction begins to occur 90–100% of the time.	Special outings or signs of affection then become contingent on how good the teen's behavior was each week.	Emotional deprivation sets in when the parents and teen stop physical affection and special outings together. Both parents and teen feel "burned" so many times that they stop trying.

Stage 5: "Second Family" Takes Over	Stage 6: Parents and Teen Get Stuck in a Vicious Cycle	Stage 7: Teen Becomes Hardened and Lacks Remorse/Empathy
If the teenager does not receive nurturance in the family, he or she will look to an adopted "second family" of peers, gangs, or drugs.	As parents see the teenager pull away, they will lecture or impose more rules, which in turn push the teenager further away until both parties get stuck in a rut and are unable to make the first move to break down the walls of emotional deprivation.	As this rut continues, the teenager becomes more and more hardened. Over time, the teenager shows an inability to show remorse or empathy and may even develop antisocial personality disorder. As an adult, the person passes these problems on to his or her children. Stage 1 begins all over again.

FIGURE 7.1. Parent handout: Timeline of the stages leading to and following emotional deprivation. From *Treating the Tough Adolescent* by Scott P. Sells. Copyright 1998 by The Guilford Press. Permission to photocopy this handout is granted to purchasers of *Treating the Tough Adolescent* for personal use only (see copyright page for details).

stuck, they needed to go back to a time before emotional deprivation set in (Stage 4). Father and son needed to reestablish the ritual of going on special outings together, regardless of how good or bad Randy's behavior was during the week. The rules and consequences would still be enforced, but their time together would be sacred. In addition, the father would have to agree to stop lecturing and telling the son how bad his friends were. If Randy missed curfew, there would be a predetermined consequence; however, tearing down Randy's friends would only push Randy closer to them. Randy would also have to realize that spending time with his father did not mean he had to choose between his friends and his father. It was a win–win scenario, because he could spend time with both. At the very least, the father and Randy could have a better working relationship without as many confrontations. This rationale made sense to both parties, and they agreed to experiment with this plan for 1 month.

In this example, the timeline in Figure 7.1 helped educate the members of this family by giving a visual representation of the current parent–teenager relationship. The timeline helped Randy and his father put the jigsaw pieces together and see how and why they were currently having problems. It also reduced blame by normalizing each person's role in the overall problem. Finally, the timeline gave the counselor and family a template to locate what stage(s) of development the father and son were stuck in, and what stage they would have to go back to in order to repair their relationship. In Randy's case, a return to special outings and a decrease in lectures by the father were needed.

Strategy 2: Opportunities to Build Trust

During focus group interviews (see Chapter 12 for a description of these), teenagers reported that hopelessness set in when their parents no longer gave them opportunities to earn back trust. When this happened, they felt that they had been "backed into a corner" and thus had nothing more to lose. Consequently, deep resentments and bitterness set in, and day-to-day interactions became increasingly negative. Without trust, it was more likely that these teenagers would be labeled as "liars," "stupid," "irresponsible," or "thieves." Whether true or not, the labels and expectations eventually became self-fulfilling prophecies and only served to confirm the parents' belief that their teenagers could not be trusted. Without continual opportunities to earn back trust, there could be no nurturance, but only lingering resentment.

CLINICAL EXAMPLE

Fourteen-year-old Tim repeatedly ran away from home and was failing in school. Over time, his parents grew so distrustful that they made the house into a virtual prison with bars and an alarm system. When this happened, a sense of hopelessness set in, and Tim felt that he had nothing more to lose. Therefore, as soon as he went to school, Tim would run away. This only reinforced the parents' belief that he could not be trusted. Without trust, there was no opportunity for Tim to improve his behavior or restore good feelings with his parents.

Reparation of trust is an extremely challenging task for the parents of a difficult adolescent. Parents often feel trapped between a rock and a hard place. They think that if they trust again, their teenager will only take advantage of the situation. When this happens, parents can become prisoners in their own home, afraid to leave the house because the teenager may do something while they are out. Parents can also become hypervigilant and constantly watch every move the teenager makes, until the teenager feels smothered and without any privacy. At this point, the parent–child emotional bond deteriorates rapidly. The parents resent having to alter their lifestyle because they cannot trust their teenager; the teenager resents the parents' constant vigilance and the lack of opportunities to regain trust.

In order to rebuild trust, two things must occur. First, the parents must be shown how to give back trust wisely and in increments. They must be shown the three possible levels of supervision (mandatory, structured, or limited) and told at which level their teenager is currently functioning. The level chosen will guide the parents in deciding how much trust to give or hold back. Second, parents must find out what issues the teenager wants to regain trust on. They usually involve freedom in various forms: extended curfew, extra phone time, more time with peers, or attendance at a special event such as a concert or sleepover. Parents can then custom-design both positive and negative consequences relating to these issues, to enable the teenager to earn back trust slowly.

Three Levels of Supervision

Parents often mistakenly see trust as an all-or-nothing proposition: They either give trust back too soon before it is earned, or become too rigid and punitive. In the former case, parents set themselves up for failure as a teenager takes advantage of trust that is given back too early. Trust has no value if it requires no sacrifice to attain. In the latter case, a teenager responds to rigidity with rebellion and defiance. This leads to a more substantial lack of trust, which leads to more defiance by the teenager, and so on.

A balance between these extremes involves consistently following through when a rule is broken, but simultaneously rewarding the teenager with trust each time the rule is followed. How much trust is given depends on which of the three levels of supervision a teen requires, as illustrated in Figure 7.2.

Using this handout as a yardstick, parents are asked to rate their teenager's current level of supervision. The teenager should not be present during this discussion, because he or she will only argue and disagree with any rating other than a Level 3. After a rating is specified, parents are given scenarios of what may happen in the coming weeks and what their subsequent responses will be, based on their teen's particular level of supervision. These scenarios serve as litmus tests to help the counselor determine whether the parents are too loose, balanced, or too strict in returning trust. This information will then help direct the counselor on how to modify the amount of trust that will be given back to the teenager. Here is one scenario that can be used as such a test:

> A 15-year-old boy asks permission to go to a party with his best friend. The party will end at 11 P.M. and he will be home at 11:30 P.M., an hour and a half past normal curfew. Should he be allowed to go and under what circumstances?

Level 1: Mandatory Supervision	Level 2: Structured Supervision	Level 3: Limited Supervision
Level 1 teenagers are not trustworthy. They refuse to complete tasks or follow rules; they do not come home on time or chronically run away. They have friends over when the parents are not at home. These teenagers require constant supervision and monitoring by their parents until they adhere to predetermined rules and consequences.	Level 2 teenagers are semitrustworthy. They comply with tasks and follow rules at least 50–75% of the time. They obey curfew 75–90% of the time and do not leave home without permission. They do not have friends over when the parent is not at home. These teenagers are required to check in at regular intervals when they go out, and they must be home at required times or risk more stringent supervision requirements.	Level 3 teenagers are trustworthy. They can regularly be depended on to complete tasks and follow rules 80–100% of the time. These teenagers obey curfew 100% of the time, and they are where they say they are going to be. These teenagers are dependable and not required to check in at regular intervals.

FIGURE 7.2. Parent handout: The three levels of supervision. From *Treating the Tough Adolescent* by Scott P. Sells. Copyright 1998 by The Guilford Press. Permission to photocopy this handout is granted to purchasers of *Treating the Tough Adolescent* for personal use only (see copyright page for details).

If this teenager is at Level 3, he is trustworthy, and the parents will ideally answer "Yes," with the stipulation that the teen must tell the parents where the party will be held. However, if the parents answer "No" at Level 3, this is an indication that they are too strict. The counselor should then help the parents to formulate responses and rules that are more in line with Level 3 behaviors.

If the teenager is at Level 2, the parents will ideally answer "Yes, but only under certain circumstances." These circumstances might include random spot checks by the parent throughout the evening to see whether the teenager is at the party. The counselor should also meet with the parents and help them to set and enforce predetermined consequences if the teen is even 1 minute late past curfew. However, if the parents answer "No" or "Yes" without any parameters, the counselor will be able to determine that the parents are too strict or too loose, and to help the parents change their position accordingly.

Finally, if the teenager is at Level 1, the parents will ideally answer "No." However, if the parents answer "Yes," this indicates a trust level that is too loose and directs the counselor to help the parents maintain a firmer stance.

The counselor can continue to give parents scenarios like the one above, until he or she is convinced that the parents understand the levels of supervision and the corresponding rewards of trust. If rewards are not congruous with a particular teen's current level, the counselor can offer suggestions that are more appropriate. In addition, parents are then told about the direct relationship between appropriate levels of trust and the parent–child emotional bond. If the trust level is out of sync with the level of supervision, the teenager will become resentful and angry, and will engage in retaliation. In turn, this can weaken or destroy any softness in the relationship.

Consequences to Help the Teen Regain Trust in Key Areas

Once the parents determine the current level of supervision, the next step is to find out what issues the teenager wants to regain trust on. These issues usually center around greater freedom, as noted earlier. The parents and counselor then custom-design both positive and negative consequences relating to these issues that will enable the teenager to earn back trust slowly.

CLINICAL EXAMPLE

Sixteen-year-old Diego ran away frequently. More than anything else, he wanted his freedom returned. To get his freedom back, he had to regain his parents' trust. His parents refused to give back this trust, because they had been burned too many times in the past. However, without an opportunity to regain trust, Diego's resentment would continue to build and the emotional bond would continue to deteriorate. The parents were faced with a predicament: How could they help Diego regain trust when he currently required mandatory supervision and was not trustworthy? With the counselor's help, they solved this predicament by balancing positive and negative consequences.

1. Diego had a history of running away as soon as he went to school. This had previously destroyed any hope of trust. To regain this trust, Diego would receive a 1-hour coupon for extra time with friends on the weekend each day he did not run away from school.

2. Diego could save these coupons and redeem them for up to 4 hours of freedom on the weekend. Since he was currently grounded every weekend and locked in the house, the coupons were a big incentive.

3. Diego was only allowed to go to a friend's house or to a movie if a parent was present at all times. As Diego moved to Levels 2 and 3 on the supervision handout, this rule could be modified accordingly.

In this way, trust was regained through the creative use of both positive and negative consequences. The positive consequences allowed Diego to earn his freedom back in increments. Finally, the different levels of supervision served as a compass to direct the parents on how tight the parameters needed to be and how much trust to initiate. The rule of thumb is to find out the areas that the teenager wants to regain trust in and then slowly give the teen ways to regain this trust, with negative consequences still in place in case of relapse.

The following points must be made clear to parents for this strategy to work. First, the parents' biggest fear is usually that if they give an inch of trust, the teenager will take a mile of misbehavior. The counselor must convince the parents that they are still "tagging" the misbehavior with predetermined consequences while simultaneously "tagging" the positive behavior to build back trust. In addition, they are using the Figure 7.2 handout as a yardstick for how much trust to give back and how tight the parameters should be. Trust is also not given back all at once, but is earned back slowly by the teen on the basis of his or her choices.

Second, the parents and counselor must anticipate and expect relapse throughout the trust-building process. When the teenager begins to build trust, he or she will relapse and go back to old habits, just as someone who is trying to give up smoking does. If the teenager relapses, the parents must simply "tag" the misbehavior and go back to the trust-building process as quickly as possible. When the parents can accomplish this goal, relapses will occur less and less often over time. This is because the teenager will continue to see that "all is not lost" and will want to regain lost trust. As stated earlier, it is critical for the counselor to make use of troubleshooting and "what if" scenarios any time things seem to be going too smooth and the teenager is regaining trust.

Finally, it is important for the counselor to keep emphasizing the central message: As soon as trust is rebuilt, both the parents and the teenager will see a change in their relationship. The relationship will become less adversarial and more nurturing. When this message is stressed, most parents will agree to use this strategy.

A majority of teenagers in my research (see Chapter 12) stated that opportunities to regain trust were the biggest reasons why they were changing their behavior and feeling closer to their parents. The teenagers could not believe that their parents were still willing to give them opportunities to rebuild trust after repeated relapses. This one factor made a tremendous impact on the teenagers and motivated them to relapse less in the future. As one teenager stated,

> "If I did bad and came home late, I was grounded the next day and lost an hour of curfew time. But after doing my time, I immediately had the opportunity to regain that lost hour if I came back on time 3 straight days. Before counseling, I would be grounded forever, and my parents would have given me the silent treatment. Now it is weird. It has gotten to the point where I do not want to disappoint them, and I feel guilty if I

take advantage of the trust they have given me. These are new feelings for me, and it is weird."

Teenagers also reported that opportunities to regain trust constituted a major difference between counseling based on this treatment model and other types of counseling that they had experienced in the past. The teen focus groups are a good example of how research informed the present model. These groups revealed that trust was a core element in altering the emotional bond between parents and teenagers. Without these focus groups, the issue of rebuilding trust might have been overlooked as a key strategy for incorporating softness back into the parent–child relationship.

Strategy 3: A New Approach to Criticism

During the focus group interviews, teenagers also reported that the parent–child emotional bond was severely damaged whenever the parents persisted in bringing up old problems or criticisms in the present. Parents would often say that they forgave, but they never seemed to forget.

When a teenager's character or personality is constantly criticized (e.g., "You will never amount to anything," "You are a failure," "You never listen"), the teen often shuts down and gives up because it seems that nothing he or she does will ever be good enough. Over time, the teenager begins to believe that he or she really is "no good," "stupid," "clumsy," or "ugly." When this happens, the teenager begins to think, "If I do not try, I cannot fail." Hence, a vicious cycle is created whereby the teenager stops trying and the parents criticize more frequently to try to motivate their son or daughter. This cycle of criticisms only leads to bitterness and severe damage to the parent–child emotional bond.

To address this problem, parents are shown the following two techniques: (1) how to "tag" a misbehavior without attacking the teenager's character or personality in the process; and (2) how to avoid criticisms when angry. Each technique is initially demonstrated and practiced without the teenager present. The teenager only needs to see the finished product; he or she does not need to witness the anger and negative affect that the counselor must wade through in the process of getting the parents to change their method of criticisms. The counselor goes through as many role plays as necessary until he or she is convinced that the parents can criticize their teenager differently.

Talking about the Misbehavior Instead of Attacking the Person

To stop critical attacks on the teen's personality or character, the counselor has to show parents a better alternative—that is, to teach them how to separate a misbehavior from the teenager's personality or character. For example, if the teenager does not complete chores, parents are told to "tag" this misbehavior without using such terms as "stupid," "worthless," or "lazy."

This is accomplished in the following manner. First, the counselor asks a parent to describe a recent argument and what was said by both parties. The counselor then plays the role of the parent and has the parent play the teenager. The counselor, as the parent, reenacts the argument and uses the same words to criticize the parent, as the teenager. This role reversal is used so that the parent can put himself or herself in the teenager's shoes. Next, the counselor conducts another role play. During this second role play, the counselor again plays the parent, but this time he or she uses helpful and constructive criticism by focusing solely on the current misbehavior without attacks on character or personality. Finally, the parent and counselor compare and contrast the two role plays and discuss why the use of constructive criticism is a better approach. The parents then play themselves and practice this approach while the counselor plays the part of the teenager. These role plays continue until both the parents and the counselor say that they are prepared to call the teenager back into the room and try the new approach "for real." The counselor will then bring up a hot topic (e.g., curfew) and watch how each parent engages the teenager. If a parent again lapses into a highly critical role, the counselor can ask the teenager to leave the room while the parent and counselor regroup and try to fine-tune this approach. A clinical example illustrates this process.

CLINICAL EXAMPLE

COUNSELOR: (*to Mike's mother*) Mary, thanks for agreeing to try this new approach to criticism. Before Mike returns, I was wondering if I could demonstrate this approach. I will play you as the parent, and you will play the part of your son. The reason for this is so that I can role-model what to do. You can feel the difference, as Mike, between helpful and unhelpful criticism. [The counselor prepared the mother and gave a rationale for why the role play was being used and why they were using role reversal.]

MOTHER: I don't know. I am not good at acting. [This is a very common response, and one a counselor will most likely have to overcome.]

COUNSELOR: That's OK, neither am I. It is just used as a practice tool to understand how to use this approach smoothly and effectively. [The counselor overcame this reluctance by downplaying the acting part and taking a one-down position.]

MOTHER: OK, I will try.

COUNSELOR: Thanks. First, can you tell me basically what happened the last time you and Mike had an argument? Can you remember a little about what you said and then what Mike said? I can use what happened in our role play and make it resemble your situation. [The counselor asked the parent for a real-life situation of past criticism. Different parents' arguments may contain different content, but the process or style of communication around criticism will be similar. Using a real-life situation increases the chances that the skills learned will be generalized to other situations.]

MOTHER: Well, Mike was late for curfew again. I was so ticked that I let him have it as soon as he walked through the door. I told him I was tired of his shit. I said that he was a disappointment and would never amount to anything if he kept this up. He said he was tired of the sermons, and said that all I do is bitch and have nothing good to say. He then walked away, and we have not really spoken since. [It is extremely difficult for parents not to criticize. Parents were often criticized by their own parents and thus have the mistaken belief that criticism will help a teenager learn right from wrong.]

The counselor then reenacted this scene, but this time the mother played the part of Mike. After this role play, the following discussion ensued:

COUNSELOR: How did you feel inside as I was talking to you? [The counselor attempted to get the mother to place herself in Mike's shoes and feel the sting of her criticism.]

MOTHER: Not good . . . it just made me angrier, and I just tuned you out.

COUNSELOR: Can you see how conversations like this one could create bitterness and distance between you and your son? [The counselor tried to connect the issue of nurturance and present-day criticism.]

MOTHER: The words definitely sting, and I am beginning to see how Mike and I have drifted so far apart. [The mother made this important connection.]

COUNSELOR: Now let's play the same scene over, but this time I will just focus on the fact that you missed curfew and recite the agreed-upon consequence of grounding. Try to bait me and push my buttons by calling me names. No matter what you do to throw me off track, I will just use deflectors like "nevertheless," and not attack you by calling you names. [The counselor outlined step by step the strategy, how it would be implemented, and how he would respond.]

MOTHER: What if Mike starts swearing and goes on and on like he usually does?

COUNSELOR: If this happens, I want you to use exiting and waiting the way we talked about earlier. Remember, you do not owe Mike an explanation or have to justify your actions. The most important thing is to practice this new approach to criticism. [The counselor integrated earlier techniques and gives the mother a concrete road map to follow.]

The mother then playfully tried to push the counselor's buttons, but the counselor focused on the consequence without criticism to Mike's character. When the mother started to attack, he role-modeled exiting and waiting, and left the confrontation before losing control of his emotions. After this role play, the mother was asked to play herself while the counselor played the part of Mike. He then tried to throw her off by swearing and demanding an explanation. When the mother started to criticize, the counselor froze the role play and offered suggestions. After three sets of role plays, the mother felt confident enough to bring Mike back into the room. The counselor then intentionally asked Mike to discuss the hot topic of curfew violations. While Mike lost his cool, the mother was prepared and was able to focus solely on his inappropriate behaviors without criticism. Mike was visibly thrown off by these new tactics and asked the counselor, "What have you done with my real mother?" The counselor ended the session by troubleshooting potential problems in the week ahead through "what if" scenarios, while the mother and Mike brainstormed solutions.

As criticism decreased by 50%, Mike and Mary reported that there was a lot less tension and that they had a better working relationship. As this continued, the counselor was finally able to get the mother and son to agree to special outings together. When this happened, both reported that they got closer and were able to talk to each other for the first time.

In addition to role plays, parents can be shown videotaped scenarios in which actors first criticize and attack a teenager's personality and then use constructive criticism to simply "tag" a misbehavior. These "before and after" scenarios can help facilitate the learning process by allowing parents to see the successful application of this strategy. Parents can even take these tapes home and review them before the next session.

As noted above in the bracketed comments on the dialogue, it is important to remember that stopping criticism is difficult for many parents. Parents who were criticized by their own parents usually have the mistaken belief that criticism will teach the teenager right from wrong. The teenager may also attack the parents' character, causing the parents to feel that they have to fight back with the same type of criticism. To counter these problems, the counselor should ask the parents to remember times when they were criticized as children or teenagers. The counselor then asks the parents to close their eyes and remember these criticizing words. They are asked to remember how the criticism made them feel inside: Did it really help change their behaviors, or did it cause bitterness and resentment? Most parents will say that criticism caused bitterness and resentment. Counselors should normalize criticism as a result of parental role modeling. Parents must also be told that if they continue to criticize, the teenager will criticize his or her own children. If this happens, the cycle will never be broken.

Finally, criticism leaves bruises beneath the skin and the heart that cannot be seen by the naked eye. A physical wound may heal, but bitter words and labels stick with a person for years and sometimes never heal. Over time, the teenager sees himself or herself as a failure and stops trying. Parents who understand this rationale may then be open to new suggestions.

Avoiding Criticism When Angry

Parents should be shown the connection between anger and criticism. Each time the parents are angry or feel personally attacked, the risk of criticism increases. To address this problem, parents are given the following two principles:

1. The counselor should repeat an earlier point by reminding parents that the teenager will purposely push their buttons during confrontations to make them angry and cause them to abdicate their authority. If the parents start to get angry and criticize, it is a clear signal to the teen that he or she is winning the argument. It is a game to the teenager, so to play the game better, the parents must not criticize.

2. The parents should give themselves permission to get angry, with one exception: No matter how angry they are, this is not a time to insult the teenager's personality and character. To accomplish this goal, parents are given the following suggestions:

a. Parents are asked to describe what they feel, but without personal attacks. Here are some examples: "John, it burns me up when I see good towels on a wet floor," and not "It burns me up when I see good towels on the floor, because you are always such a slob and so worthless," or "I get angry when you lie to me," and not "I get angry when you lie, and you are a natural-born liar. When will you ever learn?" Parents should be given a number of these examples until the point is clear.

b. After describing their anger, parents must tell the teenager the resulting consequence. Example: "It burns me up when I see good towels on a wet floor. They need to be picked up in the next 5 minutes, or you will not be allowed to go out the rest of the day, and all phone and television privileges will be taken away," or "I get angry when you lie to me. Because you lied, all phone privileges will be taken away for the next 2 days, as we wrote down in our contract."

Strategy 4: A New Approach to Praise

Praise is a sincere, positive evaluation of a person or an act. A question often asked is this: "If praise is supposed to be so helpful to teenagers, why do we have so many insecure children, unmotivated underachievers, and dropouts?" The answer lies within the way parents praise. Parents may tell their teenagers, "You are so smart," "You are so pretty," or "You did such a great job." However, these praises are not met with joy but with denial (Ginott, 1969): Teenagers will reply, "You are just saying that," or "It was luck more than anything else." The counselor needs to tell parents that this happens because a global label such as "smart," "pretty," or "great job" makes a teenager feel criticized or evaluated. In turn, this makes the teenager uncomfortable and makes him or her want to diminish such global praises; otherwise, he or she may always have to live up to these general expectations.

In addition, parents may give their teenager a "psychological sandwich"—two pieces of praise with blame in between. That is, the parents mix criticism with praise. For example, a parent may say, "I like the fact that you came in for curfew on time, but you still need to improve on your schoolwork." Whenever the teenager hears the word "but" and then a critical statement, the praise is wiped away. If this continues, the emotional bond continues to suffer, as the teenager believes that nothing he or she does will ever be good enough.

To address these two problem areas, the counselor can show the parents how to praise by simply describing the event or behavior, rather than using a global label or a psychological sandwich. For example, a parent should say, "I appreciate your helping me with the dishes the other night," rather than "You are always so helpful." The first statement signals that the teenager is helpful or improving within a specific behavior. The second statement signals that the person always has to live up to something. Therefore, the likely response to this second statement will be "No, I am not," or "I could do better."

Finally, our society has a tendency to look for the negative instead of the positive. When parents do this, they only reinforce the negative behavior. Therefore, parents are often asked to take an imaginary giant magnifying glass to look for anything positive the teen does during the coming week, no matter how small. Parents are often asked to try this homework assignment to retrain their minds to look for the positive. After these positives are located, parents can use praise without using a psychological sandwich. The parents will still "tag" misbehavior with consequences, but they will also be "tagging" the positive behaviors with a new form of praise. When they understand this rationale, many parents will agree to the experiment.

Strategy 5: Acceptance of Underlying Feelings

In the book *How to Talk So Kids Will Listen and Listen So Kids Will Talk,* Adele Faber and Elaine Mazlish (1980) make a direct connection between how kids feel and how they behave. In other words, acknowledging a teenager's underlying feelings without condoning a misbehavior can lead to a tremendous improvement in the parent–child relationship. For example, if a teenager comes to a parent and says, "I'm too tired to do the dishes," the parent can respond in one of two ways. One response may be this: "You're not tired. Quit giving excuses and get the dishes done, or you are grounded." Another response may be this: "I bet you wish that you did not have to do dishes because you are tired, but they still have to be done by 8 P.M., as we agreed." In the first response, the parent discounts the teenager's feelings and moves right into a disciplinarian role; this only leads to anger and resentment. In the second response, the parent acknowledges the teenager's underlying wish of being too tired, but still holds the teenager accountable. This second response creates an atmosphere of mutual respect, because the parent takes the time to acknowledge the teenager's underlying feelings.

This simple but powerful strategy can be used successfully to bring softness back into the parent–child relationship. Many teenagers reported in the focus group interviews that "being heard" went a long way toward increasing respect on both sides and improving their relationships with their parents. Parents also reported a difference. Parents stated that they were originally under the perception that acknowledgment of feelings was an either–or proposition—in other words, that they could not acknowledge feelings and still discipline their teens effectively. Once parents saw that they could do both, they were willing to incorporate this strategy.

To teach this strategy, the counselor must do three things:

1. Parents must be made aware of conscious or unconscious ways of responding that discount or deny a teen's feelings. The counselor presents five possible negative responses in a handout and demonstrates these responses through videotaped scenarios or role plays.

2. Parents are shown specific forms of emotional aid or ways to acknowledge underlying feelings (e.g., giving the feeling a name, listening with full attention).

3. Rules of thumb for when this strategy is appropriate and when it should not be used are presented.

Five Ways to Ignore Underlying Feelings

Each parent is given a handout (Figure 7.3) adapted from Faber and Mazlish's (1980) book. This handout outlines five ways in which parents can ignore underlying feelings. Parents are then asked to write down their reactions to the statements within each of these five areas. This is done so that parents can get a sense of how certain words and phrases can cause their teenager to feel ignored, angry, or discounted.

After the counselor goes over this handout, he or she asks the parents for any recent examples of when they used these types of responses. Once these examples are identified, the counselor will role-play each example (a parent plays the part of the teenager, while the counselor plays the part of the parent) to demonstrate the impact of ignoring the feelings. The counselor may also use videotaped scenarios of actors who demonstrate these types of responses. Parents can check out these videotapes to watch during

1. **Denial of feeling.** Parents may respond to the teenager's statement of pain or anger by simply ignoring the underlying feeling altogether. This will only lead to the teenager's feeling discounted or angry. Over time, a denial of feelings can damage the emotional bond between parents and teenager, as well as the teen's relations with other authority figures. Examples of these types of responses include "There is no reason to be upset," "You are probably just tired and blowing the whole thing out of whack as usual," "It is foolish to feel that way," and "Big deal. I would not be mad if that happened to me."

Parent's Reaction to These Statements: _____

_____

2. **Cliche or philosophical approach.** Parents may respond with a standard cliche or a philosophical approach. This only makes the teenager feel that the parents do not care or are making light of the situation. In turn, this can lead to distance in the relationship, as the teenager looks to someone else who will take him or her seriously. Examples of these types of responses include "You are still young; you have your whole life ahead of you," "I told you so," "You know, it's like my father always used to say . . . ," and "Rome was not built in a day."

Parent's Reaction to These Statements: _____

_____

3. **Pity.** Teenagers do not like to be pitied when they find the courage to express a painful feeling. Pity makes a teenager feel discounted and the pain much worse. In addition, the teenager who is pitied is less likely to risk coming back for support a second time. Examples of these types of responses include "Oh, you poor thing," "I feel so sorry for you," "My heart breaks for you, but I guess it was just meant to be," and "Oh, I feel so bad I could just cry."

Parent's Reaction to These Statements: _____

_____

4. **Minimizing the situation.** Teenagers become extremely angry and will escalate quickly when they feel that their pain is minimized. They view these responses as a slap in the face and become extremely bitter over time. Examples of these types of responses include "Come one, it can't be that bad," "I don't see what the big deal is, really," "It is not worth talking about," and "It is not as bad as you make it out to be."

Parent's Reaction to These Statements: _____

_____

5. **"The trouble with you . . ."** Parents use this statement as a prelude to negative criticism. Teenagers who hear this statement often become very angry and feel attacked. Examples of these types of responses include "The trouble with you is you never listen," and "The trouble with you is that you're always putting your foot in your mouth."

Parent's Reaction to These Statements: _____

_____

FIGURE 7.3. Parent handout: Five ways to ignore underlying feelings. From *Treating the Tough Adolescent* by Scott P. Sells. Copyright 1998 by The Guilford Press. Permission to photocopy this handout is granted to purchasers of *Treating the Tough Adolescent* for personal use only (see copyright page for details).

the week as homework, and can come prepared the next session to make changes.

CLINICAL EXAMPLE

Sixteen-year-old Tara was referred for chronic running away. In the first session, Tara reported that her mother never listened to her. Tara felt that no matter what came out of her mouth, she would receive a lecture and was judged a bad kid. It had gotten to the point where she and her mother no longer spoke. The mother denied that this was the case. Tara just needed guidance because she was "throwing her life away." The mother reported that she was frustrated and that her daughter went out of her way to spite her.

When the counselor tried to explain the concept of accepting underlying feelings, the mother stated that she had no problem in this area; it was Tara who had the problem. The counselor responded by asking the mother to look at the handout and see whether any of these responses fit how she and Tara talked to each other. (The counselor intentionally did not point the finger of blame at either the mother or the daughter. Instead, he asked from a position of curiosity to see whether there was a connection. The counselor thus made the mother the expert and took a one-down position.)

After reading each of the five possible responses, the mother was asked to write down her reactions if these statements were said to her. The mother smiled at the counselor and said, "Now I understand what you mean. I use these statements all the time, but never realized it until this moment. I think I understand how Tara feels ignored and her feelings cast aside."

The counselor then showed the mother five videotaped scenarios. Each scene demonstrated times when parents attended to underlying feelings and times when they did not. The mother had to pick out which one was which. After the mother felt confident in this task, she practiced with the counselor until she felt confident in her ability to attend to Tara's underlying feelings while concurrently "tagging" her misbehavior with predetermined consequences.

The counselor asked whether the mother would be willing to experiment with these new tools for the next 2 weeks. If the mother saw even one concrete change in behavior, she would agree to 2 more trial weeks, and so on. The mother agreed to these terms and was able to change her style of communication. Weeks later, Tara asked the counselor what he had done to change her mother. Tara stated that her mother was listening to what she had to say and was less judgmental. She added that she now wanted to "do better" so as not to disappoint her mother.

In this case, the counselor was able to change the mother's perceptions by presenting her with the Figure 7.3 handout and discussing it with her. The mother could identify the statements she herself was making through the handout and the videotaped examples. The mother was then able to draw a connection between her present relationship with Tara and a style of communication that left Tara feeling judged and unheard. The counselor was thus able to obtain a commitment to try this new approach on a time-limited and experimental basis.

Using Forms of Emotional Aid to Acknowledge Underlying Feelings

Parents often react to their teenager's statements in one of two ways: Either they will approve and agree with what the teenager has to say, or they will disapprove and tell the teenager he or she is wrong. However, there is a third way of responding that is often not used. This is a "nonjudgmental response" that contains no approval or disapproval, but simply identifies the feelings underneath the statement. This type of response gives the teenager emotional aid because it tells the teen that he or she is being heard and his or her feelings are being accepted. In turn, this leads to less misbehavior and a closer parent–teenager bond. This emotional aid occurs when one of these three techniques are followed:

1. *Listening with full attention.* It is much easier for a teenager to tell a parent his or her problems or concerns when the parent is fully listening. The television should be off, and the parent should stop whatever he or she is doing at the moment. Parents often do not have to say anything; the teen just needs to know that the parents are listening without trying to fix the problem or giving their opinion. Instead, they listen in silence and give the message that their response is nonjudgmental.

2. *Acknowledging the teenager's feelings with noncommittal words or phrases.* By using words or phrases such as "Mmm," "Oh," or "I see," a parent does not risk being judgmental or saying the wrong thing at the wrong time. For example, if the teenager comes home and says that the teacher is unfair, the parent replies with "Mmm." This gives the teenager an open door and more time to explain what he or she is thinking or feeling. The teenager may even work out his or her own solutions as the parent becomes a sounding board.

3. *Giving feelings a name.* The teenager who hears words that describe accurately what he or she is experiencing can be deeply comforted. The strength of this strategy is that even if a parent is totally off base, the teenager will correct the parent and describe how he or she is really feeling. This happens because the parent starts each statement with "It seems like ..." or "Sounds as if. ..." This allows the teenager to agree or disagree with the parent's interpretation. Another handout (Figure 7.4) can be given to parents to help illustrate this technique.

Once these techniques are demonstrated, parents are asked to practice them with the counselor through role plays until they have mastered these skills. This is done before the teenager is asked back into the room.

Teenager says:	One or two words that describe what he or she might be feeling:	Use a statement that tells the teenager what you hear him or her saying:
"School really bites. I hate all my teachers."	Angry	"It seems like you are angry with school. Is that close or way off?" "It sounds like you are angry."
"I am just so tired of all the bullshit."	Frustrated	"It seems like you are frustrated and tired. Is that close or way off?" "It sounds like you are frustrated."
"My friend is spreading rumors about me, but I don't know what to do."	Worried and unsure	"It seems like you are worried about the rumors and unsure about what to do. Is that close or way off?" "It sounds like you are worried and unsure what to do."

FIGURE 7.4. Parent handout: Giving feelings a name. From *Treating the Tough Adolescent* by Scott P. Sells. Copyright 1998 by The Guilford Press. Permission to photocopy this handout is granted to purchasers of *Treating the Tough Adolescent* for personal use only (see copyright page for details).

CLINICAL EXAMPLE

Thirteen-year-old Bill and his father rarely if ever spoke. They had once been close but were presently very distant. Bill complained that his father did not understand him and had no idea why he liked to dress in black and listened to heavy metal rock. Whenever he tried to talk, his father would immediately lecture and give his opinion without listening.

Because of the extreme emotional distance, the counselor decided to see father and son separately at first. The counselor split up the hour-long session into two parts; he worked with the father for the first half-hour and then Bill for the second half-hour. During the father's individual meeting, the counselor was able to convince the father to try to practice the techniques of listening with full attention; using "Oh," "Mmm," or "I see"; and giving Bill's feelings a name. The father only agreed to this approach after the counselor posed it as an experiment and playfully bet $10 of his own money that the father would be unable to use these strategies within the next 2 weeks. If there was no change after 4 weeks, the counselor would double his money.

The counselor then played the part of Bill and had the father practice each strategy until he felt confident in its use. Before the counselor conducted these role plays, he obtained inside information from Bill during their individual meetings. The counselor asked Bill the following question: "What would your father need to do or say in the future that would make it easier for you to talk to him?" Bill reported that his father would not lecture. Instead, he would take the time to listen, rather than being Mr. Know-it-All. The counselor then asked Bill for permission to relay this information back to his father and incorporate his suggestions into the role plays. Bill agreed. When the counselor gave this information to the father, he was surprised. The father did not know how to incorporate his son's suggestions to talk to Bill differently. The counselor role-modeled these changes by playing the part of the father while the father played the role of Bill. After several practice runs, the roles were reversed, and the father played himself while the counselor played the part of Bill. If the father started to lecture of make mistakes, the counselor would freeze the role play and offer alternative suggestions. When the father felt ready, Bill was brought into the room for an actual run-through. Below is a brief transcript of what took place when Bill and his father met to try these new strategies.

COUNSELOR: When I saw you both alone, you had in common the fact that you did not like the way the relationship was going. Dad, you felt that Bill was slipping away and shutting down, and Bill you felt that Dad lectured and did not listen to your point of view. Is that close or way off? [The counselor summarized the essence of the problem, and ended his statement by asking whether he was close or way off. This role-modeled giving feelings a name, and it gave both parties an opportunity to refute or agree with the counselor's viewpoint.]

BILL: That's right.

COUNSELOR: We have individually practiced the strategies needed to end the current "cold war" and move you both to a point where you are communicating better with one another. However, to make these changes stick, we have to practice them. Therefore, Bill, I want you to pretend you are coming home from school, and, Dad, you will practice listening with full attention, giving Bill's feelings a name, and using words like "I see" or "Mmm" before giving your opinion too quickly. I know this will be weird, awkward, and unreal, but it is meant to feel that way. Any new muscle you exercise will feel weird at first until you practice enough and it feels like nothing new. [The counselor set up the role play, gave a rationale, and informed the father and Bill that it is normal and expected for a role play to feel mechanical and weird.]

FATHER: OK, let's give it a try.

COUNSELOR: If there is a problem, or you get stuck and do not know what to say, I will be like a coach and help you get unstuck. Then you can practice these new techniques during the week. I will call in the middle of the week to see how things are going and if there are any problems. [The counselor clarified his role as a coach and let both parties know that there would be follow-up during the week.]

BILL: OK, I will go out the door now and pretend I am coming back from school . . .

FATHER: Bill, how was your day?

BILL: Not good. I just do not like this new teacher.

FATHER: Mmmm. [He successfully acknowledged Bill's feelings.]

BILL: I tried to get my point across in class, but the teacher ignored me.

FATHER: What do I do now? I want to give my opinion, but Bill will think I am lecturing again?

COUNSELOR: Try what we worked on by just starting off with "It sounds like . . ." and attach the underlying feelings that Bill may be experiencing at the moment. [The counselor played coach and helped the father get unstuck.]

FATHER: OK. This feels weird, but here goes . . . Bill, it sounds like you were feeling ignored and that your opinion was not important. [The father did a great job here.]

BILL: (*Smiling*) That is exactly how I felt, and upset also. What do you think I should do?

Bill and his father went on a little longer until the counselor asked the following question:

COUNSELOR: Bill, what was that like for you with your dad talking the way he did? [This question is used at the end of every role-play scenario, to evaluate it and help reinforce the strategies that were employed.]

BILL: A lot different than usual. I felt heard for the first time rather than lectured to. If Dad could only do that more, I think I might even ask for his advice once in a while.

FATHER: I never knew you felt quite this way. I will try this next time, but if I start on my old habits, I will need you to let me know.

BILL: OK.

In this case, the counselor was able to prepare and practice these strategies with Bill and the father individually before asking them to incorporate them. This type of preparation can increase the probability of success and limit the potential for future negative interaction and further damage to an already tenuous emotional bond. Without these new tools, the father and son would have continued their confrontations until the relationship became permanently damaged or was broken off altogether. The counselor "played both sides of the fence" and custom-fit both the father's and Bill's suggestions directly into the role plays. The counselor also explained his role as a coach and assisted the father or son if either got stuck in the role play. This type of role play is called an "enactment," because key problem issues are brought into the counseling session and modified or shaped right in the room, under the supervision of the counselor.

Rules of Thumb

Parents often ask the counselor when and where the various techniques that make up Strategy 5 should be used. The counselor should list the following rules of thumb:

1. Parents will want to know whether they should always try to acknowledge their teenager's underlying feelings, even when the teen is inappropriately swearing or threatening violence. If this happens, it is not the time to acknowledge feelings. Instead, the parents should exit and wait until things have calmed down and the teenager can make statements without disrespect.

2. These techniques should be used when a teenager appears to be hurting, upset, or angry. The negative emotions are the ones that really require this skill.

3. By acknowledging feelings, parents are not saying that they agree with the behavior. The parents are merely reflecting back the feelings. For example, a parent may not agree with a teen's statement that "School sucks." Instead, the parent simply reflects back an underlying feeling ("It sounds like you are angry with school") so that the teenager feels heard.

4. Finally, parents must resist the temptation to "make it better" or try to solve the problem instantly. The teenager may simply need to feel heard. Instead of giving advice, parents should just reflect back feelings.

Strategy 6: Physical Touch

Physical touch or small signs of affection are extremely important to the restoration of tenderness between parents and teenager. (Exceptions to this rule must be made in cases of sexual abuse between parent and child or sibling and sibling. Sexual abuse issues must be confronted directly and treated before the restoration of physical touch can be initiated.) Physical touch and signs of affection cannot be overlooked. Medical research shows that many physical problems, depression, and anxiety can be linked in part to a lack of physical touch. Dogs and cats are often used to provide "animal therapy" for the elderly and cancer patients, because their touch has led to many healing effects. Finally, studies with monkeys and human orphans have shown that a lack of physical touch can lead to disease and serious social problems (see Harlow, 1971; Skeels, 1966). The question is this: If physical touch is so necessary for survival, why do difficult teenagers and parents present such a deficit in this area? The answer to this question centers around two areas: (1) Parents often think that their teenager is too old for hugs; and (2) emotional deprivation over the years makes the teenager stiffen or push the parents away.

Parents Think Their Teenager Is Too Old

Parents often think that a teenager is too old for hugs. Teenagers often think the same thing. Fathers are often taught by their fathers that they are not supposed to hug a teenage son because he is becoming a man, or a teenage daughter because she is becoming a woman. Therefore, hugs are somehow inappropriate or no longer necessary.

When this belief is prevalent, parents must be educated that physical touch is important and necessary for emotional bonding. To support this point, counselors can provide research that demonstrates the importance of touch. I have often used the classic study by Skeels (1966) on orphaned children to convey the importance of touch. In the 1930s, one group of orphans was given surrogate mothers to play with, talk to, and physically touch. The other group of orphans was not given any surrogate mothers or any form of touch; only the basic needs for food, clothing, and shelter were met. After a period of 2 years, the members of the first group thrived in intelligence, and a follow-up study conducted 20 years later showed that most of them were married, were self-supporting, and had graduated from college. The results for the second group showed the exact opposite. Many of these orphans grew sick and died; many of those children who did survive did not progress past a third-grade education or remained institutionalized. After hearing this story, parents may be willing to reconsider the issue of physical touch.

The Teenager Stiffens Up or Pushes the Parents Away

After the counselor explains the importance of physical touch, parents may ask, "If physical touch is so important, why does my teenager hate it so much?" To answer this question, the counselor can go back to the earlier concept of "emotional deprivation." With increasing distance and hostility over the years, both parents and child have stopped practicing the art of hugging. Without practice, the teenager naturally stiffens or pushes the parents away, because the old hurts have never healed. Indeed, the teenager may no longer be used to what a hug feels like. Touch has become foreign to the teenager, and he or she no longer knows how to react. As the result of this deprivation, parents must keep trying. Otherwise, the teenager will seek this touch inappropriately through premarital sex or will pass on this lack of touch to his or her future children.

If all else fails, the counselor can use the metaphor of taking medicine. The counselor can tell the parent that, like medicine, hugs may initially "taste bad." However, sick people must keep taking medicine because it is good for them and will help them become healthy again. Similarly, hugs are necessary for emotional health; therefore, parents must keep trying to hug their teenager until they finally break down the walls and the teenager no longer stiffens or pushes the parents away.

Parents must remember that the teenager will initially be suspicious of hugs or other forms of physical touch. The teenager may think that the parents are up to no good or want something from him or her. However, if the parents keep giving hugs unconditionally, no matter how good or bad the teenager is that week, the walls will eventually come down.

Before incorporating this strategy, parents are given the following rules of thumb:

1. The parent should not try to hug their teenager in front of the teen's friends. This allows the teenager to avoid looking "uncool" in front of his or her peer group.

2. No matter how resistant the teenager is to hugs, the parents must continue to try to hug and touch the teenager. Even a gentle slap on the shoulder from one "macho" guy to another is a good thing to do, because it is still physical touch. The parent should set a goal of 1 hug a day for a week and then go up by 1 hug each week until they at least get to between 5 and 7 hugs a day. Parents can be told that a leading family counselor, Virginia Satir (1988), recommended 4 hugs per day for survival, 8 hugs for maintenance, and 12 hugs a day for growth.

3. Parents are asked to avoid hugging right after or during an argument. Both the teenager and the parents need time to "cool down." The parents are asked to hug when there is no conflict or when there are good feelings.

4. Finally, the parents are urged not to make hugs conditional upon good behavior. No matter how bad the teen's behavior has been that week, parents should be told to continue to hug. This sends the powerful message to the teenager that the parents are separating love from misbehavior.

It is important to note that if there is sexual abuse in the family, hugs will be misread by the teenager. If the counselor notices an extraordinarily bad reaction to physical touch, sexual abuse should be ruled out before this strategy is recommended further. If sexual abuse is ruled out but the teenager still has a bad reaction, the counselor might recommend that special outings be initiated first (see below) to pave the way for future hugs. For some teenagers, their emotional deprivation is too severe or they have been sexually abused by someone other than a parent. In these cases, the teenagers may not let anyone come near them. If this happens, the parents must move extremely slowly and just begin with a pat on the back or special outings.

CLINICAL EXAMPLE

Fifteen-year-old Sam was referred to counseling for sexual abuse issues. He had sexually abused the daughter of a housemother in a residential treatment facility.

His natural mother had placed him there after he had committed numerous acts of truancy and violence against the family. Sam was extremely angry with his mother, and they had not hugged or had special outings together since he was 5 years old. Indeed, Sam had little affect except anger and would not let anyone get close to him. He had no social skills and spent all of his time by himself, playing video games. Unless this isolation could be broken and the relationship with his mother repaired, San would be at high risk for another sexual offense.

Part of the treatment plan was to reestablish a nurturing bond by getting the mother to begin hugging Sam again. Sam initially refused and became very agitated whenever the mother tried to touch him. The mother also complained: If touch was so good, why did Sam pull away? The counselor then explained the concept of emotional deprivation, and stressed that Sam needed these hugs even though he acted as if he did not. Because the mother had a good rapport with the counselor, she agreed to hug Sam once a day before bedtime, whether San wanted the hug or not. In addition to this strategy, the mother agreed to make time for special outings. Later she told the counselor that doing these good deeds helped her heal and remove the guilt she had been feeling for putting him in the residential home.

Later, the mother reported that the hugs and special outings seemed to be breaking down the walls of Sam's isolation. She could tell because Sam began to smile, spent less time alone, and did not look angry all the time. Privately, she told the counselor that she was up to 4 hugs a day. Even though Sam still acted as if he did not want the hugs, his body no longer stiffened, and he even began to hug back now and then.

Strategy 7: Special Outings

Difficult adolescents and their parents often cannot remember the last time they had a special outing together or spent one-on-one time without arguing. Like physical touch, special outings are a necessity if nurturance is to be brought back into the relationship. To restore special outings, the counselor must first remove the following three stumbling blocks: (1) The parents and teenager will say that they have nothing in common; (2) the parents and/or the teenager will say that they do not have the time in their hectic schedules to go on special outings; and (3) the parents will insist that the teenager must be on his or her best behavior before a special outing can take place.

"We Have Nothing in Common"

The parents and teenager often say that they cannot or will not do something together because they do not like the same things. To counter this objection, the counselor offers three suggestions. First, going out together is reframed for each party as a way to explore the other's world by doing things the other likes. For example, a parent may have no interest in body piercing and may have a strict rule against it. However, going with the teenager to body-piercing shops does not imply consent or approval. It simply means that the parent is willing to explore the teenager's world in order to understand him or her better. By the same token, the teenager may not like going birdwatching, but will go in order to understand a bird-loving parent better. These joint activities will strengthen the emotional bond; in particular, they will help the parent understand the teenager better when the teen is in trouble or hurting. This rationale makes sense to most parents and teenagers.

Second, the parent(s) and the teenager are asked to pick a specific day and time that they will "make the time" to go out. One week a parent picks what the special outing will be, and the next week the teenager picks. Since each party gets to choose every other week, they no longer have the excuse of not going because one party never does anything the other likes. A coin is flipped to see who goes first and picks what they will be doing that week. If the teenager refuses to go at the appointed time, the parent or parents are instructed to go out with the teenager anyway. The rationale is that the teenager will probably end up having a good time, whether he or she admits it or not. The parents and teenager are also out of practice in going out. They need this practice so that these outings can eventually become fun and enjoyable. Both parties are told that they should not initially expect to have a good time, because they are not used to being together. This is a paradoxical directive designed to get the family to have a good time to prove the counselor wrong. The parents and teenager are instructed to do something social that involves talking (e.g., not going to the movies) and one that does not cost much money.

Finally, many families will say that they will plan their special outing later or wait and see how the week goes. If this happens, the special outing will not take place, because the family is not used to this kind of interaction and change. The counselor must therefore take charge by negotiating a specific time, day, and event before the parents and teenager leaves the office. The counselor must then troubleshoot and discuss all the reasons why this special outing might not take place. Alternative solutions are then discussed for every possible contingency. For example, the father in one family said this his son liked to sleep in on Sunday; therefore, a Sunday morning breakfast would fail. Based on this information, the son and father compromised and selected Sunday lunch as their outing. If this kind of troubleshooting had not taken place beforehand, this special outing would have failed.

"We Do Not Have Time"

If both parents work or there is a single parent, the reality is that the parent(s) will have fewer opportunities to spend time with a teenager. The latest statistics show that the time parents expend with their teenagers for purely sociable chatting averages only 8 minutes per day for mothers and only 3 minutes a day for fathers (Sandmaier, 1996).

If this argument surfaces, the counselor must take charge and convince the parent or parents of two things. First, the long-term costs of not spending time with a teenager will be great. Without parental time, the teenager will seek closeness through negative peer relationships or through drugs and alcohol. Second, if there is no time for special outings, the parent–child bond cannot be strengthened. As a result, the teenager will not approach the parent during times of trouble, pain, or indecision, but will instead go to his or her peer group. Time will pass quickly, and the teenager will grow up and be gone before the parents realize it. Finally, parents make the time for all types of appointments without thinking about it. Parents also often feel that they must commit themselves to large blocks of time and expense if they agree to special outings. Parents should be told that even 1 hour per week on a consistent basis is a great beginning and can make all the difference in the world. If parents are still resistant, the counselor can ask for a time-limited commitment of 1 month as an experiment to see whether special outings make a difference in the teenager's behavior.

"The Teenager Must First Be Good and Respectful"

When a child or teenager has behavior problems, special outings stop or become contingent upon good behavior. Since a teenager's functioning is based on the pleasure principle, the teen will probably misbehave at least once a week. Over time, the parents stop trying to plan special outings and make the faulty assumption that the teenager must not want them, because he or she is continuing to misbehave. Love or nurturance is no longer unconditional, but conditional on good behavior. The teenager may then grow up to be an adult who has trouble loving others because he or she will expect others to perform certain duties in order to receive love.

The counselor must help the parents separate special outings or acts of kindness from misbehavior. These two issues are separate and must be treated as such. Often the counselor must define what unconditional love consists of and how it must be separated from misbehavior. When parents understand this distinction, they are often willing to change their behavior. Once this change in perception takes place, the counselor can ask the parents to commit to the following procedures: (1) One or both parents will plan and conduct a special outing, no matter how good or bad the week was in terms of behavior; and (2) the parents will communicate to the teenager that special outings and misbehavior are two separate behaviors. In other words, the parents may not like or condone the teen's misbehavior, but they still love the teen and will prove this through special outings.

Finally, parents are told that this kind of unconditional love will initially confuse their son or daughter but will eventually lead to changes in their mis-behavior. A child who receives consistent acts of kindness and love even when he or she misbehaves will feel more secure and trusting in the relationship. This security and trust will make it more difficult to misbehave as a sense of guilt develops over time. Parents need to be told clearly that their patience will reap benefits. Parents are often burned out by the time they reach a coun-selor's office, and it takes a great deal of courage and faith for them to show acts of kindness when a teenager continues to mistreat them.

CLINICAL EXAMPLE

Sixteen-year-old Rachel was referred to counseling for committing acts of vio-lence against her mother and putting her fist through the wall at home. The mother was a single parent in the military. She was afraid to call the military po-lice because they might see the hole in the wall, conclude that she was an abusive mother, and report the incident to her commanding officer. Because of this fear, the mother did not leave the house for fear that something would happen. Over the years, a deep resentment resulted, and the mother rarely spoke to her daugh-ter. Rachel said that she in fact hated her mother and wanted to move back with her father, even though he had AIDS and had sexually molested her.

The counselor developed a good rapport with the mother. Over time, the counselor was able to help the mother stop the threats or acts of violence through the use of the bathroom strategy. For the first time she could remember, the mother felt empowered, and she trusted the counselor enough to explore un-charted territory. Part of this territory was the restoration of nurturance through special outings. The mother initially objected, stating that Rachel would first have to prove herself with a month of good behavior. However, the counselor was able to trace back and normalize a history of emotional deprivation, and to show how the mother's parents had done the same things to her. In addition, special outings would not mean that consequences would not be given for misbehavior. The mother would enforce the consequences, but special outings would be separate. The counselor also told the mother that Rachel initially would not have a good time on these outings, and that even if she did, she would not let the mother know. This was because so much emotional damage had been done inadvertently on both sides. Many special outings would be needed to break down these walls. The mother finally agreed.

The counselor asked both the mother and Rachel to specify a time, a date, and an activity that they would do together. The counselor flipped a coin to see who would decide on the activity first, with the agreement that the event would not cost a lot of money. Initially Rachel refused, but she finally agreed to go if the mother agreed to 2 extra hours a week of phone time. The mother felt that this was bribery. However, the counselor again reminded the mother privately of the years of emotional deprivation, and emphasized that they needed to get off ground zero by any means necessary. Rachel won the coin toss and picked dinner at an Italian restaurant on a Sunday afternoon. The counselor then engaged in troubleshooting to identify all the things that could go wrong ahead of time.

Some of the potential problems discussed included oversleeping, friends, an emergency call from the military that would force the mother to go in to work, and so on. After these obstacles had been discussed and contingency plans had been formulated, the mother and Rachel felt ready to take on the challenge.

This intervention was extremely successful. Within a month, Rachel was no longer asking for added phone time, but was wondering what new places they could go to each week. She even stated that it was now hard to be mean to her mother when her mother tried to be nice all the time.

INITIATING SOOTHING SEQUENCES OF COMMUNICATION

"Soothing sequences of communication" are defined as conversations in which a parent, not the teen, controls the mood, topic, and direction of the discussion. In addition, these discussions do not contain elements of criticism or attacks on the teenager's character. Instead, the parent uses one or more of the seven strategies described above (special outings, acceptance of feelings, physical touch, etc.) to initiate discussions that are nurturing and soothing rather than critical, bitter, and harsh. The focus of this section is on demonstrating the connection between parental control over the mood and topic of discussion and the initiation of soothing sequences. Once this goal is accomplished, the next section will pull everything together and demonstrate how to employ the seven strategies of nurturance to create soothing sequences of communication, using an extended case example.

Initiating soothing sequences of communication can be a challenging process. As stated earlier, difficult teenagers are more skillful than their parents in pushing buttons and controlling the mood and direction of the argument. When this happens, nurturance, in the form of soothing communication sequences, cannot take place.

CLINICAL EXAMPLE

The parents of 16-year-old Jamal tried to evoke soothing sequences of communication by reminiscing about the past and praising Jamal for his artistic abilities. Jamal, however, had a different agenda: He wanted his curfew time extended, and he started pushing his parents' buttons by swearing and threatening to run away. The father immediately became angry and forgot all about the topic of praise. Instead, the father began arguing and explaining why Jamal could not receive a longer curfew. In turn, this only provoked Jamal further and led to a bitter confrontation. In this way, Jamal, not the parents, controlled the mood, direction, and topic of discussion. As a result, a soothing sequence of communication using the nurturing strategy of praise was not possible.

The counselor saw this process unfold and asked Jamal to wait outside while he talked with his parents privately. After Jamal left the room, the following interchange ensued:

COUNSELOR: As I sat back and watched, I noticed how skillful Jamal was in pushing your buttons by swearing and running away. By doing this, he changed the entire mood and direction of the conversation. One minute you [the parents] were being so soft and sweet by praising Jamal for his artistic abilities, and the next minute he was pushing your buttons and you were trying to put out a fire. Did you notice this also? [The counselor reframed Jamal's behavior as being more skillful than his parents in the art of controlling the mood and direction of the conversation.]

FATHER: I never heard it put quite that way before. Now that I think about it, yes. We were trying to be positive as you suggested earlier, and it did not matter what we said. Jamal, as usual, had his own agenda—curfew. [The father began to see the problem from a different perspective.]

COUNSELOR: Can you give me other examples when you have tried to steer the conversation to something positive, and Jamal ends up taking the conversation into a negative or argumentative stage by pushing your buttons or changing the topic? [The counselor asked for other concrete examples to generalize Jamal's skillful ability to other conversations and settings. When this happened, the parents could see the need to change their style of communication.]

MOTHER: You know now that I think about it, Jamal does this a lot. Just the other day I tried to hug Jamal and tell him that I loved him. Instead of letting me hug him, he just pushed me away. I took this negative reaction so personally that I began to yell at him. Then Jamal began to yell at me, and it was a big disaster. [The mother gave a great example of how Jamal was again able to change the mood from a soft and soothing hug to something negative.]

COUNSELOR: That was a great example. Here again, Jamal was able to change the mood and direction of things, and you matched him mood for mood by yelling. This is in no way meant to blame either one of you. Jamal has just been able to call the shots by playing the game better and controlling the mood and direction of any soft discussion or action like hugging. He does this just to stay in charge and keep the upper hand. Would it be OK if I show you some better tools to work with to turn the tables and make you as good or better players in this game?

BOTH: Yes.

COUNSELOR: OK. We will practice together through role plays until you are both confident with these new tools. I will play the part of Jamal and do everything in my power to push your buttons, while you try to stick to your guns and not get derailed. For example, if you want to praise me, you keep on the topic of praising me no matter what I say. If I get too obnoxious, you can simply exit and wait and try again later. But here again, you are still controlling the mood, not Jamal. We will then ask Jamal to come back, and you can practice for real while I act as your coach to keep you on track. Jamal has to realize that he cannot go through life being angry and having a chip on his shoulder. He has to receive your gifts of love and softness before this wall of anger can be taken apart piece by piece. The only way this will happen is if you as parents can deliver these gifts through day-to-day conversations and actions. However, this can only happen if you do not allow your buttons to be pushed and you learn how to control the mood and direction of the discussion. [The counselor described the importance and the goal of this process: to inject nurturance into the parent–child relationship by changing the parents' style of delivery.]

In this case, the nurturing strategies of praise and physical touch could not be successfully implemented until the parents saw the connection between the delivery of soothing sequences and parental control over the mood and direction of the conversation. The counselor used concrete examples from this particular family to demonstrate this concept.

Once this connection is understood, a counselor can demonstrate this concept through role plays. The counselor should have the parents pretend that they are delivering nurturing interactions, while the counselor plays the part of the adolescent and tries to push the parents' buttons. Each time the parents fall for this trap, the counselor should freeze the role play and highlight the problem areas (e.g., the parents try to discuss special outings, but get thrown off track when the teenager swears) and then suggest concrete solutions (e.g., the parents stay on track and continue to discuss special outings). The teenager should not be in the room while these discussions are taking place; he or she will only throw the parents off track or use this information against the parents.

PULLING IT ALL TOGETHER: IMPLEMENTING THE SEVEN NURTURING STRATEGIES

Once the parents are proficient in controlling the topic and direction of a discussion, the counselor custom-fits particular nurturing strategies to the particular family. The parents are then able to mix and match the seven strategies to create soothing sequences of communication and restore nurturance. For example, one family may have an abundance of criticism but a dearth of praise, while another family may be unable to allow the teenager to regain trust or cannot make use of physical touch. Filling in the missing nurturance pieces becomes the basic work of restoring the soft side of the family hierarchy. This goal is accomplished in three key phases: (1) set-up and preparation, (2) troubleshooting, and (3) role plays and initial implementation. Clinical excerpts from the same case are used here to illustrate each phase.

Phase 1: Set-Up and Preparation

During the first phase, the counselor meets with the parents separately. The counselor goes over which of the seven nurturing strategies needs to be implemented. Getting the parents to accept the need for nurturance often takes a great deal of finesse, skill, and timing. The counselor often needs time to gain rapport or must wait until the teenager's extreme behavior is under control. As stated earlier, the timing of this discussion is contingent upon the severity of the problem behavior and the degree of emotional deprivation. If a problem is extreme, the "ace" must first be neutralized (Step 8 of the family-based treatment model; see Chapter 6) before this phase takes place. The parents are then more likely to entertain and incorporate the idea of using a soft approach.

CLINICAL EXAMPLE

Sixteen-year-old Lacy was referred to counseling for issues of chronic truancy and running away. The parents were also devout Mormons and were very upset that Lacy was dating a non-Mormon and having premarital sex. The boyfriend was physically and verbally abusive as well.

The father and Lacy had a very distant relationship and a poor emotional bond. The father described himself as a strict disciplinarian, while the mother described herself as soft and nurturing. Because of this dichotomy, it was difficult for the father to be seen by Lacy as soft. Lacy would frequently go the mother for support when she felt that the father was too strict. The mother supported the daughter instead of the father and comforted her. This split created marital tension and allowed the daughter to play one parent off against the other. Through counseling, the mother started to support the father and discipline Lacy. In response, Lacy's behavior initially became worse. She blamed her father and counselor for changing her mother; in turn, this created greater emotional distance between Lacy and her father. Moreover, the father constantly lectured Lacy on how bad her boyfriend was and told her that she needed to break up. This only pushed Lacy closer to her boyfriend. She told the counselor privately that there were times when she wanted to break up, but that her boyfriend was the only guy who seemed to care about her.

After the counselor had success in stopping Lacy's truancy and running away, the father was willing to look at the issue of nurturance. The father later reported that he did this because the counselor had been the only person who had helped his wife "get tough" and helped change Lacy's behavior, which had been going on for years. With a great deal of finesse and patience, the counselor was able to convince the father to initiate the nurturing strategies of a new approach to criticism, a new approach to praise, physical touch, and special outings.

The counselor was able to convince the father in the following manner. First, he asked the father whether he would do anything in his power to get his daughter away from her abusive boyfriend. The father replied, "Yes, anything!" The counselor then told the father the he had to "fight fire with fire." Each time he criticized Lacy's boyfriend, gave a sermon, or sounded judgmental, it forced Lacy to defend her boyfriend and run into his arms even more. The reason was that, as Lacy saw it, this boyfriend gave her unconditional acceptance and love. If she were to feel the father's love without judgment or criticism, the relationship with the boyfriend would weaken. The father told the counselor that he had never thought about it like this before, but that it made perfect sense.

The counselor then went on to use the strategy of education and normalization to explain how the father and Lacy had reached a level of emotional deprivation over the years. The counselor retraced the steps of how father and daughter had once been very close when she was a child. However, when he took a job as a truck driver, he was gone for weeks at a time. His wife grew lonely, and the daughter became her emotional support. Over time, he came home and felt like an outsider. The father also had to do all the discipline, because his wife felt that she would lose her best friend if she got tough on Lacy. As a result, the father had no time left over for softness or special outings. In turn, Lacy grew distant. As Lacy grew more distant over the years and the father saw her slipping away, he became more anxious and fearful. He lectured more, which Lacy interpreted as sermons and criticism; this only led to Lacy's growing even more distant. At this point, tears came to the father's eyes. He told the counselor that no one had been able to put into words what he had been feeling all these years. He had felt misunderstood and only wanted to get close with his daughter.

Once the father was prepared and open to suggestions, the counselor told the father than he must "fill in the softness pieces" that had been missing all these years. The father must change tactics or lose Lacy to her boyfriend; the father agreed. The counselor then gave the father the following suggestions. Since Lacy perceived the father's concern as criticism and judgment, he must avoid saying anything negative about Lacy or the boyfriend. However, this did not mean that he would condone future misbehavior or violations of the contract. The consequences would be enforced, but by the mother and not the father whenever possible. The goal was to free up the father from continuing to be seen as only a disciplinarian. The father would deal with misbehavior when necessary, but would not further damage his relationship with Lacy by giving her the traditional "deep freeze" and ignoring her for weeks on end. He would make a concerted effort to restore good feelings by looking for the smallest things to praise Lacy for each day. He would praise at least one specific action that she took each day. Finally, the father would hug her each day in private. During the hug he would tell her that he loved her. If Lacy resisted the hug, the father would still hug her. The counselor then asked the father to repeat back his understanding of what he was agreeing to do, step by step. The counselor then moved to the troubleshooting phase.

Phase 2: Troubleshooting

It is one thing to suggest a strategy and another to ensure that it is successfully implemented. As stated earlier, one of the most overlooked aspects of implementing any plan is troubleshooting. Readers will have noticed that although it is formally designated as Step 5 of the 15-step treatment plan and plays a vital role in conjunction with Step 4, troubleshooting should play a part in many other steps and strategies as well. Too often, a counselor gives a parent a specific task and is surprised when it fails; however, failure should not be surprising if no "what if" scenarios have been constructed beforehand. Nowhere is this point truer than with nurturing strategies. The reason is that both the parents and teenager have an additional layer of risk: getting hurt emotionally. Each time a parent attempts to hug the teen or to try to be soft, the parent runs a risk of getting rejected. The teenager is often afraid to risk the same rejection. For human beings, rejection can cause the deepest hurt of all. If this happens, the parent and/or the teenager may not want to try again. Both parties may also blame the counselor for making them take such a risk. The counselor must realize that he or she may be allowed only one chance, and must make the most of this opportunity by "stacking the deck" so that everyone will benefit. This is accomplished through troubleshooting, as the case of Lacy illustrates.

CLINICAL EXAMPLE (CONTINUED)

The counselor engaged in troubleshooting by first educating Lacy's father on the connection between parental control over the mood and direction of conversations and the creation of soothing sequences. The counselor warned the father that Lacy might push his buttons even when he was trying to be soft. This was because Lacy would not be familiar with this new approach, and also because she had her own agenda. Lacy wanted to be in charge and maintain her authority at all costs; to accomplish this objective, she would try to control the mood and direction of the conversation, no matter what topic was being discussed.

In addition, Lacy might fear getting too close and being rejected. If this happened, Lacy might try to push the father away first before he had the chance to hurt her. Lacy would try to make this happen by making the father agitated or angry through body language that was closed and distant, or through words that were hurtful. The father agreed that this might happen. The counselor then asked the father for suggestions of what he would do if this occurred. The father stated that he would have to realize this was happening and try not to take it personally. The father stated that he would be pressed to place the "un-" in unconditional love and show softness until Lacy knew it was for real and let her guard down. The counselor then complimented the father on his tremendous courage and commitment.

To "stack the deck" further in the father's favor, the counselor offered the following suggestion: if the father got off track, the counselor could give him the "cut sign" across his throat as a signal. The counselor would also give this same signal to his wife to use at home. The father laughed but agreed. The counselor then asked the father to go through a series of "dry runs" to practice these new skills before Lacy was asked to return.

In this case, the counselor went through a series of "what if" scenarios or events that might occur to derail the process. The counselor made the father the expert by asking him for suggestions to counter each possible contingency. In this way, the father had ownership of the plan and would be more likely to follow through with its implementation. To further ensure success, the counselor suggested a cutting motion across the throat as a visible signal to remind the father of his commitment to remain calm. Such visible signals are recommended to help a parent break old habits of communication that make soothing sequences difficult to administer. Finally, the counselor asked the father to practice a series of "dry runs" or role plays to practice these new skills.

Phase 3: Role Plays and Initial Implementation

After a nurturing strategy is selected and troubleshooting is carried out, the parents are taught how to deliver it properly through the use of role plays. As discussed earlier in this chapter, the counselor has a parent practice a particular nurturing strategy (e.g., special outings, praise, a new approach to criticism, etc.) while the counselor plays the role of the adolescent and tries to change the topic or push the parent's buttons. Once the parent is proficient in its delivery, the adolescent is brought into the room so that the parent can begin to implement the nurturing strategy.

When the adolescent is brought into the room, the counselor must often initially set the mood or tone of the discussion. This is accomplished when the counselor tries to evoke memories of the past that were soft or nurturing. From talking to the parent and adolescent individually, the counselor should have a selection of good memories to choose from. Once a tone of softness is set, it is easier for the parent to use these memories to introduce present-day nurturing strategies. If the adolescent tries to change the tone or to push the parent's buttons, the counselor must coach the parent to take charge and keep the tone of softness intact. As noted above, the counselor and parent often have a predetermined signal to remind the parent to stay on track.

If neither the parent nor the teenager has any memories of soft interactions, the counselor must get creative and ask each party a future-oriented question: What would each person be saying or doing differently if they had a better relationship? The counselor can then ask the parent to talk about these future things to set a positive tone in the room.

It is important to note that it is wise to separate parent and teenager if it looks as if they are heading for a meltdown and unable to make any progress toward nurturance. Once the parties are separated, the counselor can process what went wrong, offer solutions, and wait for a better opportunity to present itself. The counselor does not want to cause further trauma or damage to an already strained emotional bond. The counselor may have to make two or three different attempts at different times before progress can be made and negative interactions are reversed.

CLINICAL EXAMPLE (CONTINUED)

The counselor told Lacy's father that every great battle is won before the first shot is fired—that is, through careful preparation and practice beforehand. Therefore, it would be critical to go through a series of role plays or "dry runs" before Lacy's return. The counselor would play the role of Lacy, and the father could practice his delivery of each nurturing strategy. During the role play, the counselor would try every means possible to change the topic or mood of the conversation, while the father would try to hold firm by staying on track with soothing sequences of communication. If the father got off track, the counselor would use the "cut sign" across the throat. If the father still remained off track, the counselor would stop the role play and offer solutions. When the father felt confident, Lacy would be brought back into the room. The father agreed, and after several "dry runs," he stated that he was ready for Lacy.

The following is a brief transcript of the interaction between the father and Lacy. Notice how the counselor immediately set the tone of nurturance by intentionally evoking soft memories from the past. Notice also how the counselor kept the focus on the here and now, and initiated physical touch between father and daughter in order to reintroduce nurturance.

COUNSELOR: Your dad wants to talk to you. You are a teenager who is becoming a woman, and this is a weird time in your life. You need a male role model, and right now my gut tells me more than anything else you need your dad's support—not to be judgmental or put guilt trips on you, but to show love and acceptance on a day-to-day basis. You would like to be closer to your father, like it was when you were a little girl. Am I close or way off? [The counselor was evoking soft memories to set the tone and mood of discussion as soft and soothing.]

LACY: That's close.

COUNSELOR: So, Dad, I was wondering if you could talk to your daughter now and tell her how much you love her and how much you want to be there for her. Even though there have been past mistakes on both parts, you cannot change the past, only the future. There is no right or wrong way to start. There are no right or wrong words, as long as it comes from the depths of your soul. [The counselor used a spiritual reference on purpose, because the father was a devout Mormon and this fit with his belief system.] This is the daughter you love with all your heart. When you look into her eyes, Lacy knows that she is a part of you and always will be. You are her only father, and this is something in this world many daughters just don't have. [This was said intentionally to remind the father that he must be soft to offset the abusive boyfriend's influence.] Remember when Lacy sat on your lap as a little girl and you held her tight? You knew at this time that she would always be your little girl. [The counselor again evoked soft memories.] So will you talk from your heart now and tell her how you want it to be in the future? [The counselor intentionally kept the focus on here and now and on the future.]

FATHER: I will try to do what he said and show you unconditional love. This is what he asked me to do when he and I were alone. I guess the reason why I am so judgmental is that I love you too much. [The father incorporated the nurturing strategy of a new approach to criticism.] I will try to get away from the judgmental stuff and show you my love. I want to show you how much I do care, and I will try to do my best. If I can get you to sit on my lap, I would love for you to sit on my lap, like it was when you were 3 years old. I want to touch you. I want to hold you. [The father introduced the nurturing strategy of physical touch.]

COUNSELOR: Why don't you give her a hug right now? [The counselor did not miss the opportunity that the father gave him to initiate the nurturing strategy of touch right there in the office.] (*The father and Lacy hugged for the first time in years as the daughter cried.*)

In this case, the father initially agreed to soft interactions because that was what the counselor wanted him to do. Some readers may therefore conclude that the softness was not genuine. The father and daughter, however, had a long history of emotional deprivation and bitterness. The father was understandably skeptical and did not want to risk getting hurt again. With difficult adolescents, the counselor must often have to get parents to go through the motions of nurturance in a mechanical fashion before they become real and natural. The counselor may also have to warn the parents that the process will initially feel unnatural.

CLINICAL EXAMPLE (CONCLUDED)

In Lacy's case, the father was true to his word and stopped criticizing Lacy or the boyfriend; he let his wife enforce the consequences while he focused on praising Lacy on a daily basis. The father also hugged Lacy before bedtime. The father reported that this felt "weird and strange," but continued to follow through because of his trust in and rapport with the counselor. At first, Lacy was very confused by the father's actions and continued to push him away, as the counselor had predicted during the troubleshooting phase. The father was therefore prepared and kept up the soothing interactions, no matter what Lacy did or said to shake him off. Over time, Lacy began to let her father hug her without resistance, and even occasionally sat on his lap to tell him about her day. In addition, the father continued to say nothing about the boyfriend, even after Lacy said that she was thinking about a possible breakup. As the case progressed, Lacy's anger lessened and her truancy stopped. Lacy still had several relapses, but the parents were prepared, and the mother kept enforcing the consequences with the father's support. Lacy eventually left her boyfriend and started going back to school on a regular basis.

SUMMARY

In sum, a case involving a difficult adolescent like Lacy can be a success when the parents are able to balance hard and soft approaches. The counselor methodically moves from alleviating the extreme behaviors first and gaining the parents' trust to introducing the nurturing strategies that are presently deficient within the family. The counselor also helps the parents understand the connection between parental control over the mood and topic of conversation and the initiation of soothing sequences of communication. One or both parents then role-play and practice this new style of communication. The counselor acts as a coach by preparing a parent to talk to the teenager. The counselor then brings the two parties together and carefully lays the groundwork by evoking past memories of nurturance and keeping the discussion in the here and now. To increase the probability of success, the counselor troubleshoots potential problems before they occur and predicts potential negative interactions when the parent becomes more nurturing. The parent is then prepared to go the extra mile by breaking down walls of mistrust and strengthening an emotional bond. This emotional bond leads to permanent changes in behavior problems, as the teenager feels both accountable and loved at the same time. The following is a summary of the major points contained within this chapter.

1. Parents and counselors may successfully design interventions to stop the "five aces," but may fail to achieve permanent change nevertheless. Parents must be able to achieve a balance between a "hard" and a "soft" side. The hard side is maintained by the parents' ability to successfully enforce rules and consequences, neutralize the "five aces," and determine the mood and direction of confrontations. Authority, however, is also maintained by a soft, nurturing side as parents role-model empathy and nurturance with each other and their teenager. One extreme without the balance of the other can lead to serious emotional or behavioral problems.

2. When trying to restore nurturance, the counselor must carefully choose the timing for its introduction. One possible choice is to address and restore softness before behavior problems are addressed. In some cases, a teen's behavior problems are minimal, and nurturance is the only area that needs to be addressed. A second possible choice is to address and treat the hard and soft sides simultaneously. This can be done when the teen's behavior problems are first emerging or are less extreme. A third possible choice is to stop the teen's extreme behaviors first—that is, to address the hard side before proceeding to the soft side. In most cases involving difficult adolescents, this is the recommended choice for the counselor. When years of conflict and bitterness have taken their toll on the parent–child relationship, the parents feel out of control, helpless, and disempowered. Consequently, the area of nurturance cannot be addressed until the bleeding has been stopped by neutralizing the teenager's "aces" and maintaining the parents' position of authority. Only then will the parents have the necessary peace of mind and energy to bring tenderness back into the relationship.

3. Once the counselor decides on when to introduce the topic of nurturance, he or she must determine how it will be done. This is accomplished by using one or more of the following seven strategies:

- *Education and normalization.* The parents and teenager how they have reached a stage of emotional deprivation (or worse) over the years. This is done to normalize the process and reduce blame.
- *Opportunities to build trust.* Teenagers reported in focus group interviews that when they lost the opportunity to build trust, they lost hope, and resentment set in. Trust is the cornerstone of all good relationships. Parents are shown how to help their teenager regain trust while still holding the teenager accountable for future misbehavior.
- *A new approach to criticism.* Parents are shown new and better ways to criticize—ways that do not involve attacks on the teenager's personality or character, but that comment on the teen's present behavior.
- *A new approach to praise.* A teenager's self-worth is devoured by criticisms and enhanced by praise. Parents are shown a way to praise their teenager in a way that will complement the teen's behavior rather than evaluate it.
- *Acceptance of underlying feelings.* Parents are shown the direct connection between how teenagers feel and how they behave. Showing parents how to acknowledge their teenager's underlying feelings without condoning misbehavior can lead to a tremendous improvement in the relationship.
- *Physical touch.* Except in cases of intrafamilial sexual abuse, physical touch or small signs of affection are extremely important to restoring tenderness between parents and teenager. Parents are shown how to bring physical touch back into the relationship.
- *Special outings.* When a teenager or child has behavior problems, special outings stop or become contingent upon good behavior. When this happens, the relationship becomes distant and lacks a soft or tender quality. The parents and teenager are shown how to reintroduce special outings into the relationship.

4. "Soothing sequences of communication" are defined as conversations in which a parent, not the child, controls the mood, topic, and direction of the discussion. Moreover, these discussions do not contain elements of criticism or attacks on the teenager's character; instead, the parent uses one or more of the seven strategies outlined above to initiate discussions that are nurturing or soothing rather than critical, bitter, and harsh. Counselors must teach parents the connection between their control over mood and topic of discussion and the creation of soothing sequences.

5. Once the parents are proficient in controlling the topic and direction of a discussion, the counselor custom-fits particular nurturing strategies to the particular family. The parents are then able to mix and match the seven

strategies to create soothing sequences of communication and restore nurturance. Filling in the aspects of nurturance that are missing becomes the basic work of restoring the soft side of the family hierarchy. This goal is accomplished in three key phases: set-up and preparation; troubleshooting; and role plays and initial implementation. Clinical excerpts from a single case have been used to illustrate each step.

PART THREE

SPECIAL TREATMENT ISSUES AND CIRCUMSTANCES

CHAPTER 8

Working with Outsiders

"Outsiders" are defined here as people and environmental systems external to the immediate family that exert a powerful influence on the adolescent. These outsiders include (but are not limited to) peers, the juvenile justice system, foster care system, local police departments, church groups, school personnel, other mental health care providers, and probation officers. Parents may also encounter situations outside the immediate family that impede their effectiveness. Such factors include work-related stress and difficulties with extended family members. This chapter will show counselors how to take an ecosystemic approach—that is, to teach parents to work effectively and collaboratively with outside systems, and to neutralize their negative effects on both the adolescent and the immediate family.

The importance of these outside systems cannot be underestimated. (To emphasize this importance, I have made working with outsiders Step 9 of the 15-step family-based model.) As the parents lose control over the adolescent, his or her peer group begins to become more influential, acting as a substitute family unit. The counselor must help parents recognize this fact and design countermeasures to offset negative peer influences. For example, what do parents do when their teenager chronically runs away with the support of an underground network of safe houses and peers who refuse to break the code of silence? Answers to such questions must be forthcoming, or treatment will end unsuccessfully.

When a counselor sets in motion changes to parental authority, the outside environment will also react to these changes. Sometimes the reaction is positive and supportive: School personnel may begin calling the parents when the teenager is truant, or extended family members may rally in support of a single parent. Other times the reaction is negative and unsupportive: A psychiatrist may advise the parents that the counselor is wrong and residential care is needed, or a caseworker for child protective services (abbreviated in this chapter as CPS) may believe the teenager's claims of

child abuse. When teenagers feel they are losing their authority, they will often do anything to get it back, including triangulation or enlisting the support of outsiders. They may claim abuse or lie to relatives to disempower their parents; they may also enlist the support of peers or go to teachers for help.

Therefore, it is critical for the counselor to understand the environment's impact on the immediate family and on the adolescent. The counselor must be able to mediate a better fit between the family and the environment (e.g., getting the school and parents to collaborate) while simultaneously neutralizing any outside influences that might interfere with parental effectiveness (e.g., negative peer influences, unsupportive CPS caseworkers). Many family members and counselors think that outsiders will not help, so they never ask. This is a mistake. I have repeatedly found that people will help if a counselor proactively contacts these outside systems and does three things. First, a meeting must be arranged at an outsider's convenience. The counselor should be willing to meet the outsider in his or her own environment at a time that best fits the outsider's schedule. Second, the counselor should present a clear treatment plan with the outsider's role clearly specified. Third, the counselor should defer to the authority of outsiders on their own turf. For example, a counselor should first hear from teachers and guidance counselors about their points of view, before saying anything about what he or she is doing or wants to accomplish.

KNOWING THE TERRITORY

Before a counselor designs strategies to enable a family to work effectively with outsiders, he or she must first know how these environmental systems affect the family. To accomplish this goal, the counselor can use a simple visual diagram called an "eco-map," developed by Ann Hartman (1978). An eco-map is used to map out the connections between the ecological system of the family and all major outside relationships. An eco-map often has a considerable impact on family members' perception of the presenting problems. The eco-map also gives the counselor valuable information for designing interventions that take the influence of outside systems into account.

CLINICAL EXAMPLE

A single mother reported that 15-year-old Jack threatened violence whenever she attempted to discipline him. These threats of violence made her back down immediately. At this point, the mother was burned out and ready to give Jack up for

adoption. The counselor also thought that the situation was hopeless, because the mother seemed to be without any support. However, after an eco-map was diagramed, both the mother's and the counselor's points of view quickly changed. They saw that the mother had strong connections with members of her church, as well as with her sister and brother-in-law. If the mother's extended family and church group could be activated to support her, the threats of violence might stop. The counselor held a joint meeting with the mother and the outsiders, during which a plan was written to determine who would be involved to support the mother and how. After her sister's husband and two male pastors made several visits to her house, the mother only had to warn Jack that she would call these people and his threats of violence stopped immediately.

An extended case example illustrates in more detail how a typical eco-map is used to work with outside systems.

CLINICAL EXAMPLE

A single father was ordered to seek counseling because his 13-year-old son Derrick was on probation for ditching school and spray-painting graffiti on a grocery store. Since the father worked all day, Derrick would stay at home and watch television or invite his friends over. The father's relationship with the school was strained, because he felt that the teacher and principal blamed him for Derrick's truancy and poor grades. Derrick's younger brother, 9-year-old John, did not attend the session.

As the father and Derrick spoke, the counselor asked for permission to summarize the information by drawing it on a map. Derrick and the father agreed. Below is a partial transcript of what took place:

COUNSELOR: First let me draw a circle that represents your household on the chalkboard. Now I need to know everyone who is currently living inside your house. [A counselor who does not have access to a chalkboard can draw an eco-map on a piece of paper.]

DERRICK: Well, just my dad, John, me, and sometimes my dad's girlfriend. But she is only over two times a week. My friends also come and go as they please, so they kinda live there too. [The son was already describing a boundary around the household that was too open.]

COUNSELOR: Even though these other people come over a lot, we should just put people who live permanently in your house inside the circle. We will then put the other people in your lives outside this main circle. Also, please give me everyone's ages. Let me draw this, and then tell me if I'm close or way off. [The first part of the eco-map was then drawn (see Figure 8.1). Inside the inner circle of any eco-map, squares are used to depict males and circles to depict females. The age of each person is put in the middle of the circle or square, and then the family is drawn in the form of a fam-

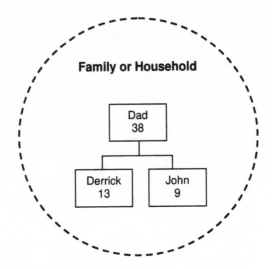

FIGURE 8.1. The basic structure of Derrick's immediate family.

ily tree to indicate relationships. Parents are placed at the top to indicate hierarchy.]

FATHER: That looks good so far.

COUNSELOR: Now let's visually see how you guys get along. Overall, how would you rate your relationship? Is it stressful or without stress most of the time? Is your current relationship emotionally distant or close? [The counselor asked these questions to get a picture of the relationships between the members of this family.]

FATHER: Very stressful, because we argue all the time, and because of this we are very distant. John and I get along fine. We are close, and he does not give me trouble. John and Derrick are always fighting, and they are distant.

COUNSELOR: OK. I will put wavy lines and arrows back and forth to show that there is a lot of stress and energy between you and Derrick and between Derrick and John. I will put double lines between Dad and John to show no stress and closeness. I will put broken lines between Dad and Derrick to show emotional distance. [The counselor then added these lines and symbols to the drawing (see Figure 8.2). In one picture, the family members could now see the quality of their relationships with one another, as well as the problem areas. A key was added to show what the lines and symbols meant. The genogram of Derrick's immediate family was now complete.]

COUNSELOR: Now I want to talk about all the people outside your household who give you stress or support. I am going to start off by putting down the outsiders you already told me about. Derrick, for you I will draw circles around your friends, your school, and your probation officer. Any others?

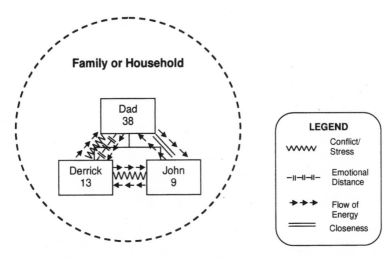

FIGURE 8.2. The complete genogram of Derrick's immediate family.

DERRICK: Yeah, put down my girlfriend, Nadine.

COUNSELOR: OK. I will add a circle that represents Nadine. Derrick, it seems that your friends are like a second family to you. Could you tell me their first and last names and their ages, so that I can draw them like I did with your household? I also want to put wavy lines between you and your friends to show any conflict and stress, or double lines to show closeness. I will also put broken lines between you and your friends to show any distance. Arrows will show a lot of energy going back and forth between you and your friends. I also want to know who the leaders are in your group.

The map of Derrick's close friends and the nature of their relationships (see the bottom left portion of Figure 8.3) was a derivative of a genogram. Like a genogram, it contained ages, lines, and symbols to indicate closeness, distance, or areas of conflict. The only difference was that the people represented were not immediate family members, but Derrick's "second family" or peer group. This map within an eco-map contained essential information that the counselor could later use to design interventions with the peer group.

The full map of Derrick's relationships outside the household (see Figure 8.3) revealed that Derrick had two friends outside his inner group who did well in school but were not close to him. This was because David, the leader of the inner group, did not like "eggheads." David was also 17 years old, 4 years Derrick's senior; this significant age difference might be contributing to Derrick's misbehavior. In addition, the map revealed a common theme of close friends who were also truant and got poor grades. The map therefore suggested that one possible intervention might be to strengthen the positive peer influences and to weaken the hold of the other friends. The counselor asked for and got the last names of

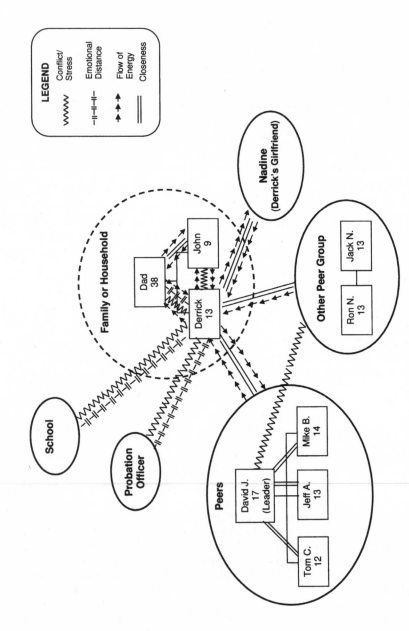

FIGURE 8.3. The family genogram combined with a map of Derrick's relationships outside the family.

each friend and how close they lived to Derrick. This was specifically done to make it easier for the counselor and father to track down these peers and their parents at a later time if necessary. Teenagers adhere to a "code of silence" and will rarely volunteer this type of information. However, they are often willing to provide it when it is drawn on a map with symbols and graphics. A counselor must gain intimate access to this territory of peers in any way possible, or run the risk of being defeated by them.

Derrick described his overall relationships with his inner peer group and his girlfriend, Nadine, as "very strong" and with no conflict. The counselor drew two lines to indicate these relationships and arrows to signify a strong flow of energy in both directions. Derrick described his relationships with the school and probation officer as distant and full of conflict. The counselor drew the appropriate symbols to indicate this.

The counselor then went on to the father's relationships outside the family:

COUNSELOR: Dad, I see your outsiders as the school and the probation officer. However, they also include your work, your girlfriend, and the court. Any others?

FATHER: Yes, my mother and father are my buddies, as well as my boss at work.

The counselor then asked the same questions as those he asked in regard to the household circle and to Derrick and his outside systems. The counselor drew lines between these outside environmental systems and the father. The father described his relationships with the school, the probation system, and the court as very stressful, unsupportive, and distant. On the map (see Figure 8.4), the counselor drew the appropriate symbols to indicate stress and lack of support. The father also stated that he put a lot of time and energy into getting these outsiders to help him, but that they gave him almost no support. To indicate these relationships, the counselor drew arrows from the father to these systems, but no arrows from these systems to the father. The father had very supportive relationships at work and with his extended family. The counselor drew two lines to indicate these supportive relationships. Arrows were drawn between the father and both these systems to show a balanced flow of energy and support. (Since Derrick's brother was so young and did not have many outside relationships, a map of his relationships was not drawn. However, if he had had significant outside relationships, these would have been included.)

After the eco-map was completed (see Figure 8.4), Derrick and the father were asked whether anything stood out. The counselor asked the family this question before offering an opinion, so as not to influence the family members' answers. After looking at the map, the father stated that he had not realized how much conflict he had with both his son and the school system. The father also had not been aware of the strong influence of Derrick's friends, or of how much support he had from both his parents and friends at work. Derrick reported that he saw that his only supports were his girlfriend and his peers.

The counselor used the eco-map to formulate the following treatment plan:

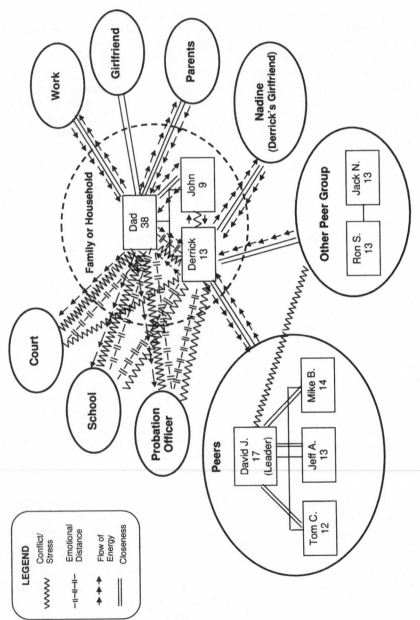

FIGURE 8.4. The completed eco-map.

1. The counselor told the father, without Derrick present, that the map showed that the father was not using the potential support of his friends at work or his parents. Instead, the father was trying to stop Derrick's behaviors all by himself. The counselor then received permission from the father to call his parents and his boss and invite them to attend a meeting with the father. The father was surprised that his boss and parents were so receptive to helping. All parties were told that each time Derrick refused to go to school or was truant, the father would bring Derrick with him to the warehouse where he worked. Derrick would then have to sit on a hard wooden pallet in the warehouse every day until he went to school and attended all his classes. The father's boss was very supportive of this plan, and even volunteered to come to the house and drag Derrick to work if he refused to go. This plan worked beautifully and empowered the father to take charge. Derrick began going to school consistently because he would rather go to school than sit on a hard pallet all day.

2. The eco-map indicated that the relationship between the school system and the father was distant and strained. The counselor set up a meeting with the school and the father to open up these lines of communication. Derrick's grandfather, who was greatly encouraged by the earlier meeting, also attended to support his son. This support inspired the father to go to the school meeting with the goal of establishing a cooperative network. He gave each teacher a typed letter outlining the treatment plan, which included a form to record daily school performance, and the father's pager number along with the request to be contacted immediately if Derrick did not show up for class. The teachers stated that they were impressed by the father's initiative and by the grandfather's support. They were excited about the treatment plan and agreed to its terms. Within this framework of cooperation and accountability, Derrick's classroom behavior and truancy started to improve.

3. The counselor observed from the eco-map that the father had conflicts with the probation department. To smooth this out, the counselor called the probation officer and outlined the treatment plan. He also gave the officer concrete examples of how the father was taking charge and being successful without becoming abusive. The probation officer was impressed by this change of events and agreed to work more cooperatively with the father. This promise was fulfilled later, when Derrick ran away and the officer supported the father by calling the police to help locate the boy.

4. In reaction to tougher sanctions, Derrick ran away to a friend's house. The counselor and father than used the "genogram" of Derrick's friends to track down where Derrick was staying. Since the grandfather was retired, he had the time to harass the parents of Derrick's friend until they refused to let Derrick stay any longer. Once his safe houses were eliminated, Derrick stopped running away.

5. Finally, it was clear from the eco-map that the father's relationship with Derrick was strained and lacked emotional closeness. The father had stated, "It is now clear why Derrick hangs out with his friends so much. We have no relationship." The counselor showed the father ways to rebuild positive feelings, and told the father that restoring nurturance would help break the stronghold of Derrick's "second family." Derrick was also required to spend time with the two friends who were academically proficient. This allowed Derrick to save face with his oth-

er friends, because he could tell them that he had to spend time with these people or be grounded. Over time, Derrick grew closer to these two friends and established a better relationship with his father. Both of these changes helped break the hold of Derrick's negative peer influences. Derrick's 17-year-old friend, David, lost interest in Derrick when he could no longer hang out at Derrick's house during school hours. This also helped Derrick stay in school.

In sum, the eco-map gave the father and counselor a visual picture of the family's connection with outsiders, and showed the counselor where to intervene. In the father's case, a dormant support system of relatives and coworkers needed to be activated, and a more cooperative relationship with the teachers and the probation officer needed to be established. The father became empowered with this new set of support systems and was able to take charge in stopping Derrick's extreme behavior. Without an eco-map, the counselor might have gotten lost within the multitude of problems. In addition, the counselor might have been unable to see the hidden resources already available to the father.

STRATEGIES FOR WORKING EFFECTIVELY WITH OUTSIDE SYSTEMS

Once the counselor has a knowledge of the family's environment, he or she must know how to intervene effectively with outside systems. Such interventions center around two areas: collaboration and neutralization. The decision of whether to collaborate or neutralize is based on the feedback received from these outside systems. For example, if outside mental health professionals attempt to undermine the treatment plan, they must be neutralized. Whenever possible, however, the counselor should mediate between the family and its environment to achieve cooperation in solving the adolescent's problem.

This section gives counselors strategies for working with outside systems to increase collaboration. Also covered are how and when to neutralize an outside influence. The following outside systems have been identified as the most important:

1. *CPS workers and police officers.* CPS workers and police officers can either make or break parental authority. Counselors thus need to know how to enable CPS or the police to empower rather than disempower parents. Disempowerment can happen when teenagers falsely accuse parents of abuse, or when they threaten or commit violent acts.

2. *Church, friends, and extended family.* Parents may not see the resources and support available to them through their religious affiliations,

friends, and relatives. This is especially true for single parents who are trying to deal with severe behavior problems alone.

3. *Other counselors, psychiatrists, or probation officers.* These outside forces can intentionally or unintentionally undermine a counselor's credibility. If this happens, parents are placed in the middle and forced to choose between treatment philosophies. In contrast, these same outside forces can also collaborate with the counselor to support parents.

4. *Peers—the adolescent's "second family."* Economic pressures, more sophisticated technology, greater mobility, and higher divorce rates have all weakened the influence of the nuclear family. As a result, the peer group exerts a greater effect on a teenager than ever before.

5. *The school system.* As stated earlier in this book, behavior problems that occur at home often occur within the school environment as well. When this happens, teachers and parents must work together to solve the teenager's behavioral problems.

Strategy 1: Working with Child Protective Services and the Police

As stated above, CPS caseworkers and police officers can be very instrumental in either the empowerment or disempowerment of parents. A teenager trying to regain control may falsely accuse his or her parents of abuse and contact the police or CPS (or have someone else do so), in the hopes that this will cause the parents to stop disciplining. Another possibility is that the teenager will commit acts of violence on people or property. The police will either support the parents by booking the teenager for assault and battery, or disempower the parents by doing nothing. These two scenarios require slightly different approaches on the counselor's part.

The Teenager or Another Person Reports Abuse

When a teenager or another person reports abuse, the counselor must act quickly. By law, a CPS worker must investigate any report of abuse. Often the particular caseworker's training, experience, and treatment philosophy will determine whether he or she supports or tries to destroy the parents' authority. Fortunately, many CPS workers now seem to understand that some teenagers will intentionally use the system to disempower their parents. It has been my experience that more and more CPS workers are willing to look at this issue before charging parents with abuse. CPS workers are trying to do what is right. They have seen some awful things and do not want to put either children or parents at risk. If a counselor takes the first step of trying to collaborate, a CPS worker will often respond accordingly.

To make this happen, a counselor *must* be proactive and contact a CPS worker or the police department on the parents' behalf. If the counselor thinks that the teenager will contact CPS, the counselor should notify the caseworker ahead of time of this possibility. A letter explaining the rationale for the procedures that will be implemented should be hand-delivered or faxed to the worker, together with a description of the intervention.

To facilitate future cooperation, the counselor should educate CPS and the police department in his or her area with a free seminar on these issues. To gain their full support, the counselor must demonstrate that the interventions of the 15-step treatment model involve no physical or mental abuse. When this fact is made clear, the CPS worker or police officer often becomes an advocate for the parents and counselor. Otherwise, problems can occur. For instance, one counselor described the bathroom strategy during a seminar. He then had a mother use the strategy the next week, but did so under the faulty assumption that the parent would never leave the child unattended. The mother, however, locked the child in the bathroom for unspecified amounts of time and left the house to go shopping. When this was reported, the CPS worker cited both the counselor and the parent for abusive behavior. This clearly illustrates what can happen if any strategy or procedure is implemented carelessly and improperly.

In sum, when abuse is reported, the counselor should first speak with the parents and the adolescent to find out what happened. If the counselor determines that no abuse occurred, he or she should advocate for the parents and immediately contact the CPS worker. Again, a letter and a description of the set of procedures used should be faxed or hand-delivered to the caseworker or the police officer. If the caseworker wants to meet with the parents before speaking with the counselor, the counselor should send a letter with the parents. After this meeting, the counselor should request a meeting with the caseworker (in writing, if necessary). Any problems existing after this meeting should be addressed by the counselor with the caseworker's supervisor.

CLINICAL EXAMPLE

Alex, a 14-year-old boy, came to treatment because of leaving his home without permission. After all other procedures had failed, the counselor implemented the bathroom strategy. It proved successful in stopping Alex from running away. Then the father had a heart attack, and the family members turned their attention to the father and often left Alex unsupervised. When this happened, Alex stayed out all night with friends. With the father in the hospital, the mother could not enforce the bathroom strategy. When the father finally returned home, the bathroom strategy lost its intended impact. Alex would either spend his 6 hours in the bathroom, or knock down the door with his shoulder and then leave the house for days at a time.

The parents were now reaching a state of hopelessness, so the counselor had to think quickly. The parents agreed to meet with the counselor one last time, because he was the only one who had had any degree of success with Alex. In collaboration with the parents, the bathroom strategy was modified in the following manner. The next time Alex ran away, he would be placed in the bathroom for 2 full days. The father was healthy again and had retired, so he could be home the entire time. The father also agreed to sleep on the couch next to the bathroom. Each time Alex ran away afterwards, the confinement would be increased by 1 day. He would get three square meals in the bathroom, but they would consist of foods he did not like. In addition, the father would replace the existing door with a metal one, so that Alex could not break down the door.

The next day, Alex told the parents of a friend that he would be locked in the bathroom for 6 days. Not knowing the truth, his friend's mother called CPS and reported abuse. However, the counselor had discussed this possibility with the parents beforehand. Because of this preparation, the parents were not upset, but calmly called the counselor and told him that they had a mandatory meeting with the CPS worker the next day. The counselor faxed the letter shown in Figure 8.5 to the parents to give to the caseworker (note, incidentally, that this sample letter can be given to parents as a handout, to show them what such a communication should include). In the letter, the counselor clearly stated the purpose of the bathroom strategy, the concept of triangulation, and future implications if the CPS worker did not support the parents. Together with the letter, he provided a copy of the handout describing the bathroom strategy itself (see Chapter 6, Figure 6.1). Within this framework, the CPS worker empowered the parents by telling Alex that she supported them. The worker also notified the other CPS workers in the office, in case others tried to claim abuse on Alex's behalf. Now that Alex's last-ditch effort had failed, he stopped running away. Once this behavior stopped, the counselor began work to bring nurturance back into the parent–teen relationship, using the procedures outlined in Chapter 7.

The Teenager Commits Acts of Violence or Property Damage

When the teenager commits an act of violence against another person or damages property, the parents frequently call the police. The police, however, may disempower the parents by choosing not to charge the adolescent. It often depends on the particular police officer, his or her philosophy, and even the particular neighborhood. If nothing happens, the teenager may begin to feel omnipotent and unstoppable. The teenager will then continue to use violence as a weapon against his parents' authority. The counselor basically has two choices when it comes to violence or destruction of property:

1. The counselor can convince the parents to take care of consequences "in-house" rather than contact the police. The rationale given is that the police may not do anything and may only make matters worse. The parents and counselor must determine ahead of time which behaviors can be handled in-

November 12, 1997

Ms. Johnson
Child Protective Services (CPS)
Address
City, State, Zip

Ms. Johnson:

My name is Dr. Scott Sells, and I am a marriage and family counselor who has been working with Alex Jones and his family for 5 months. I received a call that CPS had been contacted in Alex's case.

For the last 5 months, I have been treating Alex for symptoms that meet criteria for the DSM-IV diagnosis 312.8 (conduct disorder, adolescent-onset type, moderate). This is indicated by a persistent and recurrent pattern of behavior that violates social norms or the rights of other people. In Alex's case, he has threatened, bullied, or intimidated others; he has intentionally destroyed property; he frequently lies to avoid duties or to obtain favors or desired objects; he frequently stays out at night despite his parents' forbidding him to do so; and he has run away from home overnight several times.

In such a case, a teenager will sometimes call the police and/or CPS, or get another parent or peer to call and claim abuse, when there is no evidence of abuse. The teenager does this simply to create a crisis. Before treatment, Alex had complete power and authority over his parents. He did not go to school and ran away whenever he did not like the rules. With treatment, the parents were able to retain the power and authority needed to stop Alex's destructive behavior. However, teenagers like Alex want their authority and power back because of the freedom they once had and enjoyed. As a result, they will do everything they can to wrestle this power and authority away from the parents. One of these common methods is to get someone to falsely claim abuse. They do this because they know that the parents may be afraid of the authorities, regardless of their guilt or innocence. If this happens, the parents will be disempowered and back off from taking charge. The teenagers are then free to regain their lost authority and begin the self-destructive cycle all over again.

Therefore, if any changes are made in this case, this will not only neutralize the parents' authority, but send a powerful message to Alex that getting someone to accuse his parents of abuse works. He will then use his "ace in the hole" of running away again and again.

In sum, the parents were following my treatment procedures to the letter and are using the bathroom strategy only as a last resort. The treatment is working, and because it is, Alex has gotten a friend or parent to call CPS in a desperate attempt to disempower his parents. I have worked closely with child protective officers J. B., S. H., and P. I. on many such cases. They are in your office, and they will personally vouch for the effectiveness of this strategy and attest that it is not abusive if used properly. A parent has been with Alex at all times, and he gets three meals a day. There is no physical abuse. Enclosed is a handout describing the bathroom strategy, which has been signed by officer J. B. to indicate that the strategy has been cleared by CPS. If there are any concerns or questions, please call me on my pager at 1-800-705-2650. Thank you.

Sincerely,

Scott P. Sells, PhD
Clinical Director

FIGURE 8.5. Parent handout: Example of a letter from a counselor to a CPS caseworker. From *Treating the Tough Adolescent* by Scott P. Sells. Copyright 1998 by The Guilford Press. Permission to photocopy this handout is granted to purchasers of *Treating the Tough Adolescent* for personal use only (see copyright page for details).

house and which behaviors require immediate phone calls to the police. As stated in Chapter 6, destruction of property carries with it in-house consequences of financial restitution, while physical violence carries with it the possibility of takedown procedures and time out. The implementation of in-house consequences should be determined on a case-by-case basis. For example, a single mother with a physically large teenager and with no support systems would not be a good candidate for in-house consequences, but a two-parent family with a smaller teen and with support systems would be.

2. Parents are encouraged to call the police when they have no support or are defenseless against a violent teenager. If a police officer states that the problem is out of his or her jurisdiction, the parents should ask to speak to the staff sergeant on duty. When parents still get no response, they should ask to speak to the police chief or even threaten to notify the press if no action is taken. If the police officer tries to arrest or blame a parent, the counselor should be called as quickly as possible to advocate for that parent. Often the police fail to cite the teenager for assault or battery. In this case, the counselor should be called so that he or she can speak with the officer and advocate for the parent. The police may issue a citation, but because of the backlog of repeat offenders, nothing may happen except a "slap on the wrist." The counselors must prepare parents for this possibility, while keeping in mind that if the teenager continues to engage in this behavior, a history of citations will lead to harsher consequences in the future.

CLINICAL EXAMPLE

Fifteen-year-old Leo would consistently threaten violence to get his mother and stepfather off his back. With the counselor's assistance, his parents learned how to stop Leo by exiting and waiting, and placing him in his bedroom if he continued to follow them around the house. Leo did not like this turn of events and proceeded to kick a number of large holes in his bedroom wall.

The counselor had mentioned this possibility to the parents beforehand, so they were prepared. However, when the parents called the police, the officer said that destruction of property within the home was out of her jurisdiction. The mother than asked to speak to the desk sergeant. She told him that she would continue up the chain of command until a police officer was sent and charges filed. The desk sergeant conceded and a police officer was sent over to make a report. Since this was Leo's first offense, he received only minor punishment.

However, the intervention still had the desired effect on two levels. First, Leo knew that his parents were serious and would not hesitate to call the police if he committed future acts of violence. The probation officer strengthened this perception by informing Leo that subsequent violations would lead to more serious consequences. On a second level, Leo was held accountable for his actions by having to repair the hole in the wall himself.

Strategy 2: Involving Church, Friends, or Extended Family

Initially, parents are often unaware of the support that can be obtained from such outside systems as their church, friends, and extended family. (Note that for my purposes in this chapter, the term "church" refers to any religious organization or group—a synagogue, a mosque, a temple, etc.) An eco-map can illustrate this point clearly. Once parents see lines of conflict between themselves and so many outsiders, they begin to realize the connection between their stress level and their lack of support systems. The counselor can then explain what is involved in activating these dormant support systems.

First, the counselor asks for permission to personally contact the parents' potential outside support systems. More often than not, the counselor will be more successful than the parents in obtaining the outsiders' commitment to support the parents' initiatives. Parents may state that they have already tried and failed. The reason often given is that these potential support systems are too busy or would not like to be bothered. The counselor must counter these objections and convince the parents to try. To ease the parents' anxiety, the counselor states exactly what he or she will tell an outsider over the phone. The counselor will ask the outsider to meet with the parents to support them in solving a behavior problem. It is not a counseling session, but rather a consultation meeting to outline tactics and the roles everyone will play to help the parents solve a specific problem (truancy, violence, running away, etc.). The counselor will tell the outsider that the parents have identified him or her as a likely source of support who can be trusted. If an outsider asks about the kind of commitment required, the counselor states that this will be decided upon at the meeting. If the outsider is still not convinced, the counselor will ask for a commitment of only one meeting, so that the person can see for himself or herself. The counselor will even agree to meet with the outsider at the place and time most convenient for him or her. If distance is a problem, the counselor offers to bring the outsider into the meeting with the use of a speakerphone.

Within this framework, most parents will agree to let the counselor try. When the parents supply the counselor with the names and phone numbers of outsiders, they should also sign an agreement authorizing the release of information. If parents are still unwilling or skeptical, the counselor can give examples of other cases in which everyone was surprised at the willingness of outsiders to help, and in which this help turned the problem around. If all else fails, the counselor should bring up the subject again after trust and rapport have developed further, or after the counselor has been able to bring about small changes in the problem.

At the meeting, the counselor begins by clearly stating the purpose of the gathering: to support the parents in their efforts to regain and retain their authority with the teenager. The counselor then explains the rules and consequences that have been set up for the teenager, and clarifies the specific role each outsider can play in the process. Finally, the counselor prepares the outsiders for the probability of relapses or other problems by detailing exactly how the outsiders should handle those situations. Outsiders who are initially resistant often become energized when the intervention and their roles are clearly defined. For instance, the next-door neighbor of a single mother stated that it was not his place to interfere, and he only agreed to come to the first meeting. However, at the meeting the neighbor became active when the mother stated that his ideas were fantastic and that she would incorporate them directly into the contract. In addition, when the neighbor saw that his role was to be physically present but not to intervene directly, he changed his point of view and volunteered to come to future sessions. It is important to note that the teenager should not be present at these meetings. Only after the details have been worked through should the teenager attend.

After the meeting, the counselor engages in follow-up and works through any unanticipated glitches. Outsiders are not asked to come to every meeting, but only to help set up the plan and return if there are problems in its implementation. The counselor should be available 24 hours a day, 7 days a week until the parents get back in control of the household and the roles of the outsiders are smoothly integrated. Home visits may even be necessary.

CLINICAL EXAMPLE

A youth minister agreed to wear a beeper so that a single mother could call him if her 12-year-old son, Mark, refused to go to school. When the mother found it necessary to call, the youth minister did not return the page. Fortunately, the counselor was available as backup and quickly went to the home in place of the minister so that Mark would go to school. Later, the counselor contacted the minister and found that he had forgotten his beeper. After the minister was persuaded to always carry his pager, the intervention progressed more easily.

A longer case example demonstrates how extended family members can prove helpful even when a parent initially has doubts about this.

CLINICAL EXAMPLE

Keith was a 15-year-old boy who was referred to counseling for violence at school and truancy. The mother was a single parent who lived in the inner city and had an infant in addition to Keith. Looking at the eco-map, both the mother and the counselor realized that Keith's aunt, uncle, and grandmother were untapped resources.

The counselor asked for permission to contact these extended family members. The mother initially objected, stating that Keith's aunt and uncle had problems of their own and that his grandmother suffered from high blood pressure and stress. The counselor then tried to convince the mother to involve these outsiders, and promised that if the first meeting was not successful, he would refrain from contacting them further for a while. The counselor then proceeded to go over what he would say on the phone. The mother was still skeptical but willing to try. When the counselor called the extended family members, he found that all were willing to come; in fact, they wondered why they had never been asked before. A meeting was set for the next week.

During the meeting, hidden family dynamics emerged. The aunt and grandmother stated that Keith's mother babied him and was not tough enough. The mother agreed, but stated that she was all alone. At this point, the counselor expanded on the theme of feeling isolated; he then clarified how each family member could support the mother in specific ways. This would empower the mother to get tough when she needed to be, but would allow her to continue the nurturing relationship with Keith as well.

The uncle volunteered to go to school with the mother if Keith was truant or became violent with a classmate. Keith was very invested in looking good in front of his peers and would not want his mother and uncle sitting next to him during each class. The aunt agreed to accompany the mother to inform the school of this plan and help enlist their support. Finally, if Keith refused to do his homework and the mother was too tired to argue, the uncle, aunt, or grandmother would come over and make Keith sit at the kitchen table until he finished his homework. With this plan, the mother had the backup she needed to stop these behaviors. The family members liked their roles, and within 2 months Keith's problems ended.

Strategy 3: Collaborating with Other Counselors, Psychiatrists, and Probation Officers

Often the most difficult challenge facing the counselor is not the family being treated, but the conflicting messages the family members receive from other mental health care providers. (I discuss probation officers along with mental health care providers in this section, because probation officers often serve as *de facto* counselors for families with difficult adolescents.) For the same problem, a client may receive a different treatment approach from every professional he or she consults. For example, a violent teenager may be treated with medication from a psychiatrist, "boot camp" tactics from a probation officer, and/or family intervention from a marriage and family counselor. The treatment process can look more chaotic than the adolescent being treated.

The family is then caught in the middle and forced to choose among different approaches. When this happens, the counselor must take charge and either collaborate with these outside forces or neutralize their influence. When possible, it is wise to try collaboration before proceeding to neutralization, since there is strength in numbers. With a difficult adolescent, the counselor and parents can use all the help they can get.

Techniques for Collaborating with Outside Professionals

The counselor will be able to enlist the help of outside professionals by means of the following five primary methods:

1. The counselor finds out who the key professionals are through an eco-map and initiates contact with them immediately. This is done to lessen the possibility that these professionals will undermine the counselor's treatment plan. It is important for the counselor to explain the treatment plan to these outside professionals before the parents do. Otherwise, the parents will give their "spin" on the plan, and without the entire picture, the other professionals may tell the parents that they disagree with the plan. The counselor's expert status is then placed in question, and treatment can fail.

2. The counselor takes a one-down position, checks his or her ego at the door, and meets each of the other professionals on the other's turf. This can keep the other off the defensive and increase the probability of success. When the treatment approach is explained, a resistant professional may suddenly become cooperative. The counselor states that he or she needs the help of all the other professionals involved to change the teenager's behavior. This attitude will prove more productive than an attitude of "This is what you need to do." The counselor may be saying the same thing, but *how* the message is delivered can make all the difference in the world. In addition, during initial contacts, the counselor should ask the other professionals for their opinions about the case before giving his or her own. This too is done out of respect and in the spirit of collaboration.

3. As with other outside forces, the roles of each professional must be defined in detail. The counselor and the other professionals must also clarify what each of them will tell the parents. Deciding who is going to say what and when is critical to treatment success. If a family member states that another professional has recommended a particular course of action, the counselor should tell the family member that it is standard policy to check with that other person. This limits the parents' or teenager's ability to triangulate or play one professional off another. A teenager or parent may intentionally try to "divide and conquer" by saying that other professionals have said that the counselor is incompetent or doing a poor job. If this happens, the counselor must not overreact, but should simply touch base with the other professionals. Open communication can put an immediate stop to such tactics.

4. Treatment philosophies must be agreed upon or integrated. For instance, a counselor and a psychiatrist must agree on a systems theory framework that involves the parents taking charge. If this does not happen, the

family may get confused and choose the path of least resistance, or the one calling for the least parental involvement. For example, parents were asked by one counselor to take charge in getting their son to stay in school. When they began to do this, their marital tension increased, so they looked for an alternative. When another counselor told them that this was the wrong approach and that the son needed residential care, they were more than willing to switch rather than continue in their state of anxiety.

5. Leverage from outside professionals must be utilized whenever possible. Depending on the nature of the offense, the court system and probation officers can have a significant impact.

CLINICAL EXAMPLE

In the case of 15-year-old Daniel, who refused to come to treatment, the counselor simply picked up the phone and spoke with his probation officer. Since the probation officer and the counselor had a very collaborative relationship, the probation officer immediately called Daniel and told him that he had no option but to continue with counseling. If Daniel still refused, the officer would recommend additional community service and more mandatory probation meetings. Daniel returned to counseling the next week.

A more detailed example illustrates how a counselor was able to use the leverage of a psychiatrist to achieve treatment aims.

CLINICAL EXAMPLE

Twelve-year-old Rosa was diagnosed by a psychiatrist as having attention-deficit/hyperactivity disorder (ADHD). She was placed on Ritalin, but continued to exhibit behavioral problems in school and poor grade performance. After careful analysis, the counselor wanted to try a different approach. This involved Rosa's being weaned off Ritalin and the parents attending school with Rosa if she did not comply with her teacher's requests after two warnings.

The counselor had a thorough knowledge of this family's eco-map and noted that the parents had complete trust in the psychiatrist. Therefore, the counselor realized that he needed the blessing of the psychiatrist before the parents would agree to a change in treatment. With this in mind, the counselor scheduled a meeting with the psychiatrist before sharing his proposed change in treatment with the family.

During this meeting, the counselor took a one-down position and told the psychiatrist that he *needed* his help and support. The counselor said that it was not his position to agree or disagree with the diagnosis of ADHD. However, since Rosa was still having behavior problems and poor grades, the counselor wanted to propose a change in tactics as an experiment. If the plan did not work, they would go back to the original plan. The counselor then proceeded to outline his treatment plan and, in the spirit of collaboration, asked for suggestions. The psychiatrist liked the plan and the fact that it required an increase in parental involvement. However, he cautioned that the parents were firmly entrenched within the theoretical framework that Rosa's ADHD was primarily biological. Consequently, he thought that the parents might balk at the idea of weaning Rosa off Ritalin. As an alternative, the psychiatrist suggested that he tell the parents he would continue Ritalin only if the parents gave the counselor's plan 100% effort. This would give the counselor the added leverage he might need to get the parents motivated.

The counselor thanked the psychiatrist for his input and incorporated his suggestions into the treatment plan. The two professionals then decided who would say what and when to the parents. It was agreed that the counselor would initiate the plan with the parents and tell them that the psychiatrist was in full agreement. The counselor would then have the parents call the psychiatrist the next day to explain how continuing Ritalin would be contingent upon their 100% effort. The psychiatrist would then become the "bad guy," leaving the counselor neutral and his rapport with the parents intact. In addition, there was an explicit agreement between the counselor and the psychiatrist that if the family tried to triangulate them, each would call the other to confirm or deny what was supposedly said about the other.

This case was successful because the counselor knew the eco-map territory of this family and the influences of outside professionals beforehand. He considered the possible reverberations of his treatment plan across these outside systems, and had the foresight to collaborate and seek the necessary agreement. This proactive stance diminished the possibility that his plan would be undermined. The counselor also integrated the psychiatrist's ideas directly into the treatment plan, and the two professionals clarified their roles in order to present a unified front.

Techniques for Neutralizing Outside Professionals

The counselor will be able to neutralize the effects of outside professionals when necessary by means of the following five methods:

1. If the parents are caught in the middle between professionals with different philosophies, the counselor should openly acknowledge their dilemma. The field of mental health is very confusing, and professionals have many different treatment approaches. Ultimately, the decision should come down to the effectiveness of the counselor's treatment approach as opposed to that of the other professional. After a reasonable period of time, the parents should ask themselves the following question: "Is the teenager doing noticeably better since beginning the present treatment?" The rule of thumb is that if improvement is not perceived in 1 month's time, a different approach should be tried. The counselor can also ask the parents: "If the approach you

are currently using is not working, do you think we should try something different?" In this way, the counselor does not take a defensive stance, but raises the appropriate questions to help the parents draw their own conclusions.

2. Parents are informed that they cannot commit themselves to following conflicting treatment approaches simultaneously and expect to achieve a positive outcome. One treatment may work, but it cannot be successful if it is in conflict with another. The counselor must take a stand and ask the parents to choose one approach or the other. If the parents choose the other approach, the counselor should not take it personally. Instead, he or she should tell the parents that the door is always open if they are not satisfied with their results in the future. The counselor should even ask permission to call in a month to check in. This will allow the parents to save face in case the other treatment approach fails.

3. The counselor points out actual moments of success that have been achieved with his or her treatment approach. Even though parents may have achieved some of their desired outcomes, they will often focus on the negative or on what they failed to accomplish. The counselor must gently point out specific elements of the treatment approach that have led to positive change, with concrete examples to make this connection. If relevant, the counselor also reminds the parents how other treatment plans and professionals have failed to stop the behavioral problem. This helps the parents look at the bigger picture and make an informed decision based on concrete evidence rather than misperceptions.

CLINICAL EXAMPLE

Eighteen-year-old Kim was referred to counseling for anorexia nervosa. During the course of treatment, the counselor was able to convince the parents to stay at the table until Kim had eaten a complete meal three times a day. When this happened, Kim's menstrual cycle returned for the first time in 2 years, and an analysis of her diary revealed a 70% decrease in her preoccupation with food.

Nevertheless, Kim was in a fragile state and just beginning to solidify these new changes. The counselor recommended that Kim attend a local college rather than an out-of-state school. Both Kim and her parents disliked this suggestion and felt that Kim was strong enough to return to school. The counselor knew that arguing would be futile and predicted that Kim would relapse in the first semester. The counselor persuaded Kim and her parents to sign a contract pledging that Kim would return home if her weight dropped by 10 pounds. The student counseling center would monitor her weight on a weekly basis and report the results directly to the parents.

As the counselor predicted, Kim did relapse. However, the school counselor got involved and told the parents that anorexia nervosa was a disease. She also told the parents that the original counselor did not know what he was talking about, and that, as a disease, anorexia nervosa needed to be treated in a hospital under the care of a psychiatrist. At this point, the parents were caught in the middle and did not know which treatment philosophy to follow. The original counselor acknowledged this dilemma and asked to see the parents and Kim at least one more time before they committed themselves to a new treatment approach.

During this session, the parents lamented Kim's relapse and said that the situation seemed hopeless. They focused on all the things that had gone wrong over the last 2 months, but failed to acknowledge the previous summer's successes. After the counselor let each parent vent, he gave them several concrete examples of how Kim had been successful and which specific treatment elements had led to this success. The counselor reiterated how happy Kim had been over the summer, and stressed the fact that her weight had steadily increased because the parents had held her accountable. The reasons for the relapse were that no one at school was able to hold Kim accountable and that she was not yet strong enough to stand on her own. As a result, the counselor maintained that the parents should go back to what was working, rather than rush into another treatment approach that was unproven. The counselor added that he would withdraw from the case if the parents did not see the same changes in 1 month's time. One month out of Kim's entire lifetime was not too much to ask, especially considering that the approach had a proven track record of success. In addition, if the parents chose hospitalization, they might have to pay thousands of dollars out of pocket with no guarantee of success. The parents said that they could not argue with this reasoning and agreed to try the counselor's approach again for 1 month.

4. The counselor can use his or her experience and insight to predict future outcomes if another treatment approach is selected. This is a very powerful technique, and one that can give the counselor instant credibility or expert status. If the counselor's predictions come true, the parents are often willing to return the teenager to the counselor's care with a firm commitment to follow the treatment plan fully and without question.

CLINICAL EXAMPLE

The parents of 16-year-old Missy were caught in the middle between professionals with different philosophies. On one hand, the psychiatrist recommended hospitalization and medication. On the other hand, the counselor recommended that the parents take charge to stop the behavior. The parents wanted to try both approaches and see both the psychiatrist and the counselor. The counselor told the parents that he would be setting them up for failure if he supported this plan, and asked them to choose one approach or the other.

The parents understood this rationale and chose to try the psychiatrist's approach. The counselor told the parents that although he did not take their decision personally, he would be remiss if he did not explain the risks involved. He predicted the following outcomes: (1) Missy's running away would stay the same or worsen; (2) Missy would make a temporary change in a locked hospital unit, but it would be short-lived; (3) when Missy returned home, there would be a 1-

to 2-week "honeymoon" period before the behavior problems returned. The reason was that the hospital staff and locked facility would have made the change, not the parents. Therefore, Missy would have no more reason to respect the parents than when she first entered the hospital.

After predicting these future events, the counselor asked the parents to consider this option: If his predictions came true, would the parents come back and try his treatment approach? The counselor would not say, "I told you so." Instead, the counselor and parents would roll up their sleeves and get back on track as quickly as possible. The parents felt that this was a very fair proposal, but that it would not be needed. They believed that hospitalization would "scare Missy back into obedience." Besides, they knew of no one who could predict the future.

When Missy returned home from the hospital, she relapsed in precisely the same way that the counselor had predicted. The parents could not believe the accuracy of the prediction and time frame in which the relapse occurred. The parents then went on to tell the counselor that even though he did not have an MD, he was the one they wanted to go with because everything he said came true.

This technique worked because of three important factors. First, instead of getting defensive or argumentative, the counselor recognized the parents' dilemma and put the ball back in their court. Second, the counselor did not try to get into a contest over who was the better mental health care provider. Instead, the counselor proved his worth through the age-old saying that "seeing is believing." Predicting the future accurately was the most powerful way in which he could prove both his knowledge and his skill level. In the United States, an MD or a PhD somehow automatically signifies that a person is more competent and skillful than someone with a lesser degree. To counter this misperception, counselors must often prove themselves through accurate predictions. Finally, the counselor made it clear that if the parents came back, there would not be any "I told you so" comments. This allowed the parents to save face and provided an easy route for them to reenter treatment.

5. Finally, the counselor of the parents may need to ask the outside professional to remove himself or herself from the overall treatment plan. If the counselor does this, the parents' prior consent must be obtained. Needless to say, asking an outside professional to "back off" should be done in a respectful manner, or egos will get bruised and tempers will flare. The counselor may need to give concrete examples of how the family has been placed in the middle. If all else fails, the counselor may need to go over the outside professional's head and speak to his or her supervisor. The counselor then tries to convince the supervisor to give the treatment plan a chance.

Strategy 4: Working with Peers—
The Adolescent's "Second Family"

Today's adolescents are so deeply defined by their peer networks that working with the parents alone is rarely enough to effect change. The disintegration of the family has allowed the peer group to become a powerful influence. Busy parents now spend 50% less time with their children than they did 20 years ago (Nagel, 1996). Within this changed social context, it becomes critical for the counselor to integrate the teenager's peer network into the overall treatment process. This is accomplished through both indirect and direct interventions. For example, strengthening the parent–child bond through nurturance can indirectly weaken negative peer influences, as the adolescent can now rely on the parents for part of the support he or she needs. Direct interventions include actually bringing the teenager's friends into treatment or having the parents contact the parents of their teenager's peers to form a collaborative parental community.

Indirect Peer Group Interventions

Parents must be educated on the connection between nurturance and the amount of influence a peer group can have on their teenager. In general, the less nurturing there is between parents and child, the greater the influence of the peer group. However, if parents provide nurturance without discipline, the result may be similar: The teenager may act out and follow a negative peer group. Without a balance of both, the teenager may rely on the peer group for guidance and structure. Parents can be given the following scenario to explain this important point:

"Imagine for a moment that your teenager has a choice between two families. In the first family there are rules, restrictions, and adults who always seem to point out the negative or sermonize on what you are doing wrong. At the same time, there is a lack of special outings, good times, hugs, or trust. Or the family has plenty of good times but lacks rules and restrictions.

"In the second family, your teenager feels accepted for who he [she] is, maintains trust, experiences a lot of good times, and enjoys special outings. In addition, this family may not require the teenager to follow any rules or accept responsibility for his [her] actions.

"If you were your teenager and you had to choose, which family would you want to be with the most, and which family would have the most influence on your heart and your mind? The first family represents your immediate family, and the second family represents your friends and peers."

After hearing this scenario, many parents will say, "I never thought of it like this before," and begin to gain insight into this connection. With this knowledge, parents are shown how to bring what is missing back into their teenager's life. For example, if the parents have many rules but no special outings, the counselor introduces the strategies outlined in Chapter 7 to restore nurturance and good feelings between parents and teenager. If the parents are overprotective and smothering, or if they lack rules, the counselor uses the strategies outlined in Chapters 4 and 6 to provide limits and structure. In both cases, the goal is simple: indirectly lessening negative peer influences through the use of these direct strategies. The first case example below shows the counselor how limits and structure can indirectly limit peer influences, and the second case example shows how nurturance can have this same effect.

CLINICAL EXAMPLE

Ray, 15-year-old boy, was referred to counseling for violence at school, shoplifting, car theft, and truancy. During the first session, Ray reported that his mother "needed to get her own life." For the past 5 years, since her divorce, she had not dated or gone out with friends, instead, she followed Ray around the house, wanting to know what he was going and where he was at all times. Ray thought his mom was lonely, because she always wanted to go out and do things with him rather than with people her own age.

The mother reported that she needed to watch Ray all the time because his problems warranted such vigilance. Whenever she backed off, Ray would take advantage of the situation and get in trouble. The mother admitted that it was difficult to provide consistent structure and discipline, and reported that if she got too tough, Ray might get angry and withdraw his support, friendship, and love. The mother acknowledged that this possibility was too threatening, because without Ray she did not have a life.

In addition to this information, the counselor discovered that Ray's peer group was very negative and highly influential. The probation officer reported that Ray was heavily involved in gang activity and used drugs and alcohol within this group. He was put on probation for grand theft auto after he and his friends were caught stealing a car. Ray and his friends did not have much respect for authority and exhibited no remorse for the crime.

To counter these problems, the counselor collaborated with the probation officer, and together they designed a plan to empower the mother. They met with the mother while Ray waited in the other room. Together they wrote out a contract of rules that addressed truancy, school violence, threats of violence, and disrespect. If Ray missed one class or was violent, the teacher would call the mother, and she would go to school wearing pink curlers and fuzzy slippers. If Ray refused the mother access to the classroom or continued to violate these rules, the probation officer would authorize detention for 2 days for the first offense, 4 days for the second offense, 6 days for the third offense, and so on. If Ray committed any acts or threats of violence against the mother, the probation officer would authorize detention according to the same schedule. For each day Ray did not violate these school rules, he would receive a coupon worth 1 extra hour of phone time.

The probation officer and counselor combined their expertise and resources to give the mother the backup she needed. Ray valued his freedom and phone use above all else. Detention was used therapeutically because it was implemented to back up the mother's rules and consequences, rather than being directly imposed by the probation officer. With this support, the mother was willing to get tough with Ray even though he might withdraw his love temporarily, because she was accountable to the counselor and probation officer if she did not follow through.

Two very important changes happened indirectly as the result of this new structure and discipline. First, the mother no longer had to be vigilant with the son. She now had the support she needed to be free to pursue outside interests, such as dating and going out with friends. This provided Ray the space he needed to move past the individuation stage in his development. Second, Ray's negative peer group began losing its appeal. Ray quickly got tired of losing his freedom for detention and his phone privileges for disrespect. He made the connection that hanging out with his friends did not help his cause; it only helped him to continue to get into trouble. In addition, Ray finally understood that "being good" got everyone "off his case." This had always been his goal, but he had never known how to achieve it. Ray began to gravitate toward friends and activities that did not break rules or commit crimes, because he had changed and was behaving differently.

In sum, Ray's peer group lost its negative influence as the direct result of changes made within the immediate family environment. When Ray's household environment took on limits and discipline, so did his peer environment. These parallel patterns can be defined as "isomorphic," as they have the tendency to recur across different settings and can work in either a positive or a negative direction, depending on the particular behaviors exhibited. In Ray's case, the parallel patterns started off negative, but quickly changed to positive as the mother created an environment of structure and discipline.

CLINICAL EXAMPLE

Fifteen-year-old Jackson was referred to counseling for violence and truancy. During the first session, the counselor asked Jackson what he wanted to get out of counseling. Jackson's answer was simple and straightforward: "Since I was 10, my mother and I have stopped talking and we never do anything together. I would like my mom and I to learn to love each other again. We seem to have forgotten how." Jackson also stated that his friends had become family to him, as he felt they were the only ones that cared and took the time to understand him.

The mother, a single parent, later confirmed Jackson's perceptions and said that since Jackson was 10, they had had one argument after another. She could not remember the last time they had hugged each other or had a special outing together. The relationship had recently been strained even further with the introduction of Darryl, the mother's new boyfriend. Jackson did not like Darryl and was extremely jealous of the relationship. The mother stated that she used to spank Jackson until he reached 10 years of age; after that, he became too big to spank. However, she did not have any alternative form of discipline. Her method went from spankings to threats and the withdrawing of affection. Further probing revealed that the mother would repeatedly make a conditional promise of nurturance. If Jackson was respectful and well behaved the entire week, they could have a special outing together. However, Jackson always fell short of this goal. Consequently, the divide between Jackson and his mother became greater over the years as nurturance and tenderness left the relationship. The message to Jackson was clear. Love and nurturance were tied conditionally to good behavior.

In addition to this information, the mother confirmed that Jackson's peer group was extremely influential. He spent more time with his friends than at home. He loved his friends and was very protective of them. If the mother criticized them, Jackson would become extremely agitated and at times violent.

To counter these problems, the counselor helped the mother in the key area of restoring nurturance unconditionally. This was done concurrently with the restoration of structure and discipline. First, the counselor drew the mother's eco-map and identified neighbors, cousins, and church members who could support her in times of crisis. With the mother's permission, each of these people was contacted and asked to attend a network meeting. A total of 12 people showed up to support the mother. At the meeting, each outside member's role was clarified as the mother collaboratively developed a written contract of rules and consequences. With this support, the mother was able to regain and maintain her authority to stop Jackson's two "aces" of truancy and violence.

Second, while these extreme behaviors were being stopped, the counselor introduced strategies to help the mother restore nurturance to the relationship. The counselor used education and normalization to show the mother how she and Jackson had gotten stuck in Stage 6 of the emotional deprivation timeline (see Chapter 7, Figure 7.1). Jackson sought nurturance from his "second family" of peers as a normal reaction to years of bitter confrontations and a fear of rejection. Next, the counselor showed the mother how she had inadvertently placed conditions on her love by making Jackson earn his special outings through good behavior. The mother was shown how to separate softness from misbehavior. She was asked to go on special outings with Jackson regardless of his behavior that day or week.

Finally, the mother was educated on the direct connection between the current lack of nurturance and Jackson's need to go outside the home to get these basic needs met. Jackson reported that the special outings each week brought them closer together. When Jackson was hurting or needed to talk, he now felt that he could come to his mother. The mother reported that Jackson even allowed her to hug him each day. In turn, his relationships with friends began to grow more positive as he began going to school each day and felt closer to his mother.

Direct Peer Group Interventions

Negative peer influences may also be neutralized by working directly with the peer group itself. This can be accomplished in one of three ways:

1. The counselor can show parents how to establish what is called a "phone tree." A phone tree consists of the names and phone numbers of the parents of each of the teenager's friends. With these numbers, the friends' parents can be called any time there is a problem (e.g., the teen is cutting or skipping school) or a need to verify information on a party, a sleepover, or a particular meeting time or place. Parents can then give their phone tree to other parents to establish a community network. With an established network, any parent can activate the phone tree to report a problem, such as an unsupervised party or substance use. Parents are told that without a network of their own, they will be defeated by the code of silence that surrounds their teenager's peer group. Parents are often surprised by the willingness of other parents to collaborate. With strength in numbers, previously reluctant parents are suddenly willing to get involved. This is especially true when parents can be assured that their anonymity will be protected. In other words, one set of parents will tip off another set about something they heard or saw. Parents can then act on this information without revealing the source. To get other parents' phone numbers, parents must be both creative and direct. Creatively, they can write down a name and number left on scratch paper or thrown in the trash. The information is then recorded in a logbook. Directly, the parents can mandate that they must meet all their teenager's friends and receive the friends' parents' names and numbers before the teen is allowed to go out.

2. As described in detail in Chapter 6, the parents must be prepared to "poison" their teenager's "safe houses" if necessary. One reason a teenager can run away from home is often that he or she can stay with friends. Many times, the parents of these friends do not know that the teenager is staying over or think that the teenager has permission to sleep over. In other cases, through lies or half-truths, the teenager may be able to convince a friend's parents that he or she has been abused. To counter these problems, the parents must do everything in their power to find these safe houses and ensure that the teenager will no longer be welcome there. (See Chapter 6 for specific strategies.)

3. Finally, it may actually be necessary to bring members of the teenager's peer group into treatment. Usually the leader of the peer group is the most charismatic but also the most disturbed teenager of the group. He or she establishes the behavior patterns for the others. If these patterns are dysfunctional, the teenager is stuck. Once in the group, the teenager is implicitly forbidden, under the threat of ostracism, to develop interests or values out-

side the group. The counselor must often get the peers' direct approval before they will allow the teenager to comply with treatment requests.

CLINICAL EXAMPLE

Fourteen-year-old Todd was referred to counseling for chronic truancy. Todd's house was designated as the "fun house," because his peer group would skip school and stay there during the day. Every intervention failed to stop Todd's truancy until the counselor asked to meet Todd's friends. Todd was told to tell his friends that the purpose of the meeting was not to conduct counseling, but to get their ideas on how to get everyone off Todd's back. Since they were his best friends, they might have the best ideas on how this should be done.

At the meeting, the counselor explained to the peers that Todd needed to attend school to get everyone off his case. The "evil judge" was about to lock up Todd for violating probation, and Todd's father had just informed him that the neighbors would now be watching the house closely during the day and calling the police if anyone was there. The police would then come and arrest anyone who was there illegally for trespassing. The counselor asked Todd's peers for suggestions to keep this from happening.

Todd's friends then let him off the hook by saying that they could go to another house if they wanted to ditch school. In addition, if Todd tried to ditch school, they would tell him to go to school now that they realized how high the stakes were. The counselor even got a commitment from three of the friends to call the counselor's beeper and leave a voice mail message if Todd refused to go to school. The counselor would then try to reason with Todd, with the understanding that it was still his choice whether or not to go to school.

With his friends' approval, Todd soon returned to school on a regular basis. The friends even agreed to come back for one more visit in 3 weeks to evaluate how Todd was doing and offer other suggestions if needed.

This case was successful for the following reasons. First, Todd's friends were not asked to come into the office for counseling; instead, they were asked to serve as a panel of experts to help Todd solve a specific set of problems. This made the friends feel important and gave them a sense that they were helping Todd. Many adults never take the time to ask teenagers for their opinion. When one does take the time to do this, they are often flattered and willing to help. Moreover, by incorporating their expertise into the treatment plan. Todd's peers essentially gave him the "thumbs up" to follow the counselor's suggestions. With this approval, Todd did not have to risk the pain of ostracism from the group.

Second, the counselor skillfully played the game of "good cop" versus "bad cop." The counselor played the role of "good cop" and teamed up with Todd and his peers to design strategies to defeat the "bad cops," or the judge and nosy neighbors. A bonus is that changes in one member of the system can have a pronounced ripple effect on its other members. When Todd stopped being truant, some of Todd's friends soon followed suit.

It is important to note that when a counselor is seeing peers, a teen's confidentiality must be protected. Before seeing the peer group, the counselor gets approval from the teenager on the topics that can be discussed. The topics should be strictly limited to specific problems (e.g., truancy). The counselor should never discuss issues relating to the family, or personal thoughts and feelings that the teenager has shared in confidence. In addition, if the counselor sees any of the teenager's friends, boundaries must be respected at all times. Issues discussed in one counseling session should not be discussed in another.

Strategy 5: Working with the School System

A counselor cannot rest until parents are collaborating with the school system. Teachers and parents are often isolated and view one another with mutual suspicion. Many teachers feel overworked and unappreciated. When a teenager acts up and they have to babysit, teachers become resentful and often blame the parents for the teenager's problems and poor grades. By the same token, parents regularly complain that the teachers are either too strict or too lenient, or that they do not understand their teenager's particular difficulty. Each side blames the other, but there is a lack of communication between the two systems. The teenager is no longer accountable for his or her behavior because one hand does not know what the other is doing. If this stalemate persists, the teenager will continue to have problems in school but will maintain his or her authority. To break the stalemate, the school personnel and the parents must meet and work together as a team. This collaborative process is outlined in detail in Chapter 6; readers are asked to refer to the discussion of parent–school collaboration within the section entitled "Ace 2: Truancy and Poor School Performance."

SUMMARY

To be truly effective, a counselor must adopt both a family systems approach and an ecosystemic approach. Ecosystemic interventions change the parents and adolescent in relation to their interactions with outside systems. If the counselor can effect change only within the family system and not the outside environment, treatment may fail or the adolescent may relapse once treatment is concluded. This is because the whole (the environment and family system) has a greater impact than the sum of its parts (the adolescent, the parents, and outsiders as individuals). Hence, outside forces are as powerful as, or in some cases more powerful than, the immediate family itself. If these outside systems cannot be persuaded to collaborate with the overall treatment, they must be neutralized through direct or indirect interventions. A counselor must be willing to leave the comfort of his or her offices and be a guest within the outside system. This may mean keeping early morning appointments at the school, meeting with church leaders after services, or meeting with a psychiatrist for 15 minutes during his or her lunch hour. When the counselor is willing to "go the extra mile," the family and its outside systems are often willing to follow. The following is a recap of the major points contained within this chapter:

1. "Outsiders" are defined as people and environmental systems external to the immediate family that exert a powerful influence on the difficult adolescent. These outsiders include peer influences, the juvenile justice system, local police departments, church groups, school personnel, child protective services (CPS) workers, other mental health care providers, and probation officers. Parents may also experience outside problems and stress at work or with extended family members, which can impede their effectiveness.

2. Before the counselor designs strategies to work effectively with outsiders, he or she must first know how these environmental systems affect the family. The counselor can use a simple paper-and-pencil visual diagram called an "eco-map." The eco-map was developed by Ann Hartman (1978) and is used to sketch the ecological system of the family with all significant outside relationships.

3. Once the counselor has intimate knowledge of the environmental territory, he or she must know how to intervene effectively with these outside systems. Interventions center around two areas: collaboration and neutralization. The decision of whether to collaborate or neutralize is based on the feedback received from these outside systems. If outside systems attempt to undermine the treatment plan, they must be neutralized quickly; however, this should only be done as a last resort. Whenever possible, the counselor should mediate between the family and its environment to achieve cooperation in solving the adolescent's problem.

4. The following outside systems have been identified as the most significant in work with difficult adolescents and their families:

• *CPS workers and police officers.* The CPS and the police have the potential either to empower or to disempower parents. Counselors need to know how to help CPS workers and police officers support rather than disempower parents whose teenagers falsely accuse them of abuse or commit violent acts.

• *Church, friends, or extended family.* Parents may not see the hidden resources available to them through these outside systems. This is especially true for single parents, who often feel alone and without support.

- *Other counselors, psychiatrists, or probation officers.* These outside forces often intentionally or unintentionally undermine the counselor's credibility by disagreeing with the treatment plan. The parents are placed in the middle and forced to choose between different treatment approaches.

- *Peers—the adolescent's "second family."* Economic pressures, technology, mobility, and divorce have seriously weakened the influence of the family, so that the peer group exerts a greater effect on a teenager than ever before. A counselor must know how to neutralize negative peer influence and to harness the potential power of peers to help the teenager and/or the family.

- *The school system.* Behavior problems that occur at home also occur in the school environment. When this happens, the counselor must be skilled at intervening with school personnel to establish a collaborative link between parents and the teachers.

CHAPTER 9

Single-Parent Families
Sharing Parental Responsibility

The single-parent family is emerging as a prominent unit in U.S. society (Zastrow, 1996). Because most single-parent families are female-headed, and women generally have lower earning capacities than men do, the probability of task overload increases: Maintaining the household and caring for the children constitute one job, and income production represents another (Lindblad-Goldberg, 1989). As a result, the traditional notion of an executive hierarchy in which two parents are in charge has to be adapted accordingly. Such essential parenting functions as setting limits and providing nurturance to a child often have to be compromised, because a single parent does not have the emotional reserves available. Consequently, the parental responsibility may have to be shared with one or more children, usually the oldest. The implication of this situation is that the counselor must involve the designated child when setting up rules and consequences in the household. However, this arrangement can become problematic if the teenager with the behavioral problem is the designated coparent. It is extremely difficult for a single parent to apply consequences to a teenager who often both provides emotional support and helps maintain the household. This arrangement places the teenager in an extremely powerful position that is incongruent with his or her developmental level. However, other alternatives are often far too threatening for a single parent who is overworked, overstressed, or depressed. The following strategies are suggested for work with single-parent families.

STRATEGY 1: WORKING BOTH SIDES OF THE FENCE

During the engagement phase (Step 1 of the 15-step family-based model), it becomes even more critical for the counselor to "work both sides of the fence" and generate meaningful goals for both the difficult adolescent and the single parent. In particular, the needs of a difficult adolescent who is in a designated authoritarian position must be addressed, or any plan of action can be undermined. The counselor sees the adolescent individually and asks, "How can I be helpful to you?" or "Is there something you would like me to go to bat for with your parent?" The counselor thus creates an alliance with the adolescent so that he or she is part of the treatment plan. The adolescent will now have a sense of ownership of the treatment process, and can brainstorm concrete solutions and his or her own set of consequences if rules are violated in the future.

CLINICAL EXAMPLE

Fifteen-year-old Stan was the oldest of four children and created the most problems for his single mother. The mother reported that Stan was deeply involved with a gang and frequently left his 5- and 6-year-old siblings unsupervised. Stan was also failing school and refused to comply with requests for help unless he felt "in the mood." Stan and his mother always fought, and she felt that Stan could not be trusted. In this brief transcript, we see how the counselor was able to ask Stan questions in such a way as to convert him from an enemy to an ally.

COUNSELOR: How can I help make your life easier at home? [The counselor asked what he could do to be of service to the teenager. This was a different twist, because other counselors had always made him feel blamed and treated him as if he were the "bad seed."]

STAN: (*Moving forward in his chair*) No one has ever bothered to ask what I want. Weird. I guess to get my mom from hassling me all the time. [Stan began to open up and show interest.]

COUNSELOR: What would your mom be doing or saying differently if she were no longer hassling you? [This question forced Stan to define "no hassling" into concrete behavioral terms. This would make it much easier to formulate a treatment plan.]

STAN: I guess letting me go out with my friends without so much hassle, and telling me once in a while that I do a good job and not nagging me so much. Nothing I do ever seems good enough. [Stan was starting to get at the heart of the real issue: He felt unappreciated and unloved by his mother. The counselor tracked this and tried to check out this perception in the next question.]

COUNSELOR: Am I hearing you right? At times you feel that your mom does not really understand you and appreciate how much you try. Her nagging stings your heart, because you want to get close, but you feel she constantly pushes you away. Is that close or way off? [The counselor tried to summarize the underlying issue that was keeping this teenager so angry and hurt. He ended the statement with the question about being close or way off, so that Stan could easily agree or disagree with the counselor's perception of the problem.]

STAN: You got it! When I was 10 years old, these people came and took us away to these foster homes, because Mom used drugs all the time. When she did get us back a year later, things changed between us. We stopped talking, and she hovered over me like all the time, not letting me do anything. I just had to bust out, you know. [The counselor struck gold. Not only did he tap into the underlying issue, but he was able to get the teenager to open up about how and why the relationship between mother and son had become so strained.]

COUNSELOR: What might have happened is that your mom came back and got scared. She thought that she might lose you again. As a result, she was afraid to let you out of her sight for fear they might take you away again. And even now when she nags and sounds angry, I bet it is because she might be scared she is losing you all over again to your friends or the streets. She feels helpless to stop it. [The counselor reframed the nagging and anger by weaving them into the underlying theme of being scared and helpless. If this was a correct perception, the teenager would become softer and move toward helping the mother.]

STAN: (*Becoming tearful*) I never thought about it that way, but I can see where you are coming from. But how do we get back to connecting again? The walls are so thick. [Stan now wanted to become part of the solution process and to find a way to reconnect with his mother. His perceptions were beginning to change as he began to see the anger and nagging from a different point of view.]

COUNSELOR: Well, here is what we do. Let me meet with your mom alone and try to soften her up before the three of us meet. I will ask her for one or two suggestions that would make things run smoother at home. In addition, I now realize that I have to work with her on nagging less and connecting with you in a softer way. How does that sound? [The counselor gave a concrete description of his proposed approach to treatment and the supporting rationale. Most importantly, he framed treatment as a way in which both parties would get their needs met. This created a cooperative working relationship between mother and son.]

STAN: Good!

COUNSELOR: One more thing. Please help me do a better job. What do you think your mom will say if I ask her what you would be doing or saying differently to make the household run more smoothly and give her peace of mind? [The counselor framed the teenager as an "expert" who could come up with suggestions that could change the family. The teenager thus became an ally rather than an enemy.]

STAN: I think she would say coming home when I am supposed to, and helping her out with my brother and sisters more. [The teenager gave the counselor the road map of what needed to happen. In addition, the teenager could take partial ownership of the treatment process and could work toward a solution.]

The counselor then obtained more details on how Stan would come home on time and exactly what he would be doing to help his mother with the other children. Next, the counselor met with the mother individually and used the same types of questions to outline her side of the treatment plan. Consequently, when the counselor met with the mother and son together, they had in essence already developed the treatment plan. The discussion at this meeting was devoted to the process of combining the mother's and son's ideas into one written treatment plan. In this way, the counselor successfully worked both sides of the fence by incorporating the goals of both parties into a single contract.

This strategy works well because the counselor sees both parties individually rather than together; this prevents yelling, blaming, or accusations that would only further damage an already tenuous relationship. If either the parent or the adolescent needs to vent any anger, it can be done without the other party present. After this venting takes place, the counselor moves quickly into a series of questions that force both parties to come up with their own custom-designed solutions. This promotes ownership and cooperation. Also, the counselor has the opportunity to find underlying themes and past events that have caused present-day damage in the relationship. When this happens, the counselor can find an acceptable way of reframing the issue to the clients so that they can see the painful events differently and begin to repair the relationship. In the example above, the central themes were abandonment and feeling left out. Knowledge of these core themes provided the counselor with a road map to address these issues.

STRATEGY 2: JOINT DETERMINATION
OF RULES AND CONSEQUENCES

A single parent is often so overworked that the household lacks any rules or sense of order. Consequently, an adolescent's behavioral problems are often a reflection of this disorganization. If rules and consequences are determined with the aid of a coparenting adolescent (whether or not this is also the difficult adolescent), the household can become more organized. A cooperative coparenting adolescent can decrease the anxiety and tension within the household and can give the single parent the time and energy needed to take charge. The behavioral problems of a difficult adolescent may also subside.

The counselor meets with the parent and the coparenting adolescent together. They become the executive system, which will determine rules and consequences without the other children present. This meeting acknowledges the special relationship between the single parent and the coparenting teenager within the household.

However, for this plan to work, the single parent must also outline clear parameters for the teenager's assumed role as substitute parent. This includes defining when the mother expects the adolescent to function as a substitute parent (i.e., specific times and situations), defining when the adolescent is relieved of this burden, and listing the teenager's responsibilities in that role. This clear definition must then be communicated to the other children, with the parent's expectations that they will accept the coparenting adolescent's authority in the parent's absence. If there are problems while the parent is at work, the parent should meet privately with the parental child for a debriefing when he or she returns home. The parent, *not* the adolescent, should then administer the predetermined consequences. In effect, the adolescent monitors the other children's behavior but does not administer punishments. Otherwise, resentment and bitterness will develop between the siblings; the adolescent could also physically hurt the other children in a heated argument. Parental administration of consequences prevents a power struggle between the siblings, while allowing the parent to retain ultimate executive authority.

CLINICAL EXAMPLE

The mother of 13-year-old Nick reported that he refused to do chores and would terrorize the rest of the siblings by threatening violence when the mother left for work. The oldest daughter, Mandy, was the designated parental child but was ineffective at stopping her brother's behavior. However, when the techniques described above were implemented, the mother told Nick that Mandy was in charge during her absence. If Nick continued to refuse to do chores or threaten violence, Mandy would no longer try to stop him. Instead, Mandy would write down what Nick did and debrief the mother privately when she returned from work. The mother would then administer the consequences and not his sister.

The consequences were as follows: Nick would have to complete any undone chores under his mother's supervision and would lose the privilege of going out on the weekend. Since Nick valued his freedom, this was a harsh penalty. In addition, if Nick threatened violence, he would be placed in the bathroom for double the time it took the mother to get home from work. The problem behaviors stopped immediately. The mother thus clearly defined the role of her daughter as the substitute parent while still retaining her ultimate authority as parent.

In the example above, Mandy's role as the parental adolescent was clarified to each of the other children. This immediately took the pressure off Mandy and decreased the risk that the other children would resent her. Mandy was now there to monitor while the mother backed her up, so that Mandy did not feel she was shouldering all the responsibility. The ultimate result was a household that ran more smoothly. An arrangement like this one also allows the coparenting adolescent time to pursue other interests that are more congruent with his or her developmental level. These include dating, going out with friends, and pursuing outside activities (e.g., sports or clubs).

It is important to note that the difficult adolescent may still refuse to cooperate. When this happens, the counselor must go directly to Strategy 4 (see below) by enlisting members of the community to help the mother. In addition, the counselor may need to be part of that community network by assuming a pseudoparental role until the problem behaviors are under control. This role involves home visits and being on call 24 hours a day, 7 days a week.

STRATEGY 3: EMPLOYING THE ASSISTANCE OF OTHER CHILDREN

When a single parent or parental child is overworked or overwhelmed, the counselor can bring in the other children to assist them with the executive functions. The single parent and counselor meet with all of the children in a family meeting to brainstorm solutions to each problem. Each possible solution is written down, evaluated for its potential effectiveness, and prioritized. The tasks and roles of each family member in solving the problems are then defined. This plan is often effective when each family member is labeled as part of the problem and is asked to work collaboratively to find a solution.

The parent still retains his or her executive authority through final approval or veto power of any plan developed. However, this process shifts the focus off the difficult adolescent as the only problem and expands this definition to include other family members. When this happens, the difficult adolescent (as well as the coparenting adolescent, if this is a different child) and the single parent may feel less overwhelmed. This is because they now have the support and cooperation of other family members.

CLINICAL EXAMPLE

One mother was severely depressed and overwhelmed. She blamed her oldest child, Phil, for all her problems. Phil was in a gang, used drugs, and was constantly in trouble at school. Further inspection revealed that the home environment was extremely disorganized, with no rules or consequences. Instead of focusing exclusively on Phil's problems, the counselor convinced the mother that she needed to be supported more by everyone in the family. The mother agreed. Everyone in the family was then asked to brainstorm ways to make the household more efficient. From this meeting, chores were divided up equally, bedtimes were negotiated, mealtimes were designated, and special outings with the mother were planned.

As a result, the household became more organized and less chaotic; the mother felt less overwhelmed and depressed; and Phil was no longer seen as the sole problem. This allowed the counselor to use Step 11 in the family-based treatment model (restoring nurturance and tenderness) to change the parent–adolescent communication from one of blame to one of understanding and mutual respect. Over time, Phil's behavioral problems began to lessen.

When roles are clarified and everyone has rules and consequences, it is less likely that one child will be singled out and treated differently. This is an important concept, as adolescents are particularly sensitive to the idea of "fairness." If they perceive that other children are receiving preferential treatment, resentment will build, and the teenagers will rebel. It is therefore critical that all children have rules and consequences appropriate for their particular developmental level. For example, time out for a 4-year-old should be administered for shorter periods of time and should be implemented for different behaviors than time out for a 13-year-old should be. Adolescents should be told these differences so that they understand why their siblings receive punishment tailored for their particular chronological age.

STRATEGY 4: COMMUNITY FAMILY COUNSELING

Finally, if all else fails and the difficult adolescent continues to have behavioral problems, the counselor must look to extended family members or the community. This approach is similar to the network therapy approach developed by Speck and Attneave (1973), whereby a single parent's entire social network (family, friends, neighbors) is gathered together to help the parent watch over the problem adolescent. Once a support system is created, there is always someone to call for backup when there is a problem.

The goal of this intervention is to support the single parent's executive authority. These outside people are invited to the meeting and, with the parent, outline rules and consequences. (See Chapter 8 for a description of how to initiate and conduct such a meeting.) The single parent still retains his or her executive authority and veto power, but is no longer isolated. The support roles of these outside members are clearly defined, and everyone engages in troubleshooting to identify possible problems.

CLINICAL EXAMPLE

Fourteen-year-old Lewis refused to go to school in the morning. The mother was ineffective in getting Lewis to attend, and he refused to negotiate a compromise. The mother had a next-door neighbor who was a police officer, but she had never considered the idea of asking him for help. With the mother's permission, the counselor called and invited the neighbor to come to the next meeting. At the meeting, the mother and neighbor met with the counselor privately to outline the following plan of action: The next time Lewis refused to attend school, the mother would give him 10 minutes to get ready. If Lewis refused or was still in bed after 10 minutes, she would call the neighbor. The neighbor and the mother would then take Lewis to school by force. If he was truant, the neighbor and the mother agreed to sit with Lewis in class and accompany him between classes. The neighbor would wear his police uniform. Lewis tested this consequence once, but never again. The mother became empowered by her neighbor to exercise her executive authority and stop the behavior.

If there are no outside supports available, a counselor must sometimes support a single parent in a pseudoparental role until the behaviors are eliminated on a permanent basis.

CLINICAL EXAMPLE

In one case, the counselor was on call 24 hours a day and went to the home on several occasions to support the mother when she enforced consequences. During one visit, the mother discovered marijuana in 13-year-old Chris's room, but was very hesitant to call the police. With the counselor's assistance, the mother did call the police and have Chris arrested. The mother thus gained the confidence she needed to make changes in the future.

This kind of hands-on support has usually never been experienced by a single parent and is often the basis for turning things around. The parent is so appreciative of this support that he or she may become energized to do whatever is necessary to take charge, as a more detailed case example illustrates.

CLINICAL EXAMPLE

A single mother came to the first meeting extremely angry and hostile. She told the counselor that all her previous counselors and probation officers had made her feel that she was a bad mother. She belonged to a church, but even her pastor and fellow church members told her that the problems were her fault. She stated that she was attending the meeting only because she was ordered by the court to do so. She also wanted the counselor's help to get her two problem children (Dale, 14, and Geoff, 12) placed in residential treatment. She was tired of "getting the runaround" from professionals, with no help from anyone. The mother reported that her oldest son, Dale, held knives to her throat and threatened to kill her while she was sleeping. Geoff regularly told her to "fuck off" and constantly skipped school. Both Dale and Geoff would bring their friends over and destroy the household. Her youngest son, Kenny, was now copying Geoff by swearing at her and refusing to do time outs. The boys' father lived out of state and refused to help.

From this description, the counselor stated that the mother was not to blame. Rather, she had not received the support she deserved. The mother breathed a sigh of relief and said simply, "Thank you." The counselor then went on to describe a concrete treatment plan that included the following steps.

1. The counselor would meet with the entire family at the mother's house after work, to see what she had to put up with and talk with each of the children individually.

2. The counselor would personally contact the father by phone to see whether Dale could visit or live with him, to give the mother some respite.

3. The counselor would collaborate with the probation officer and advocate for the mother's needs.

4. The counselor would be on call 24 hours a day, 7 days a week to come to the house if a crisis took place. A "crisis" was defined as destruction of property, physical violence, or any incident in which the police or child protective services were called for any reason.

5. The counselor would arrange a meeting with the mother's pastor and other church leaders to formulate a plan to support the mother and be available in case of future crises.

The mother was skeptical, because she had received so many broken promises in the past, but reported that the plan at least looked good on paper.

When the counselor went to the home, he tried to persuade Dale to help determine rules and consequences jointly with the mother. However, Dale refused to cooperate and told the counselor to "fuck off." Later, Dale threatened the mother with a knife. As planned, the mother paged the counselor. The counselor went to the house, and they called the police. This only agitated Dale further, and he started destroying property. The counselor then called the probation officer, who came over to the house as well. With the probation officer and counselor present, the police officer arrested Dale. This was the first time this kind of action had been taken.

Once Dale and the police officer left, the counselor had a meeting at the kitchen table with the mother and the probation officer. He stated that due to the seriousness of the threats, Dale's violent history, and his refusal to cooperate, the mother needed respite from Dale for safety reasons. The probation officer agreed and came up with the following plan: The son would either be placed in a "boot camp" institution or go live with the father. The probation officer would personally call the father with this ultimatum. The mother began to cry and said that she was finally getting the help she needed. She also no longer felt that the probation officer blamed her. The next day, the father was contacted; rather than see his son go to the youth camp, he agreed to fly down to get him. However, the probation officer made it clear that if he attempted to return the son because he was having problems, Dale would be arrested and placed in the camp.

While this was taking place, the counselor moved quickly to mobilize the church forces. The church members agreed to meet the next day. At the meeting, the counselor formulated terms for implementing the bathroom strategy for Geoff, should he continue to miss school, swear, or threaten violence. The mother did not have a solid bathroom door, so the church agreed to provide funds to purchase the door. One of the church members even offered to install the door. If the mother tried to place Geoff in time out and he refused, she would go down the phone list of church members at the meeting until she found one who was available. That person would come to the house to help the mother place Geoff in time out. If no one was available, the mother would call the counselor. Geoff would be told up front that if he refused to go to time out, he would be required to be in time out for as long as it took for the church member or the counselor to arrive. Everyone present then engaged in troubleshooting; all the potential things that could go wrong were discussed and worked through.

As predicted, the church members only had to come out to the house twice before Geoff's extreme behaviors stopped. The mother was so relieved and so grateful for the counselor's support that she committed to changing her behavior. This included taking her sons on special outings, looking for positives, ending lectures and sermons, and energizing herself by going out with a friend at least one night a week. Over time, the mother fulfilled each of these commitments.

This case was successful for the following reasons. First, the counselor enlisted outside forces to assist the mother. He played the role of mediator and took charge of the meetings with a concrete set of procedures to stop the extreme behaviors. He clarified everyone's roles and encouraged everyone to envision potential future problems. This made the mother feel less blamed and more energized to initiate both positive and negative consequences. Second, the counselor was willing to "go the extra mile" by being available to the mother 24 hours a day, 7 days a week, until the mother was strong enough to take charge on her own. Finally, the counselor broke down the multitude of problems into "bite-sized" pieces and prioritized them from most to least severe. He then methodically developed a plan of attack to solve each problem.

SUMMARY

The interventions described in this chapter—working both sides of the fence, joint determination of rules and consequences, employing the assistance of other children, and community family counseling—can be used as effective adjuncts to the family-based model. They incorporate the strengths rather than the deficits of a single-parent family constellation, and they make use of alternative supports when the family is stressed by developmental and external changes. However, it is important to note that these interventions are not always effective. If a single parent abdicates his or her parental role through alcoholism, drug addiction, depression, or desertion, the adolescent will continue to have problems. If this occurs, the counselor must quickly try to activate a support system, utilize residential treatment to give the parent temporary respite, or work with the adolescent on an individual basis to teach him or her better coping strategies.

CHAPTER 10

Divorce and Stepfamily Problems

Difficult family issues such as divorce and stepfamily problems pose special challenges for the counselor. In both of these areas, a difficult adolescent often takes advantage of the situation by playing one parent or parental figure off against the other to undermine their joint authority. In the case of a particularly difficult divorce, the parents are so often angry with each other that they cannot work collaboratively to solve their son's or daughter's problems. In the case of a stepfamily, an adolescent and stepparent are often at odds with each other and fail to establish a working relationship. The biological parent is then forced to take sides as the adolescent's behavioral problems escalate. The aim of this chapter is to describe the special treatment issues associated with these family constellations, and to provide specific strategies to stop adolescent problems within these settings. Two case examples are used to clarify specific points and concepts.

THE EXCEPTIONALLY DIFFICULT DIVORCE: STRATEGIES FOR CONDUCTING A CONTROLLED ENCOUNTER

A divorce becomes even more difficult than usual when the parents cannot control their disputes and place the children in the middle of their heated arguments, unresolved conflicts, and hostilities (Isaacs, Montalvo, & Abelson, 1986). One or both parents may use the children as pawns by telling the children negative things about the other parent or trying to recruit them to turn against the other parent. For an adolescent with severe behavioral problems, an exceptionally difficult divorce presents several distinct advantages. If the adolescent's parents are not communicating at all or are only exchanging hostilities, they cannot exert joint authority or be in charge of their teenager's behavior. For example, if the adolescent does not like the rules of one household, he or she can easily move into the other household. This scenario can repeat itself over and over again, because the parents are unable to communicate, work together, or agree on a plan of action. As a result, the adolescent never has to work through any rules or consequences that he or she does not like. The parents will eventually stop trying to enforce consequences for fear that the teenager might move away or form a special alliance with the other parent. Since one parent can continue to blame the other, neither has to take responsibility for solving their teenager's problem. The adolescent can now "divide and conquer" the parents, because they are themselves divided in anger and unable to conquer their teenager's difficulties.

For the present treatment model to be effective under these circumstances, the counselor must have the skills necessary to bring the hostile parents together in a "controlled encounter." Otherwise, no matter how sound an intervention may be, it will be ineffective because the parents will be unable to enforce it. A "controlled encounter" is defined as a structured mediation meeting between two warring parents, in which the counselor takes charge and negotiates concrete ways in which the parents will reorganize their relationships with each other and their children (Campbell & Johnston, 1986). The counselor may have to meet first with the parents individually to convince them of the importance of attempting a controlled encounter. Parents must also perceive the counselor as a person who is neutral and does not take sides. They must be convinced that the counselor's concern about the well-being of the difficult adolescent and any other children is his or her number one priority. Conducting a controlled encounter involves the following three strategies: (1) establishing ground rules, (2) having parents talk directly through the counselor, and (3) finding a workable topic. Each of these strategies is outlined below, with a case example to clarify key points in the use of all three.

Strategy 1: Establishing Ground Rules

The counselor must give each parent concrete examples of how their teenager has been able to play one parent off against the other. In addition, the counselor must demonstrate how the parents' continued hostility has helped their teenager misbehave and maintain authority. Finally, before beginning the meeting, the counselor must carefully outline the purpose and goal of a controlled encounter. The counselor must tell the parents before the meeting begins that they are in charge and can call a time out immediately if either party strays from the topic or begins to verbally abuse the other. In addition, "hot" topics such as money or visitation will not be discussed until later. The discussion will focus strictly on their teenager's misbehavior, rules and consequences to stop this behavior, and specific ways in which the parents can exert joint authority. The parents are reassured that this will be different from past dialogues, because the counselor will not permit runaway hostilities. These ground rules have to be agreed upon and repeated by both parents before the controlled encounter can begin. If there is no agreement, parents are told that they can return later when their teenager's behavior worsens.

Strategy 2: Having Parents Talk Directly through the Counselor

At this stage, the counselor does not allow the adolescent to be present, because he or she will probably try to derail one or both parents. In addition, no attempts are made to get the parents to talk directly to each other, because they are already on such unfriendly terms. Instead, each parent is asked to direct responses to the counselor, who will then filter or reframe that response to the other parent. This is done to increase the likelihood that each message will be heard. Problems and goals are then prioritized, and the top three problems are selected for attention.

Strategy 3: Finding a Workable Topic

The counselor's most difficult and challenging responsibilities are to find at least one area of agreement to start from and to keep the parents on task. This is difficult because one or both parents will try to make cutting remarks to the other or undermine the other's authority. To counter these moves, the counselor must be ready to call a time out quickly, or even to separate the parents temporarily to let them vent their hostilities individually. This may have to be done before the encounter can be resumed.

The counselor must constantly bring both parents back to the key issue of the adolescent's problem and remind them of the possible future consequences if they cannot work together. Finally, the counselor must be willing to block out 2 or more hours of time for this meeting, because it may take that long to get the parents to agree on any one issue. The parents must leave the meeting with the sense that progress has been made and that no further hard feelings have been created. Otherwise, the counselor may never get a second chance.

CLINICAL EXAMPLE

In the case of 16-year-old Don, the parents had not spoken to each other for over a year. Whenever the father tried to enforce rules and consequences, Don called his mother and told her how unfair the father had been. The mother than told Don that it had been the same in her marriage with his father, and invited him to come to her house to live. Once he was there, the mother encouraged Don not to visit his father. The father eventually became so frustrated that he stopped trying to contact the son.

Don was brought to counseling because he had been arrested for possession of marijuana and for breaking and entering into a house. The mother was concerned, but blamed the father for her son's current difficulties. The counselor spent the first three meetings engaging the mother and convincing her to let him contact the father. The rationale was that previous counseling attempts had been unsuccessful and that she and her son wanted the court system "off their backs" as quickly as possible. In addition, if these problems persisted, Don would probably go to prison and would not have a chance to go to college. The counselor described in detail the contents, process, and rationale of a controlled encounter, and gave the mother the option of not having to continue if it was not helpful the first time. The mother agreed with this rationale. The counselor then met with the father twice to convince him, using the same rationale.

Before the controlled encounter began, the counselor repeated the ground rules. He also stated that yelling made him nervous and gave him stomach cramps; he asked the parents to stop yelling if he called for a time out. The parents felt concern for the counselor and stopped quickly whenever a time out was called. The counselor then asked for a picture of their son and taped it to an empty chair. He told them that Don was the reason for this meeting. If the parents deviated from this mission or became hostile in any way, the counselor would respectfully call their attention back to their son's picture and remind them of what would happen to Don if he went to prison. This process was extremely helpful in keeping them on track.

The counselor then established rules and consequences, assisted the parents in changing their methods of confrontation, and helped them to troubleshoot potential problems. The parents agreed that Don's failure to find employment caused him to have too much idle time and to get into trouble. It was also determined that Don cherished his car, and that continuing to give him money for gas helped prevent him from looking for work. After much discussion, the mother agreed to let the father come by and demand Don's car keys if he did not have at least six new job applications filled out every day. To ensure his accountability further, Don had to have a list of the places he visited and the managers he talked with. The mother and father both agreed to call these places to spot-check whether the son had actually talked with these managers. The father also agreed to take Don on weekends to help him look for a job. The father would stand in the background to watch how proficient Don was in asking for an application and applying for a job; the father would then give the son pointers.

Finally, the parents role-played how they would talk to each other on the phone in a cordial manner, and decided which topics to stick to and which to avoid. All possible future problems with this were then reviewed, and solutions were agreed upon. Once this task was a success, the counselor would start addressing the issues of Don's drug usage and stealing. It is important to note that the counselor had to start where the parents were in terms of a mutually agreed-upon topic in order to built momentum and instill hope. With success established, more difficult issues could then be addressed and solved.

In this example, the counselor successfully brought the parents together in a controlled encounter to begin to solve Don's behavioral problems. The counselor had to take total charge of the session and stop the proceedings immediately if any fighting or verbal barbs arose. Otherwise, the session would have become so emotionally charged that the parents would have been unable to work together. The counselor avoided "hot topics" and found one issue that the parents could agree upon.

It is important to note that some controlled encounters will fail, regardless of the strategies used. This is because many divorced parents abhor each other to such a degree that, simply to spite each other, they will agree to nothing. When this happens, the counselor must predict what will happen in the future and leave the door open for a return to counseling when these predictions come true. The counselor may also have to report these findings to the court and let the court decide on custody issues. Often one parent sees the "bigger picture" better and is more cooperative than the other parent. The counselor may have to submit an evaluation to the court to advocate a change of custody to the parent who has the best interests of the teenager in mind. However, this should only be done as a last resort. Whenever possible, the counselor should remain neutral and try to get the parents to work collaboratively.

STEPFAMILY ISSUES: STRATEGIES FOR ADDRESSING UNREALISTIC EXPECTATIONS

One of the greatest challenges to a stepfamily is that it faces two developmental life cycle transitions simultaneously: It faces the stresses and strains that accompany the formation of a new family, while still attempting to operate as if it has a set of traditions, rules, and roles that has existed since the birth of the oldest child (Kleinman & Whiteside, 1979). For instance, if the tradition of one household was that the father did all the disciplining, then this may be the unspoken expectation of the paternal figure in the new stepfamily. However, the other household may not have followed the same tradition. If these traditions are forcibly combined in the new stepfamily, resentments and anger will surface and will inevitably cause problems. Members of blended families often fail to realize that it takes an average of 2 years to stabilize and develop a new culture of rules, traditions, and roles (Crosbie-Burnett & Ahrons, 1985).

Often members of stepfamilies base their behavior on unrealistic expectations, and thus increase the chances that problems will develop. Some of these unrealistic expectations include the following: (1) The stepparent and the children will instantly experience a loving relationship; (2) the rules of one household will be used in exclusion to those of the other household; (3)

children will not need to mourn the loss of their former family unit, and they will not experience loyalty conflicts between their biological parents; (4) the parent–child relationship needs to take precedence over the new spousal relationship; and (5) the stepparent can discipline the children just as the biological parent would, without repercussions or resentment from the children. When biological parents or stepparents behave in accordance with any of these expectations, problems can develop in the children. The following strategies are suggested to address such problems, and a case example is used to highlight these strategies.

Strategy 1: Using a Nonblaming Educational Approach

The best initial strategy is to use a nonblaming educational approach to inform the family of the special problems and needs of a stepfamily. The counselor tells the parents that they did not receive a training manual or handbook on what to expect when they joined two separate households together. Therefore, many of the problems that they experience are the normal results of a difficult blending of two separate families. The spouses may not realize that their couple bond is fragile because they have had to go directly to the stage of parenting (Crosbie-Burnett & Ahrons, 1985). Therefore, they must give their relationship special attention and spend "quality time" alone together, without always wanting to put the children first or feeling guilty about what their children have been through. The children may continue to remind them of this, but their parenting skills will suffer unless their spousal bond is strong. Fortunately, most parents understand this rationale and will agree to have at least one night out alone together per week, regardless of the children's behavior.

Strategy 2: Having the Biological Parent Enforce Consequences

In order for a stepparent and an adolescent to have a "working relationship," it is important to have the biological parent administer the discipline and enforce the consequences whenever possible. The adolescent has not yet had time to develop an emotional bond of trust and respect with the stepparent. This relationship can become even more tenuous when the stepparent tries to enforce rules or consequences; the usual result is that the teenager resents the stepparent for overstepping his or her role. When this happens, it becomes difficult or impossible for the stepparent and teenager to form the connection necessary to build a healthy relationship. The counselor tells both parents and the teenager that this foundation must be established before a loving relationship or friendship is possible. This is an important concept, because it takes the pressure off both parties to experience "instant love" within a short period of time.

Strategy 3: Clarifying the Stepparent's Role

Once the biological parent agrees to administer the discipline, rules and consequences are outlined and written down in a contract format so that the roles of both the biological parent and the stepparent are clarified. For example, if a stepmother is home alone with a teenage stepson who breaks a rule in the contract by not doing his household chores, the stepmother should not get into a confrontation with the teenager. Instead, she should wait for the father to return home. At that time, the two parents will go behind closed doors so that the stepmother can debrief the father. Then the father, not the stepmother, will enforce the predetermined consequence. Resentment and unnecessary confrontation between the stepparent and teenager are thus carefully avoided; as noted above, this prevents damage to a relationship that is fragile to start with.

To maximize the effectiveness of this strategy, the parents must agree that consequences do not have to be administered immediately after a rule is broken. They will be just as potent at a later time, as long as the parents are consistent and the consequences are administered by the biological parent. The rules and consequences must be outlined in a written format and in clear detail. This is particularly critical in a blended family, where there is often confusion regarding disciplinary procedures. If a negative behavior that is not covered in the contract occurs, the stepparent should wait until the biological parent returns home so that they can privately determine the consequence. The biological parent still administers the consequence, but the stepparent is included in the decision-making process. In addition, the parents should understand that the stepparent will become more directly involved in the future administration of rules and consequences, once a better working relationship has been established with the adolescent and any other children.

Strategy 4: Adapting Step 6 (Changing the Timing and Process of Confrontations) for a Stepfamily

Once roles and rules are clarified, the counselor uses the same principles as outlined in Chapter 5 to change the timing and process of confrontations. The only difference is that special care needs to be taken in removing the biological parent from being caught in the middle of confrontations between the stepparent and teenager. This should be done in the following manner.

First, outside the presence of the teenager, the counselor must educate the stepparent on how the game is played. A typical stepparent tends to take a teenager's manipulation personally, particularly when the relationship is already strained. Therefore, any confrontation will be amplified to a greater degree. The stepparent must learn through concrete examples how the teenager "pushes buttons." The stepparent is a target not because of who he or she is as an individual, but simply because he or she is the stepparent. This perspective may help the stepparent not to take the attacks so personally.

Second, the counselor, must teach the biological parent these confrontational dynamics and persuade him or her to take a more active role. As noted earlier, this means that the biological parent, not the stepparent, must be the one to confront the teenager. Often a stepparent engages in confrontations with a teenager only because he or she feels that the biological parent is ineffective or unable to enforce rules and consequences. If this occurs, the counselor must convince the biological parent of the importance of being in charge, and must show him or her how this will remove the stepparent from a confrontational role.

Finally, the counselor shows the stepparent how to take a supportive role in helping the biological parent confront the adolescent. This support can take the form of secret signals between the parents, as described in Chapter 5. Other means of support include verbal praise and going out on dates to replenish both parents' energy.

Strategy 5: Understanding the Adolescent's Developmental Needs

Both the biological parent and the stepparent must understand the developmental needs of an adolescent as he or she begins the process of separation and individuation. The adolescent may still require special outings with both parents, but will also need time with peers. In addition, the biological parent and teenager need to have special outings together; otherwise, the adolescent may resent the stepparent if he or she feels that the stepparent is monopolizing the biological parent's attention and causing a reduction in the teenager's time alone with the biological parent. The counselor must convince the stepparent of this special need and share the implications if it is not met. The stepparent and teenager may also need to spend time alone together, to get to know each other in a nonconfrontational setting. At the same time, the parents need to acknowledge the teenager's need for independence and not require him or her to participate in every family activity.

CLINICAL EXAMPLE

In the case of 13-year-old Carol, the presenting problems were breaking curfew and not following rules. Further assessment revealed constant conflict between Carol and her stepfather. Each time the mother asked Carol to follow a rule, she would argue until the stepfather got frustrated and attempted to take over. The mother would then tell her husband that he was being too tough. Carol continued to misbehave and show no respect for the stepfather. The stepfather complained that there were no rules and that the mother was unable to enforce any consequences. The counselor met with the parents alone, and together they outlined the rules and consequences in a contract form.

The counselor showed both parents how the stepfather was placed in a confrontational role, and how the mother needed to get tougher yet remain nonreactive. The counselor then played the part of the daughter, to teach the mother how to deliver the consequence while the stepfather refrained from intervening. The stepfather also came up with a nonverbal signal to alert the mother when she needed to be tougher; in this way, the stepfather was able to support the mother indirectly and without confronting the daughter. Over time, the stepfather and Carol were able to develop a better relationship.

SUMMARY

Issues relating to divorce and stepfamilies create particular challenges for a counselor. In the case of a divorce that is even more difficult than usual, the ex-spouses are often so hostile to each other that they are unable to communicate, cooperate, or agree on a plan of action in regard to their children; this state of affairs exacerbates the problems of a difficult adolescent, because the adolescent can "divide and conquer" the parents. Three strategies for conducting a "controlled encounter" between warring parents are presented: (1) establishing ground rules, (2) having parents talk directly through the counselor, and (3) finding a workable topic.

In a stepfamily, if a stepparent and teenager are to establish a positive relationship, the biological parent must possess the ability to enforce rules and consequences. If the stepparent attempts to take this role, resentment and conflict will appear, and the biological parent will be caught in the middle. This will cause tremendous stress on both the new spousal bond and the stepparent–adolescent relationship (both of which are tenuous to begin with). Also, parents must be familiar with the common myths regarding blended family interactions and must learn how to deal with them. Two households joined together by marriage will each come with distinct rules, parenting styles, and traditions. These previous histories must be reviewed so that roles and boundaries for the new family can be clearly defined. Five strategies for helping members of a stepfamily address unrealistic expectations are presented: (1) using a nonblaming educational approach, (2) having the biological parent enforce consequences, (3) clarifying the stepparent's role, (4) adapting Step 6 (changing the timing and process of confrontations) for a stepfamily, and (5) understanding the adolescent's developmental needs.

CHAPTER 11

Alcohol and Drug Use
"I Don't Have a Problem"

Research shows that there is a high correlation between other behavioral problems in adolescents and the use of drugs and alcohol (Liddle & Dakof, 1995; Miller, 1992). As a result, the counselor must be skilled in applying the 15-step treatment model to a family suffering from these particular problems. Most adolescents do not see the use of drugs or alcohol as a problem, and therefore do not want to attend a traditional Twelve-Step program such as Alcoholics Anonymous or Narcotics Anonymous (Loeber & Schmalling, 1985; Schmidt, Liddle, & Dakof, 1996). Even if adolescents do attend these programs or are required to do so by court order, the prognosis is likely to be poor if they do not see drug or alcohol use as a problem (Swadi, 1992).

As a result, it is suggested that adolescent substance use may best be addressed through the implementation of creative consequences: Parents clearly define abstaining from drug or alcohol use as a rule for the teenager, and design a set of severe consequences if the rule is not obeyed. The consequences must be painful enough to make the adolescent choose giving up drugs or alcohol over suffering the consequences. The adolescent does not have to agree that his or her substance use is a problem; rather, the teen only has to realize that continuing the behavior is more trouble than it is worth.

Parents, on the other hand, must see drug or alcohol use as a problem, since they are the ones who are responsible for initiating the consequences. If not, the counselor can use the tactic of reasoning that the parents can be held accountable if the police find illicit drugs in their house or if probation or child protective services become involved. However, if parents model deviant behavior or misuse drugs or alcohol themselves, the adolescent is more likely to exhibit the same or similar behavior (Brown, Mounts, Lamborn, & Steinberg, 1993). If this happens, the adolescent has no positive role model and no reason to comply with any consequences for drug or alcohol use. In these cases, the counselor may first have to treat the substance-misusing parent(s) before initiating a treatment plan for the adolescent.

CLINICAL EXAMPLE

The mother of 13-year-old Shawn brought him to counseling because she suspected that he was selling and using marijuana. Large amounts of money were missing; Shawn was ditching school; and he was leaving home without permission at all hours of the night.

At the first session, the counselor suspected that the father was using drugs or alcohol: The father was unable to sit still, was extremely agitated, and had dilated pupils. The counselor also observed parental and marital discord. The mother openly stated that they did not agree on how to parent, and added that she disliked her husband as a person. Neither parent would allude to the fact that one or both parents had a drug or alcohol problem. When Shawn was seen individually, he admitted that he "used and sold pot occasionally," but he did not see pot smoking as a problem. Furthermore, Shawn stated that his dad used cocaine and drank on a daily basis; therefore, why should he stop using if his dad continued to "party"? Shawn told the counselor that no one could stop him from using pot.

Two days later, Shawn decided to test this theory. The mother phoned the counselor and told him that she saw a bag of marijuana in the middle of Shawn's bed with a note attached. The note stated, "Mom, this is my pot and you or that crazy doctor will never stop me from enjoying it when and where I want. Ha ha. Just try and stop me." The counselor asked whether he could come over to the house and offer suggestions; the mother agreed. When the counselor arrived, the mother told him that her husband was drinking at a bar and that Shawn was nowhere to be found. The mother then began to cry and proceeded to reveal a long history of her husband's drug and alcohol misuse. He was intoxicated so often that he could not be counted on for parental support or guidance. The mother also stated that she was on the brink of divorce.

The counselor suggested the following interventions. He found out that the mother had an extended family support system, consisting of her parents and a brother who was a judge. The counselor then convinced the mother to phone her brother and parents immediately for support. The rationale was that unless the mother took a stand now, Shawn would win, and he might use harder drugs in the future. In addition, the mother could be prosecuted if drugs were found in her home. "Taking a stand" consisted of the following actions: phoning the police, filing charges, and asking her brother to come to the house for support. As the police and brother were arriving, Shawn returned home. He looked shocked as he was handcuffed. Shawn even spit in his mother's face as he was being placed in the police car. The police told the mother that the amount of marijuana was small—not enough for Shawn to be charged with a felony. However, the mother's brother (the judge) used his influence to hold Shawn in detention.

Armed with this success, the mother became stronger. As she did so, she demanded that her husband seek help for his drug and alcohol problems. At first, the husband refused. In response, the mother threatened to move out of the home and into an apartment. The husband thought at first that this was just another bluff, because his wife had threatened this move many times before. However, this time the wife had her family's support, and she began to pack. When this happened, the husband finally agreed to an inpatient program and a Twelve-Step program. Over time, the parents were able to exert joint authority, and Shawn's marijuana use and problem behaviors improved.

There appeared to be a direct connection between the changes in Shawn's parents and Shawn's reduction in marijuana use and other problem behaviors. When the father became sober, he was a more effective parent; in turn, the mother felt supported, and the marriage improved. This improvement helped reinforce the father's desire to continue his aftercare treatment. This type of direct connection is supported by a recent study that revealed a significant association between improvement in parenting and a reduction in adolescent drug use and other behavior problems (Schmidt et al., 1996). Finally, all of these changes came as the result of the counselor's ability to mobilize and engage the mother's support system. The mother no longer had to do all the work alone and had the backup she needed to make the difficult changes necessary. The importance of multiple systems in the battle against adolescent substance use is addressed below.

A prevalent idea is that substance misuse is an individual problem and is therefore best addressed on an individual basis. This viewpoint has merit when an adult or even an adolescent views substance misuse as a problem. Twelve-Step programs such as Alcoholics Anonymous or Narcotics Anonymous have shown great success in the treatment of substance use problems. However, as stated earlier, most adolescents do not view substance use as a problem, and they are often still anchored in their families. Because of these factors, the parents must take charge of seeing that something is done. Once this goal is accomplished, an individual Twelve-Step program may be incorporated into the overall treatment plan. These tenacious problems often require a multimodal attack, in which many systems work collaboratively with the parents (e.g., teachers, probation officers, juvenile court judges, extended family members). Solving a teen's substance use problem can be accomplished through the following four strategies: (1) determining the extent of the adolescent's drug or alcohol use and monitoring this behavior closely through random drug screens or sobriety tests; (2) mobilizing multiple systems to empower the parents; (3) implementing specially designed consequences to force the teenager to choose between substance use and freedom; and (4) addressing and solving other family and environmental issues that help maintain the adolescent's substance use.

STRATEGY 1: DETERMINING THE EXTENT OF THE ADOLESCENT'S SUBSTANCE USE

The counselor's first step is to determine the extent of the adolescent's drug or alcohol use. By talking with the adolescent privately, the counselor may be able to ascertain how much of a substance is being used and how often. However, since the adolescent may not answer honestly, it is important to verify these statements with actual random drug tests (or, in the case of alcohol, sobriety tests—see below). After giving their consent, parents must agree not to inform their teenager of a test ahead of time. Since there are ways to contaminate the results of tests for illicit drugs (e.g., using certain herbal supplements), such screening must be random to ensure accuracy.

If parents object to drug testing on the grounds that it violates their teenager's privacy, then the parents are not ready to take charge. The counselor will have to convince the parents that such testing must be performed before proceeding further in treatment. Frequently, the court will order random drug tests for teenagers, with the results submitted directly to a judge or probation officer. If no such court order exists, the counselor may want to request one so as to have the leverage necessary for parental or adolescent compliance.

Since alcohol does not stay in the system long enough to be tested as illicit drugs are, different methods of detection must be used. The simplest is for parents to perform the same field sobriety tests that the police use when evaluating potentially intoxicated drivers. Another option is for the parents to purchase a Breathalyzer to determine more objectively whether their teenager has been drinking. Regardless of the type of substance used, the consequences of being found using the substance will be determined beforehand, so that the parents will not be forced into a power struggle with the teenager. If the adolescent refuses to take the test, then guilt will be assumed and the agreed-upon consequences will be imposed.

Parents are instructed that they are not to apply any consequences unless the adolescent refuses to take a test or unless there is absolute proof that alcohol or drugs are being used. Otherwise, it is not fair to the adolescent, who then feels set up to fail. Random room searches for drugs or alcohol can also be initiated, but only when the adolescent is present. This allows the adolescent to maintain his or her privacy and to feel less violated and more respected.

STRATEGY 2: MOBILIZING MULTIPLE SYSTEMS

Mobilization of outside support systems is important, because parents want to know that the counselor is not asking them to do all the work by themselves. As was the case with Shawn, parents often require the support of out-siders to stand firm and not waver when the adolescent tests the waters. There is power and strength in numbers. The parents will need this power and strength to resolve a difficult problem like drug or alcohol use. This is because a sudden withdrawal of any addictive or pleasurable substance will often lead to an initial extreme reaction; without leverage or support, parents may im-mediately back down out of fear, guilt, or anger.

In addition, an adolescent may try to "divide and conquer" by going to someone outside the immediate family for support.

CLINICAL EXAMPLE

The parents of 16-year-old Juan failed to notify or work collaboratively with their extended family. As a result, when the parents tried to ground Juan for the use of cocaine, he immediately ran to his grandparents' house and told them how he was being abused and grounded for no reason. Without an understand-ing of the overall picture, the grandparents immediately took Juan's side. The grandparents told Juan that he could move into their house. This position caused extreme bitterness and anger between the grandparents and Juan's par-ents. Juan then moved into his grandparent's house and continued his cocaine use unchecked.

Counselors must understand such dynamics and immediately move to mobi-lize or neutralize these outside forces, using the procedures described in Chapter 8. The roles of all the various systems involved must be clarified. The counselor must act as a mediator by bringing all of these outsiders together in the same room to work collaboratively with the parents in formulating a plan of action. All of this is done without the adolescent present. Troubleshooting must then be used in anticipation of the adolescent's negative reactions. If an outsider is not "on the same page" as the parents and other outsiders are, he or she must be neutralized, or the plan can easily unravel.

CLINICAL EXAMPLE

Seventeen-year-old Seth was referred to treatment for his alcohol dependence. The mother was a single parent who stated that she was "scared to death" of Seth's size and strength. In response to this problem, the counselor assembled all of the mother's sources of support in one room. These included her neighbors, her minister, her parents, and her sister.

At this meeting, the following plan was initiated, with the role of each member clearly outlined. If Seth came home intoxicated, the mother would exit and wait, and would phone her minister, neighbors, and parents. They would then come to the mother's home and stand behind her as she required Seth to submit to a Breathalyzer test. If he refused or failed the test, the following consequences would be enforced. Since Seth valued his weekends and the use of his car, the car keys would be taken away immediately. Friday night, Saturday, and Sunday would be spent with the minister at a shelter for the homeless. If Seth was drinking and driving or became violent, the police would be called and charges would be filed. Seth would not get his car back until he remained sober for a week and performed his community service with the minister. If the behavior happened again, the penalty would be extended to 2 weekends of community service with no car. If it happened a third time, the consequence would be extended to 3 weeks, and so on. Furthermore, if the alcohol intoxication continued a second and third time, it would be obvious to everyone that Seth had a problem. At this point, Seth would be offered a choice: either to enroll in an inpatient program and a Twelve-Step aftercare program, or to continue to have his freedom and car use restricted.

The mother's sister immediately objected to this plan, calling it harsh and unfair. With the counselor's subtle guidance, other members in the room were quick to neutralize the sister's objections. They asked her to try the plan as an experiment. If the plan did not work in a month, they would consider an alternative. In the meantime, everyone asked the sister whether she would agree not to harbor Seth or listen to his complaints while the plan was being implemented. The sister agreed.

The mother stated that she was nervous about Seth's getting violent, but she was ready to initiate the plan with everyone's support. The mother was also relieved that she did not have to do all the work herself. Seth tested the plan the same week. The counselor was called and went to the mother's home; the other outsiders arrived at the house as planned. The intervention was successful, and Seth gave his car keys to his mother without a fight. After a third violation, Seth grew tired of losing his freedom and being treated like a "baby." He decided to take the option of inpatient alcohol treatment rather than to continue to lose his freedom. Over time, Seth conquered his alcohol addiction and remained a consistent participant in a Twelve-Step program.

In this case, four important things happened concurrently. First, the mother was able to become a firmer disciplinarian through the support of outsiders. This support increased her power and authority as a parent. When this happened, the mother was able to enforce the necessary consequences to stop Seth's alcohol use. Second, the roles of all outsiders were clarified; the minister, neighbors, and parents each knew when to come to the house and how to empower the mother. Third, the sister's threat to unravel the plan was neutralized in a respectful manner. The other outsiders asked the sister for her permission and approval to initiate the plan. Finally, the consequence was custom-designed to make continued alcohol use a hardship on Seth. The consequences made Seth accountable for his actions and led him to seek treatment. Without this multimodal attack, Seth's alcohol dependence would probably have continued.

STRATEGY 3: IMPLEMENTING SEVERE CONSEQUENCES FOR DRUG OR ALCOHOL USE

Since adolescent drug and alcohol use occurs most frequently within peer groups, it is very likely that the peer subsystem will influence an adolescent to continue the behavior. In addition, the freedom to see friends, especially on weekends, is something that the adolescent will not want interrupted or terminated. Therefore, a teenager who remains drug-free and sober may be given the freedom to see anyone he or she wishes. However, if test results are positive, the adolescent is grounded and forbidden to have any contact with friends (except at school) until the test results are negative or until he or she has abstained from substance use for a specified period of time.

If grounding is not effective, the counselor can recommend that the parents use one of the other consequences described in Chapter 6. For one 16-year-old who tested positive for marijuana use, grounding simply did not work; however, when the parents pawned his compact disc collection, he immediately stopped using marijuana for fear of losing his stereo system. The limitations of this strategy are that once the random drug or sobriety tests stop, an adolescent may return to his or her previous behavior, especially if the teen did not see it as a problem in the first place. Therefore, depending on the case, the parents may need to continue with surprise spot checks or random testing to keep the adolescent on the alert.

CLINICAL EXAMPLE

Sixteen-year-old Savannah was referred to outpatient counseling after five attempts at inpatient care (four stays in an inpatient hospital and one in a "boot camp" setting) to stop her alcohol and methamphetamine use. By the time Savannah began counseling, she was unable to sleep, had severe weight loss, and was prone to violent outbursts. In addition, she was suicidal, ran away continually, did not attend school, and had threatened her father and stepmother with a knife.

Savannah was tiny in stature (4'11"), but her father was extremely afraid of her angry outbursts. This was ironic, because the father was a Special Forces captain in the Army. The stepmother reported that she would have to take over, because the father would back down any time Savannah yelled. This only caused further resentment and tension between the stepmother and Savannah. In addition, the father thought his wife was too hard on Savannah, and the stepmother had reached the point of considering divorce.

Savannah reported that she did not have a drug or alcohol problem, and that even if she did, she would be able to stop. According to Savannah, all she needed was for everyone to "get off her case" and let her do as she pleased. If not, "people would be sorry." Savannah had proven this statement the previous week by attempting to cut her wrists with a kitchen knife when she was not allowed out of the house to see friends.

With such a multitude of problems, the counselor did not know where to begin. Although he wanted to address the drug and alcohol issues first, he knew that this would not be possible until he got the threats of violence and suicide under control. So he started off with a 24-hour suicide watch for Savannah. With this intervention, Savannah would be watched continuously until the danger passed (see Chapter 6 for more details). Getting the father to agree, however, took considerable skill and finesse. The counselor pointed out that since other outside experts had failed to stop the problem, the father was Savannah's last hope. Otherwise, she would be likely to die from a drug overdose within a year. The counselor also told the father that he would be available 24 hours a day, 7 days a week for consultation and home visits until the father was successful. After the counselor addressed a lengthy list of "what if" scenarios, the father agreed to his treatment plan. The bathroom strategy was also incorporated to secure Savannah at night and prevent her from running away. The takedown procedure was described and role-played ahead of time.

The counselor had to make several home visits, but within 1 week's time, Savannah was begging to be removed from the 24-hour watch. In addition, the father became hopeful once he saw that he could control Savannah's violence in a nonabusive fashion. He also learned how to recognize when his buttons were being pushed, how to exit and wait, and how to stay short and to the point. With this renewed energy and early success, the father was ready to tackle the drug and alcohol problems.

Eager to end the 24-hour watch, Savannah agreed to the following terms: random hair tests for drug use weekly, and filling out four job applications per day (under the supervision of the father) until she obtained a job. If Savannah's test results were positive, she would be confined to the house and placed on 24-hour watch until she submitted a "clean" drug test. The father, stepmother, and counselor then engaged in troubleshooting to review everything that could go wrong. Savannah did relapse several times over the course of counseling; however, each time there were no guilt trips and no disappointment expressed. The father simply enforced the consequence, with the intention of getting back on track as quickly as possible. The stepmother and Savannah even became closer as the father took charge and the stepmother was no longer seen as the sole disciplinarian. Savannah eventually found a job and felt proud of herself. This increase in self-esteem helped her stay sober, as did becoming friends with people through work who were positive influences. The more time Savannah spent with her new friends, the less time she spent going out with her old friends who were still using drugs.

STRATEGY 4: ADDRESSING OTHER FAMILY AND ENVIRONMENTAL ISSUES

For consequences to be successful, parents and teenagers must successfully complete the other steps of the family-based model. While the parents closely monitor the ongoing drug or alcohol use, the counselor must simultaneously work with the family to alter parent–child interactions and address other family or environmental problems. This is because drug or alcohol use is often a symptom of other problems (Steinglass, 1987). It is often a teenager's best way of coping within the family or the larger environment, as two examples illustrate.

CLINICAL EXAMPLE

A case in point involved 14-year-old Joshua, who was unable to tell his father how he felt unless he was drunk. For Joshua, alcohol served a problem-solving role by helping him to be assertive in his communication with the father. Therefore, if the counselor had not helped the father and son change their communication patterns without the use of alcohol, there would have been no reason for Joshua to give up drinking.

CLINICAL EXAMPLE

All but one of 15-year-old Eric's friends used cocaine. Eric was concerned that if he stopped using cocaine, he would lose the majority of his friends. Therefore, it became clear that Eric's cocaine use served a purpose greater than the enjoyment of the drug itself; It also provided him with admission and perceived acceptance into a powerful peer group. Therefore, unless this problem could be solved by other means, there was no reason why Eric should stop using cocaine. With this knowledge, the counselor held a meeting with Eric and his one friend who did not use drugs.

With the counselor's assistance, Eric and his friend brainstormed ways they could stay sober by putting themselves in situations where they could meet new friends. This list included sports, extracurricular activities, and double-dating. Eric initially maintained his association with his former peer group and had several relapses. However, while this was happening, he began to make new friends through dating and school activities. Once this new social environment was firmly in place, Eric no longer needed the cocaine; his usage decreased, and he eventually remained drug-free.

SUMMARY

For the 15-step model to be effective in a case where adolescent substance use is a problem, the counselor must first help parents closely monitor their teenager's substance use, with the understanding that alcohol or drugs are often used to solve or cope with other problems both inside and outside of the family environment. Otherwise, once the monitoring stops, the adolescent will have no reason not to return to drug or alcohol use.

The teenager's family and social environment must also be modified in such a way that the continued use of drugs or alcohol is no longer needed;

this is often a challenge for even the most experienced counselor. In addition to helping the parents implement stringent consequences for substance use, the counselor must address other behavior problems (e.g., depression, running away, and violence) while also organizing many different systems (e.g., the family, school, and peers). This is not impossible, but it is difficult.

The counselor must have the ability to divide multidimensional problems into workable and solvable components that can then be prioritized. As one problem is solved and then another, the momentum intensifies, and the parents' confidence in the counselor grows stronger (as it did in the case of Savannah, above). When this happens, the parents may now be willing to make the investment of time and energy necessary to tackle the more difficult problem of substance use. Many counselors make the mistake of taking on this giant problem too early in the treatment process. The parents may not yet possess the strength, determination, or trust in their counselor that comes from solving less extreme problems. As a result, interventions to stop the drug or alcohol problem can fail. The counselor must first know the territory (i.e., must understand how the drug or alcohol use solves other problems) and then mobilize both parental and outside forces. Usually this opportunity only arrives after helping the parents achieve victory over other presenting problems.

PART FOUR

RESEARCH FINDINGS
AND FUTURE IMPLICATIONS

CHAPTER 12

Process–Outcome Research and the Family-Based Model

Refining and Operationalizing Key Theoretical Concepts

The aim of this chapter is to show how I used the process–outcome research method of "task analysis" (Rice & Greenberg, 1984) to create the 15-step family-based model for difficult adolescents.* I describe how I used video-taped counseling sessions and focus group interviews with both counselors and clients to shape and refine the model itself. The findings from these sessions and interviews served as feedback to clarify and strengthen the theoretical concepts developed in earlier phases of the research. For example, in the focus group interviews, parents reported that disrespect was an "ace" that neutralized their effectiveness. This information led to a change in the original model and the addition of disrespect as one of the "five aces." This chapter also shows how concepts drawn directly from this model can be operationalized and tested for effectiveness via outcome measures. Finally, future implications of this type of process–outcome research for family therapy and other mental health fields are discussed and highlighted.

CURRENT CHALLENGES AND CONTROVERSIES IN MENTAL HEALTH CARE RESEARCH

Ready or not, our field is caught up in a health care revolution that demands accountability. Health care insurers require demonstrations of our services'

---

*I would like to give special recognition to Dr. Neil Schiff and Jay Haley for their review of and help with this chapter. They are among the first to open up their videotape library for the scrutiny and analysis of an entire case study. Because of their foresight and vision, as well as their help and guidance, this research was possible.

effectiveness with particular problems and treatment populations. Many counselors write books and articles that claim effectiveness, but fail to demonstrate the processes and empirical outcomes that back up such claims. This lack of accountability and credibility gives little comfort to third-party payers, legislators, students, or fellow professionals. The problem can be traced to three main causes: (1) treatment models with procedures that are abstract, generalized, and difficult to implement; (2) outcome studies that answer the question "Does it work?" before answering the question "How does it work?"; and (3) a failure to combine process and outcome research to create, refine, or operationalize treatment models.

Treatment Models That Lack Specificity

Most treatment models either lack specificity or contain procedures that are abstract, generalized, and difficult to implement. A particular model is often employed because it is popular at the time, because it fits with a particular counselor's treatment philosophy, or because it mirrors the philosophy of the school where the counselor received his or her training. In an article on research into the effectiveness of marital and family therapy, Pinsof and Wynne (1995) conclude that "in almost all of [this] research, it is impossible to know what actually occurred in counseling" (p. 606). This should certainly concern counselors as the 21st century approaches. Without the specification of key concepts, it is difficult if not impossible to assess what takes place in any particular counseling session so that its effectiveness can be determined. Counseling then becomes a mystical process behind closed doors, rather than a systematic one that is well articulated. Under these conditions, it is not surprising that third-party payers are leery about funding undefined and untested treatments.

Outcome Studies That Fail to Account for Their Results

The majority of current research consists of comparative/competitive or "who won" studies, which pit one treatment approach against another (e.g., cognitive therapy vs. structural family therapy with depressed women aged 19–35) but fail to specify what factors within the model were associated with improvement and deterioration. Without this information, the study may have little relevance for an individual counselor. The counselor reads that one treatment approach is better than another, but has no idea what particular techniques might be responsible for the superiority of the first approach. Outcome research without process research is therefore minimally informative.

In a review summarizing trends in theory and research from 1980 to 1987, Bednar, Burlingame, and Masters (1988) stated that 140 family counseling studies revealed a virtual absence of treatment variables drawn from systems theory literature. The reviewers concluded by saying that rigorous experimental outcome research was premature for a field that had yet to operationalize its essential theoretical concepts. Wynne (1988) reached a similar conclusion:

> The term "research" is often understood by psychotherapists as referring to confirmatory studies, such as comparative studies of the outcome of the two methods of counseling. In sharp contrast to this usual view, at the present stage of development of the family therapy field, a strong emphasis should be given to exploratory, discovery-oriented and hypothesis-generating research, rather than primarily or exclusively to confirmatory research. (p. 251)

Before a particular counseling model can be applied, the concepts must be operationally defined. Outcome studies that answer the question "Does it work?" before answering the question "How does it work?" are suspect and premature.

Failure to Combine Process and Outcome Research

Once investigators have an idea of how a model performs through process research, they must conduct outcome studies to determine whether the model does work. Often one step is conducted without the other. If the outcome studies fail to show effectiveness, this is invaluable feedback. It informs the researchers that parts of the model are not working or that this particular model does not work with a particular problem (e.g., alcohol or drug use, depression, psychosis) or treatment population (e.g., adult, individual, child). The researchers are then forced to reevaluate the model to strengthen or revise it in specific ways.

GOALS AND OBJECTIVES OF MY PROJECT

To address these challenges, I focused on the following two objectives in my research: (1) developing a treatment manual, and (2) combining process and outcome research. This section describes how focusing on these areas addressed each of the research gaps noted above.

Developing a Treatment Manual

Before embarking on this project in 1994, I realized that I had to address each of the above-described research gaps. First, I had to provide counselors with a road map of step-by-step procedures, techniques, themes, and therapeutic maneuvers. This was needed because current books and articles on treatment with difficult adolescents often lacked specificity. The current treatment models (i.e., multitarget ecological treatment, functional family therapy, social learning counseling, strategic therapy, and structural therapy) articulated key theoretical concepts (e.g., hierarchy, boundaries, power, ecosystems, coercive interaction patterns), but failed to provide readers with a step-by-step account of how and when these concepts should be implemented. In addition, there was an abundance of "who won" studies with difficult adolescents (e.g., Chamberlain & Rosicky, 1995), but these studies lacked relevance for the individual counselor because they failed to provide information on the specific treatment components that affected change.

With such a challenging population, I wanted to be able to tell a counselor what to do and when to do it if A, B, or C should occur. For example, what should the counselor do the next time the parents refuse to take charge? Can he or she choose from a menu of creative and innovative techniques? Although I realized that there is no magic formula, I needed a more explicit road map to increase my chances of helping the counselor succeed and keep one step ahead of the cunning adolescent or resistant parent.

Second, the treatment manual also had to be flexible enough to be customized to meet the needs of individual clients without stifling the flexibility, innovation, and creativity of the counselor. My goal was not to produce a rigid application of treatment, but to give guidelines that were systemic yet adaptable enough to encompass novel situations and circumstances. For example, what does one do with a single mother who cannot take charge because she has no support systems? Or with an adolescent who is protected by a highly dysfunctional set of peers? Many manuals feature a simplistic, "one size fits all" approach that is simply unrealistic with difficult adolescents. A counselor only has to be around them for a short time to realize that creativity and quick thinking are essential qualities for success.

Finally, I felt that the manual itself had to emerge directly from an intensive case-by-case study of counseling sessions and focus group interviews with both clients and counselors, rather than strictly from a literature review in the library. As stated earlier, many family counseling models have yet to operationalize essential theoretical concepts or to map out these concepts in clinical practice rather than in a laboratory setting. As a result, I felt that theory had to be linked directly with clinical practice.

Combining Process and Outcome Research

To accomplish my second goal, I used a "task analysis" method (Rice & Greenberg, 1984) to conduct the process research portion of the study, and then I used outcome measures to test the key theoretical concepts that emerged. A task analysis methodology would help me discover key moments of change within counseling sessions from an intensive analysis of videotaped interviews and self-reports from clients and counselors. The characteristics of these moments of change could then be written up as hypotheses and tested through outcome measures. Results from these outcome measures would then be used to clarify or strengthen these moments of change. For example, pretest measures supported the hypothesis that difficult adolescents and their parents enter treatment with severe conflict and a lack of nurturance. This outcome data strengthened the need for the procedural step or restoring nurturance and tenderness within the 15-step model. Elsewhere, my colleagues and I have discussed the benefits and procedures of blending qualitative process research and quantitative outcome research within the same study, and have described how these two methods can reciprocally help clarify, strengthen, or refine key theoretical concepts (see Sells, Smith, & Sprenkle, 1995).

DEVELOPMENT OF THE 15-STEP MODEL: A TASK ANALYSIS APPROACH

In this section, I illustrate through sample flow charts and coding manuals how the 15-step family-based model was created. The entire process can be referred to as "discovery-oriented" because the key concepts were generated not from a review of the literature, but directly from an intensive study of clinical practice cases. The research consisted of the following five phases: (I) creating idealized performance models, (II) creating revised performance models, (III) broadening the range of application, (IV) consolidating the theoretical yield, and (V) combining process and outcome research.

Phase I: Creating Idealized Performance Models

During the first phase of the project, I went to the library and located books and articles that outlined theoretical concepts and treatment procedures for difficult adolescents (i.e., teenagers between the ages of 12 and 18 who meet the DSM-IV diagnostic criteria for either oppositional defiant disorder or conduct disorder).* I extracted the major concepts from this literature and

---

*The books and articles under study came from structural, strategic, solution-focused, and multidimensional treatment models (i.e., Fishman, 1988; Haley, 1976, 1980; Keim, 1996; Liddle, 1995; Madanes, 1991; Minuchin, 1974; Minuchin, Montalvo, Guerney, Rosman, & Schumer, 1967; Price, 1996; Selekman, 1993). Other treatment models were not selected because they were not theoretically congruent with the 15-step family-based model or a systems theory framework. All of the models selected for review were theoretically congruent with a family systems perspective.

placed them into a spreadsheet format. I combined these spreadsheets into three idealized performance models—what should theoretically happen throughout the treatment process. The key concepts were then placed in a step-by-step treatment or laid out within the literature. The process of consolidating the many different concepts on spreadsheets and arranging them in the three hypothesized series of optimal procedural steps was like taking hundreds of tiny puzzle pieces and trying to place them together in the proper order, with little to go on except similar shapes and colors. The three idealized theoretical models corresponded to three separate stages consisting of "markers"—clinically significant events appearing to change the course and direction of the treatment process. Each of the models is described and illustrated below, to show the step-by-step process by which the models were created.

Model 1/Stage 1: The Parents Decide Whether or Not to Take Charge

According to the literature, the first stage of treatment seems to begin with the counselor's calling the parents to set up the first appointment and to end with the adolescent's functioning without behavior problems. There also appears to be a proverbial "fork in the road," at which point the parents choose to accept or not to accept a position of changing their teenager's problem behavior. Which road the parents choose often seems to depend on the quality of the parents' rapport with the counselor and on whether or not the counselor is seen as a credible expert. Once the decision is made, a series of steps should follow. If the parents refuse to take charge, the teenager or other outsiders will take charge, and treatment will end unsuccessfully. If the parents do take charge, the counselor will assist the parents through a series of steps to keep the parents in this position of authority, troubleshoot potential problems with interventions, and stop the teen's extreme behavior problems.

Each step within each of the three idealized models was operationalized in terms of observable behaviors. These behaviors were then defined in a coding manual format. For example, the concept of "presession preparation" (Step 1 of the first model) was defined in the following manner:

Step 1: Presession Preparation

Before the first session, the counselor personally contacts the parents and explicitly asks them to come in with their son or daughter to help him or her with the identified problem by providing information and guidance that only they can provide. They should not be asked to come in to have "therapy," because few people want "therapy." Following this same rationale, members of the extended family (including other siblings, grandparents, etc.) are also asked to attend.

This observational code is defined with statements made by the counselor to the parents asking them to come in with their teenager "to help the teenager with his [her] problems by providing valuable information to the counselor." Everyone in the family, including other siblings, is asked to attend.

Model 1/Stage 1 is illustrated in Figure 12.1.

Model 2/Stage 2: Therapist and Family Deal with Crises and Relapses

It appears from the literature that Stage 2 begins with a relapse of the difficult teenager and ends with the parents' weathering the storm by devising a plan to prevent further relapses. There are basically two reasons for this relapse. First, once the teenager is functioning without problems, the parents are lulled into a false sense of security. They think that these changes are permanent. However, the teenager is not likely to hand over his or her power and authority without a fight and at least one major relapse to test the waters. The teenager wants things to return to the status quo. A teenager functioning without behavior problems has not yet had enough time to realize that most of his or her needs can be met through good behavior. For many teenagers, being "good" is a change in identity and feels awkward and different. As a result, the risk and temptation for at least one major relapse are high.

Second, the teenager's problem may be a conscious or unconscious attempt to shift the focus off more threatening issues in the family, such as marital conflict, depression, or substance misuse. If the parents or other family members remain focused on the teenager's problem, other issues are not addressed. Consequently, every time the teenager begins to function normally and without problems, the family becomes unstable and other problems surface. The adolescent must again function incompetently and relapse, to shift the focus off these other problems so that the family can restabilize. This cycle will repeat itself again and again until the underlying family issues are solved or resolved.

These two reasons may be occurring separately or together. The teenager will probably always want to test the waters, regardless of whether or not there is a connection with other family issues. The counselor can spot whether such a connection exists if other family problems surface immediately or soon after the behavior problems are solved.

In either case, the parents' reaction to the relapse is usually negative. They feel personally betrayed and take a "here we go again" attitude. When this happens, the parents' inclination is either to remove the teenager from the family and place him or her in an institution, or to feel apathetic and give up. At this point, the counselor must take charge and somehow convince the

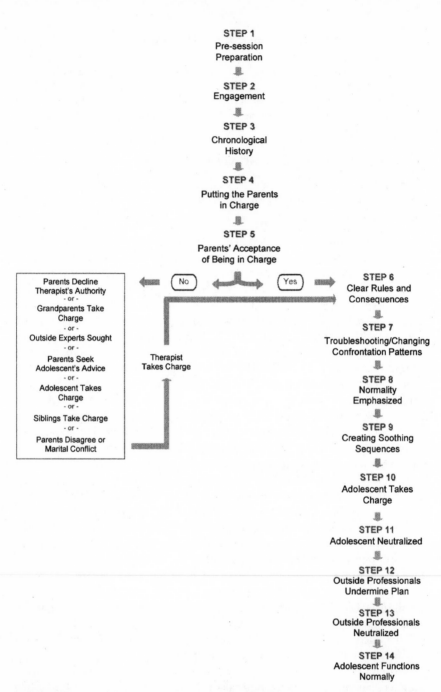

FIGURE 12.1. Model 1/Stage 1: The parents decide whether or not to take charge. The steps of this model are illustrated to show what the family will go through, depending on whether the parents choose to take charge or refuse to accept this responsibility. Each step is operationalized within a coding manual format in terms of observable behaviors. Stage

266

parents to stand firm and not give up. Instead, they must devise a plan of action to address the present relapse and prevent further relapses from occurring in the future. The counselor must try to prevent institutionalization; otherwise, the parents risk starting from scratch when the teenager finally returns home.

Model 2/Stage 2 is illustrated in Figure 12.2.

Model 3/Stage 3: Peace Sets In and Teenager Moves into Adulthood

It appears from the literature that Stage 3 begins when the adolescent continues to test the limits, but does so in a way that is not extreme (not, e.g., violence, running away, truancy, etc.). The stage ends when relapse ends on a permanent basis. The adolescent is then able to move freely through the developmental stage of individuation by leaving home and becoming an adult.

In essence, at the end of Stage 1, the parents survive the initial onslaught of the hurricane and briefly experience calmness in the eye of the storm, but do not buckle or fold when the hurricane resumes its gale force winds in Stage 2. In Stage 3, the parents survive the hurricane and can finally enjoy the fruits of their labor, as the hierarchy is permanently reversed and they maintain their authority even when it is tested. As a result, calmness and peace set in within the household on a consistent basis. The teenager is now free to shift his or her time and energy from trying to maintain power and authority to pursuing employment, dating, sports, and/or college, and eventually leaving the home to become an adult. It is important to note that this disengagement from the family is also contingent upon the resolution of underlying family issues. Otherwise, the teenager will be unable to disengage from the family and will display self-destructive behavior that prevents him or her from leaving home to become self-supporting.

Model 3/Stage 3 is illustrated in Figure 12.3.

---

1 begins with the therapist's calling the parent to set up the first appointment in Step 1 and ends with the adolescent's functioning without behavioral problems in Step 14. Concepts within Model 1 were drawn directly from the literature (i.e., structural, strategic, solution-focused, and multidimensional). For example, the concept of the parents' taking charge emerged directly from the structural and strategic writings about hierarchy (Minuchin et al., 1967; Minuchin, 1974) and power (Haley, 1980; Madanes, 1991). The concept of engagement in Step 2 emerged from the work of Liddle (1995). The concept of how outsiders neutralize the parents' or therapist's authority emerged from the descriptions of conducting a multidimensional assessment within the Liddle (1995) article and the writings of Haley (1980). In addition, the creation of soothing sequences or the restoration of nurturance originated in the writing of Keim (1996).

STEP 1
Relapse of
Adolescent

↓

STEP 2
Parents Feel
Personally Betrayed
-or-
Adolescent Placed In
Institution Outside Family
-or-
Parents Feel Apathetic
Or Hopeless

↓

STEP 3
Therapist Takes Charge

↓

STEP 4
Parents Define Goal

↓

STEP 5
Clear Rules and
Consequences Outlined

↓

STEP 6
Preparation

↓

STEP 7
Troubleshooting

↓

STEP 8
Adolescent Functions
Normally

↓

STEP 9
Second Relapse;
Institutionalization
Prevented

FIGURE 12.2. Model 2/Stage 2: Therapist and family deal with crises and relapses. The steps of this model illustrate the onset of Stage 2 with the adolescent's relapsing and the actions that follow to prevent institutionalization or a future relapse. Stage 2 ends after the parents implement their plan of action and another relapse is prevented. Each step is operationalized within a coding manual format in terms of observable behaviors. Many key concepts in Model 2, such as relapse and the therapist's taking charge, emerged from Haley's (1976, 1980) work. Other concepts, such as preparation and troubleshooting, emerged from the work of Madanes (1991). In sum, Haley's work provided the framework of Model 2, while Madanes's work helped fill in the missing pieces.

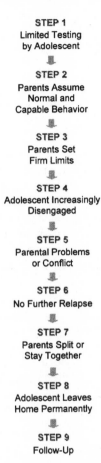

FIGURE 12.3. Model 3/Stage 3: Peace sets in and adolescent moves into adulthood. The steps of this model illustrate the onset of Stage 3 with the adolescent's continuing to test limits, but in a way that is not extreme (not, e.g., violence, running away, truancy, etc.). The stage ends when a state of nonrelapse continues and the adolescent is free to move through the developmental stage of individuating from the family by eventually leaving home and becoming an adult. Key theoretical concepts in Model 3, such as disengagement and parental problems, emerged from the work of both Haley (1980) and Minuchin (1974). The overall process of leaving home and pursuing adulthood came from Haley's (1980) work.

Phase II: Creating Revised Performance Models

When Phase I was completed, I began Phase II by following Rice and Greenberg's (1984) recommendation to acquire and analyze videotapes from "expert clinicians regarded by colleagues, trainees and clients as being instrumental in facilitating substantial amounts of positive client change" (p. 291).

I analyzed each videotaped counseling session and created a description in coding manual format and a performance model diagram to accompany each session. Each procedural step was a "marker," or series of interventions hypothesized to be optimal for promoting change.

After each tape was completed, I compared the performance model diagram and the coding manual with the appropriate portion of my three idealized models to locate similarities and differences. If a marker in a model based on an actual counseling session was similar to a marker in an idealized model, the matching idealized theoretical concept was strengthened. If there were discrepancies or new discoveries, I made revisions accordingly. For example, after the first videotaped session was analyzed, one marker closely matched the idealized model's concept of engagement. This idealized theoretical concept was therefore supported and strengthened. In contrast, a new concept also emerged from this session—one that involved the parents' redefining the son's problem behavior. This led me to include the new procedural step of defining and redefining the problem in the revised performance model.

This process of shifting back and forth between analyzing actual videotapes and revising models continued for each videotaped treatment session. A final revised performance model emerged at the conclusion of Phase II; this model contained both original theoretical ideas and new and exciting discoveries from the videotapes. Below is a brief description of each part of Phase II, together with several performance model diagrams to demonstrate the research process. The final revised performance model is also illustrated, to highlight the developmental steps in creating the 15-step family-based treatment model.

Part 1: Acquiring Videotapes of Expert Clinicians

As stated earlier, an intensive study of videotaped treatment sessions conducted by expert clinicians is an ideal approach. This is because most process researchers select the work of student counselors or counselors who are not regarded as experts in the model under investigation (Mahrer, 1988; Rice & Saperia, 1984). A closely related issue is a lack of "treatment integrity," or the failure of counselors to adhere to the guidelines specified within the treatment model (Pinsof & Wynne, 1995). It becomes increasingly difficult to locate key moments of change when one is uncertain whether change is even occurring or whether the treatment model guidelines are being followed.

To address these problems, I asked Jay Haley, the founder of strategic family therapy, if I could analyze videotaped counseling sessions that he felt were instrumental in facilitating significant amounts of positive change. After hearing about the project, he consented and suggested an intensive, beginning-to-end analysis of a 28-session case involving an 18-year-old male who exhibited extreme behavior problems (i.e., threats and acts of violence).

Haley stated that this case contained all the essential theoretical concepts and procedures for promoting change in difficult adolescents, and that it was therefore representative of how to work with this population. In addition, Haley stated that the counseling was successful in this case, as indicated by an annual follow-up for 10 years that showed no relapses or return to previous problem behaviors. The adolescent had since graduated from college and was functioning successfully as a high school art teacher.

Neil Schiff was the counselor in this case, while Jay Haley supervised each session from behind a one-way mirror. Both Schiff and Haley are considered by colleagues, trainees, and clients to be the leading experts in treating difficult adolescents and their families.

Part 2: Constructing a Performance Model from an Analysis of Videotapes

Briefly, a performance model was constructed from an intensive analysis of all 28 sessions. Each videotaped session was transcribed; the markers were operationalized within a coding manual format; and the procedural steps were illustrated on a schematic diagram. Each code was accompanied by an actual transcript from the session to support the inclusion of that particular code. For example, the marker of "task check" emerged from the third session and was operationally defined in the following manner:

Step 3: Task Check

The counselor asks the parents and the adolescent whether the teenager and/or the parents completed the tasks assigned at the end of the last session. After giving a task, the counselor should always ask for a report at some time in the next interview. In this way, the teenager and parents are accountable for completing each task.

This observational code is defined as one or more statements by the counselor asking the parents and the teenager whether the tasks assigned at the end of last session were completed.

Sample Dialogue from Session

Time: 3 minutes and 30 seconds into video session

67   Ther: Well I'm delighted that you had some more normal
68   moods, but I'm disturbed about you crashing, and I wish, I
69   hope that there's something we can set up that will alleviate
70   the pain associated with that. Anyway, let me go on a bit and
71   then come back to this. Did you register for a course?

Figure 12.4 is the performance model diagram that emerged from the third counseling session. Notice that the parents vacillated between taking

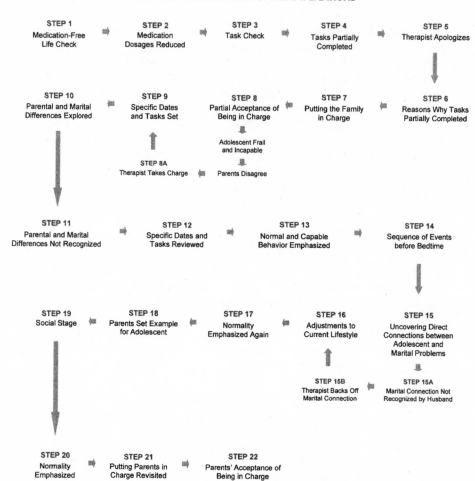

FIGURE 12.4. Session 3 of counseling: Videotape-based performance model diagram.

charge and refusing to take charge in Steps 8, 21, and 22. In response, the counselor asked the parents in Step 8A to take charge and set tasks with specific time frames for completion. Notice also how the parents struggled with defining their son as frail, incapable, and not responsible for his extreme behavior under Step 8. The counselor countered by redefining the adolescent as normal, capable, and responsible for his actions in Steps 13, 17, and 20. The counselor also emphasized the normality of the son in Steps 1 and 2 by convincing the parents to decrease the son's medication. As stated earlier in this book, the use of medication can result in an adolescent's being labeled as a chemically imbalanced mental patient, rather than as a misbehaving teenager responsible for his or her own behavior. This theme of emphasizing normality, capability, and responsibility also emerged in later sessions and was influential in the construction of Step 3 (parental empowerment) and in Step 2 (defining and redefining problems) of the family-based treatment model.

Part 3: Informant Verification

After each session was analyzed, the coding manual and diagram for that session were sent to both Neil Schiff and Jay Haley. I interviewed each clinician by phone and asked whether he agreed or disagreed with my conceptualization of each procedural step contained in the coding manual. If there were discrepancies, the concept was modified accordingly. For example, Schiff and Haley both stated that a third relapse was avoided due to Schiff's use of "troubleshooting," whereas I described the same event as "problem solving." The concept was then modified to fit the definition of "troubleshooting" and operationalized according to Schiff's and Haley's descriptions. The term "informant verification" refers to the extent to which a set of meanings held by multiple observers are sufficiently congruent that they describe the phenomenon in the same way and arrive at the same conclusions (Goetz & LeCompte, 1984). I used informant verification to assess the reliability of the codes; that is, I checked to see whether Schiff, Haley, and I independently described the codes in the same way and arrived at the same conclusions.

In addition to checking reliability, these interviews helped shape the final revised performance model by expanding my conceptual definitions and highlighting key interventions that promoted optimal change. These brainstorming sessions by telephone generated rich clinical data. For example, we discovered that the use of role plays or "dry runs" was essential to prepare the parents for future confrontations with their teenager. A turning point in the case came when the father asked his son to return the house keys and move out because of his extreme acts of violence. Schiff prepared the father for this critical confrontation by playing the part of the son while the father practiced his delivery of what he would say. We all felt that this preparation was key to the father's ability to take charge. These valuable discussions led to the creation of role plays or "dry runs" as a strategy or mini-step in the larger step of troubleshooting.

Part 4: Comparing the Videotape-Based Performance Models with the Idealized Models

After the videotape-based performance model diagram for each session was further refined on the basis of my telephone interviews with Haley and Schiff, I compared it with the approximate portion of the three idealized models. If there were similarities, then the idealized theoretical concepts were validated. On the other hand, if there were discrepancies, I made revisions accordingly. I demonstrate this process by providing and discussing three diagrams: one for the idealized Stage 1 model, or Model 1 (Figure 12.5A); one for the videotape-based performance model for Session 1 of counseling (Figure 12.5B); and one for the revised performance model for Session 1 that resulted from my integration of these two models (Figure 12.5C).

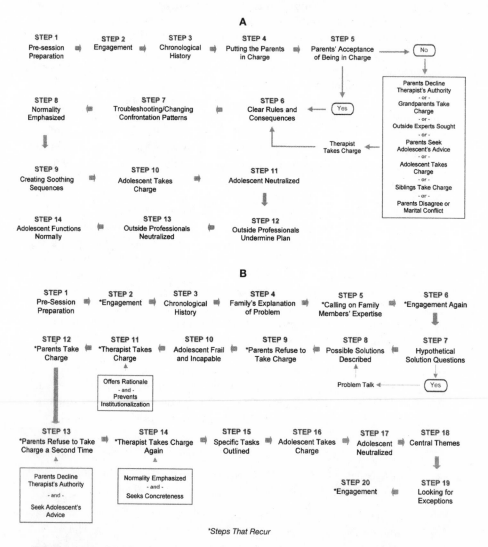

FIGURE 12.5. (A) The idealized Stage 1 model (Model 1). (B) The videotape-based performance model for Session 1 of counseling.

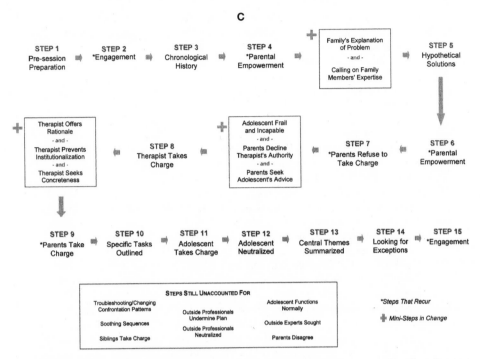

FIGURE 12.5. (C) The revised performance model for Session 1 of counseling, based on my integration of the models shown in A and B.

Comparison of Session 1 and the Idealized Model

Notice how the first three steps within the Session 1 videotape-based performance model were identical to those of the idealized model. From this point on, however, there were discrepancies and similarities. Step 4 (family's explanation of the problem) and Step 5 (calling on family members' expertise) of the Session 1 model did not occur anywhere within the idealized model. Thus, these concepts were organized under Step 4 of the revised Session 1 model under the broader category of parental empowerment. This was done because calling on the family's expertise and asking them to define the problem were both strategies designed to empower the family members to solve their own problems. The two models were similar with regard to the parents' decision to take charge or not to take charge. As a result, these concepts in the idealized model were substantiated.

An exciting breakthrough came with the discovery that two key procedural steps recurred throughout the counseling session. The Session 1 videotape-based model indicated that the parents vacillated between assuming and refusing authority throughout the counseling session. In addition, engagement was not a one-time step and continued to surface throughout the first counseling session. The idealized model made it appear that certain steps occurred only once throughout the counseling process; however, the Session 1 model indicated the opposite. Counseling with a difficult adolescent was discovered to be a very fluid and circular process, as key steps continued to resurface again and again. These repeating patterns made it easier to identify steps that were optimal for change.

Other discrepancies between the models centered around the use of solution-focused hypothetical and exception questions, as well as the concept of revisiting central themes. As I continued to make revisions, these steps were rearranged under broader categories. For example, the use of solution-focused questions was classified in Step 5 of the final revised performance model (clear rules and consequences outlined) when analysis showed that the counselor used these types of questions as a way to define rules and consequences clearly.

The revised Session 1 performance model that resulted from comparing the Session 1 videotape-based model with the idealized Model 1 thus retained the idealized concepts from Model 1, but added the following new components: *recurrence of empowerment; recurrence of parents' taking charge; recurrence of engagement; hypothetical solutions; looking for exceptions;* and *summarizing central themes.* Steps within the idealized model that were not observed or that were still unaccounted for after my analysis of Session 1 were listed next to the revised performance model, in the event that they arose in future videotaped sessions.

In sum, each cycle of looping back and forth between the idealized model and a videotape-based performance model both clarified and further operationalized existing theoretical concepts. The process also uncovered new and exciting discoveries. The process could be compared to the work of an anthropologist who has books and ancient descriptions of a particular population, but goes to the ruins of this civilization to discover new artifacts that both confirm and deny these original writings. These artifacts not only lead to an expansion and clearer definition of these original writings, but also generate new and exciting discoveries.

Part 5: Constructing the Final Revised Performance Model

After analyzing all 28 taped sessions and comparing the results with the three idealized models, I constructed a final revised performance model by integrating all of the preceding models and noting similarities and discrepancies. Steps that were similar in concept were placed under one main category. For example, several revised performance models contained steps that pertained to seeking concreteness, outlining specific tasks, and setting specific dates. Each of these described the same basic process of outlining clear rules, consequences, and task procedures. Consequently, these steps were integrated under one main category called Step 5 (clear rules, tasks, and consequences out-lined).

Another interpretation of this process is that "mini-steps" were united into one main step. For example, executing role plays or "dry runs" and constructing "what if" scenarios were the mini-steps the counselor took in conducting the larger step of "troubleshooting." These mini-steps were particularly helpful because they represented the step-by-step procedures used to achieve the end result. This process of integrating smaller, related steps under one main category continued until one final revised performance model remained. Figure 12.6 is an illustration of this final model. The question mark next to Step 8 in Figure 12.6 indicates that although the concept of soothing sequences was contained within the idealized models, it was not identified in any of the 28 taped sessions. This step was implied during several of Schiff's interventions, but without the clarity needed to make these observable actions into a distinct step. As a result, further investigation was needed.

Phase III: Broadening the Range of Application

After Phase II was completed, the next phase was to take the final revised performance model and test its procedural steps in the field with a variety of different counselors, clients, and behavior problems. The goal was to fine-tune the model by pursuing any anomalies or new ideas resulting from a broader range of its application. If anomalies were discovered, the revised model was modified accordingly. I continued this process until analyses of the focus group interviews and the videotaped sessions failed to provide any new information.

It is important to note that this does not mean that no additional discoveries can be made in the future. If a variety of counselors in different parts of the United States or other countries use this model with a larger sampling of difficult adolescents, additional concepts may well emerge. The idea that any treatment model can be theoretically saturated and produce no new concepts is naive and misleading. One of my hopes in writing this chapter is that other counselors will utilize this model and provide feedback on whether or not new discoveries are made that require further refinement. Thus, this model should be seen as a work in progress, rather than as the definitive treatment model for difficult adolescents. Readers should refer to my Website (www.difficult.net) for further inquiries on this issue.

It can be argued that the real work of model building began during Phase III, as the process of enrichment and elaboration of the treatment steps through a broader application unfolded. In developing the 15-step family-based model, I started with the three idealized models and moved in a progressive fashion toward more intricate models that more closely reflected the complexity of working with difficult adolescents. The basic steps in creating

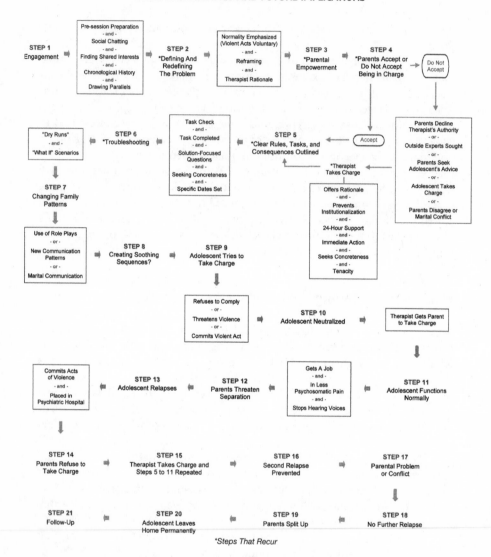

FIGURE 12.6. Final revised performance model.

the performance models of Phase III were similar to those outlined for Phase II. The differences between this phase and Phase II included (1) the analysis of sessions by four counselors involving a variety of cases, rather than the analysis of one case by two expert clinicians; and (2) qualitative focus group interviews with clients, to gain access into their thoughts about the use of this treatment model.

Description of Counselors, Clients, and Target Problems

A team of four counselors was selected to implement field testing of the final revised performance model from Phase II. The counselors included three recent graduates of an MSW program with 3 to 7 years of experience, and a supervisor with a PhD and more than 10 years of experience. Over a 2-year period, 83 difficult adolescents and their families were seen for a minimum of five sessions. The average length of counseling was 10 sessions.

Most of the adolescents treated were males (78.9%), with an average age of 15 years ($SD = 1.5$). Over half of the adolescents (52.2%) had a history of fighting or assault; 56% had a history of stealing or shoplifting; 43.5% were truant from school; 39.9% had drug or alcohol problems; 39.1% had problems with running away; and 8.7% had been charged with property damage, use or possession of weapons, or sexual abuse. These percentages reveal that the majority of the adolescents had multiple problems. The demographic data showed that 54% of all families served had an income between $10,000 and $35,000. A majority of the adolescents had numerous stays in detention, prison, and residential treatment ($M = 2.1$ stays). These adolescents were also multiple offenders, having an average of 3.3 arrests each.

As the descriptions above indicate, the three counselors selected were recent graduates with only limited experience in treating difficult adolescents. The adolescent population was primarily characterized by severe conduct problems and low-income households. This use of inexperienced counselors and a population of difficult adolescents was an intentional choice, for two reasons. First, I felt that the applicability of the model and the ease of its implementation might be better understood under these conditions. If inexperienced counselors were successful as demonstrated through pre–post outcome measures, a case could be made that the treatment model was prescriptive and highly applicable. In addition, if the model was effective in producing change with extremely difficult problems, it might result in even greater success with less severe cases and families with greater economic and social resources.

Second, I felt that anomalies or unsuccessful change episodes would be more revealing. Since the counselors were rather inexperienced, they might make mistakes on the most basic of steps. In turn, these mistakes would force me to make each treatment step clearer, more concrete, and more user-friendly. In addition, unsuccessful change episodes would be much more common and challenging with extremely difficult adolescents from families with limited economic and social resources. This would force me to become more innovative with the treatment steps. An example of this was the development of neutralizing the "five aces," in which a creative menu of strategies was outlined to help struggling counselors stop extreme behavior problems.

Treatment Integrity

As stated earlier, a major problem in research is whether or not the counselor treating the case is actually following the steps of the treatment model (Wynne, 1988). I addressed this concern in two ways. First, each counselor was given the final revised performance model to read and memorize like a play book before entering the first counseling session. Each was then asked by the supervisor to demonstrate each step through role plays. If there were problems during implementation, the supervisor would stop the role play and model the correct procedures. In addition, the supervisor observed each counselor through a one-way mirror during the first three sessions and once a week afterwards, to ensure that the treatment steps were being followed fairly closely. Videotapes of the sessions were also analyzed.

It is important to note that the training and role playing did not require a rigid application of each treatment step; they were demonstrations of general guidelines. This forced the counselors to hone their skills of creativity and intuition. In addition, the model was still a work in progress, and many steps either had not yet been developed (e.g., restoring nurturance and tenderness, neutralizing the "five aces") or were not yet concretely defined (e.g., troubleshooting, working with outsiders). These gaps revealed the weaknesses and the strengths of the model, and showed me where it needed to be revised or more clearly defined.

Focus Group Interviews

As also stated earlier, clients' thoughts and feelings about counseling are as important as observable behaviors, since a comprehensive process analysis requires both (Pinsof, 1988). For instance, comparisons of how differently family members view treatment provide valuable information about practice effectiveness as a prelude to clinical-trial outcome research (Gurman, Kniskern, & Pinsof, 1986).

To address this issue, the procedures from an earlier study (Sells, Smith, & Moon, 1996) served as a template for conducting client interviews. In this earlier study, my colleagues and I used ethnographic interviews that immediately followed counseling sessions to elicit the clients' thoughts and feelings about their sessions. Since one goal of the present project was to tap into these same areas, procedures from this earlier study were replicated during this phase of the project. Each counselor asked each client a series of questions at the end of every third session; I felt that this time frame would give interventions a chance to prove successful or unsuccessful. The answers revealed a wealth of information on what clients perceived as effective and ineffective interventions, important counselor qualities, and recommendations for future counseling sessions. The following eight questions were asked:

1. Could you tell me in detail all the things that have been most helpful so far?
2. What are the most helpful things I have done or said as your counselor so far?
3. Could you tell me in detail all the things that have been least helpful so far?
4. What are the least helpful things that I have done or said as your counselor so far?
5. What needs to be done in the future to make your sessions more useful or helpful?
6. How would you describe to a friend what we do here or the approach that I am using?
7. What are all the things you like about it?
8. What are all the things you dislike about it?

Each interview was either audiotaped or videotaped and then transcribed. Major themes were uncovered from these interviews and coded in the same manner as they were from the videotaped treatment sessions. These codes were then compared with the idealized models and the final revised performance model for discrepancies and similarities.

Several very interesting findings emerged that helped refine and shape the 15-step model. For example, interviews with 37 teenagers revealed that they saw the opportunity to regain trust as one of the most important things needed to improve future counseling sessions. These teenagers reported that when they lost the opportunity to rebuild trust, they lost hope, and resentment set in. Before these interviews were conducted, the area of trust was not looked at as an intervention; after the interviews, it was made one of the seven strategies for restoring softness and nurturance between parents and teenager. I then field-tested the concept and closely analyzed the videotapes when this marker was being used by the counselors. We also conducted more focus group interviews with both teenagers and parents to locate any further inconsistencies. Each new set of information led to additional refinements of this strategy or mini-step. For example, we found that parents must give trust in increments proportional to the level of supervision (mandatory, structured, or limited) at which a teenager is currently functioning. The level chosen should guide the parents on how much trust to give and how much to hold back.

Explanation of Anomalies

The most important action of this step was the intense scrutiny of instances in which the model did not appear to work for clients. Whenever this happened, I looked for potential explanations of the anomaly by asking the following four questions:

1. Was the counselor marker or the concept poorly defined?
2. What factors could account for the anomaly?
3. Did something specific the counselor did or said account for the intervention's not being effective?
4. Were there particular characteristics of the client that seemed to make the counselor's intervention particularly difficult or impossible?

One of the anomalies that emerged from this analysis is presented below, with Figure 12.7 illustrating the mini-steps uncovered.

Discovering the Mini-Steps of Setting Clear Rules and Consequences

During the analyses of two different videotaped sessions, I found that the procedural step of setting rules and consequences did not appear to be working. This was indicated by the fact that the parents failed to follow through with rules and consequences that were outlined with the counselors the week prior. After considering the answers given in this case to the four questions listed above, I began to find reasons for this anomaly. First, both counselors outlined the rules, but only in very vague terms. The rule of showing respect, for example, was not operationally defined by listing concrete behaviors considered "disrespectful," such as swearing and refusing parental requests. In addition, consequences were not clearly de-

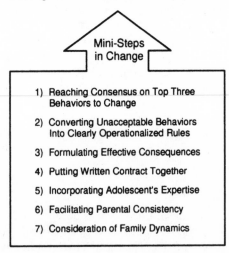

FIGURE 12.7. Mini-steps of setting clear rules and consequences.

fined. One consequence might be grounding, but there was no discussion of when the grounding would occur, how long it would last, or who would enforce and monitor it.

Second, the counselor markers for this step were poorly defined. The two counselors had to be shown the strategies or mini-steps involved in helping the parents operationalize specific rules and consequences. The seven strategies shown in Figure 12.7 were developed from observed mistakes made by the counselors and from focus group interviews with clients and counselors.

After the counselors were trained to implement these seven strategies successfully, analyses of later interviews with the same families revealed that the rules and consequences were enforced. In addition, parents reported that a clear road map of rules and consequences enabled them to be more effective as parents.

In sum, an intensive analysis of videotaped treatment sessions and focus group interviews enabled me to create and fine-tune the 15-step family-based model. The idealized models and the final revised performance model revealed the steps themselves, but its broader application revealed the strategies or mini-steps needed to achieve each major procedural step. At the end of Phase III, the 15-step family-based model emerged. Figure 12.8 illustrates not only the 15 procedural steps, but the mini-steps or specific strategies that can be used to generate change within each step.

Phase IV: Consolidating the Theoretical Yield

In this section, I summarize some of the major ideas that emerged to expand my thinking about treatment with difficult adolescents. I highlight key moments of discovery throughout the three previous phases that shaped the 15-step family-based treatment model. Of particular interest is the discovery of what I call "mini-steps"—that is, the strategies a counselor must engage in to accomplish a larger goal. For example, it was discovered that to restore nurturance and tenderness (Step 11), a counselor may have to employ as many as seven different strategies.

It is important to note that the concepts outlined here are not altogether new. Many of them originated from the three idealized models, which in turn were derived directly from the literature, as described earlier. Concepts such as engagement, parental empowerment, and relapse have been in the field for a long time. What is new is the way these concepts and the steps related to them are mapped out. The task analysis methodology allowed me to gain an in-depth clinical understanding of the "what, when, why, and how" of interactions between difficult adolescents and their families. The patterns and themes that were identified provided a much clearer road map of the com-

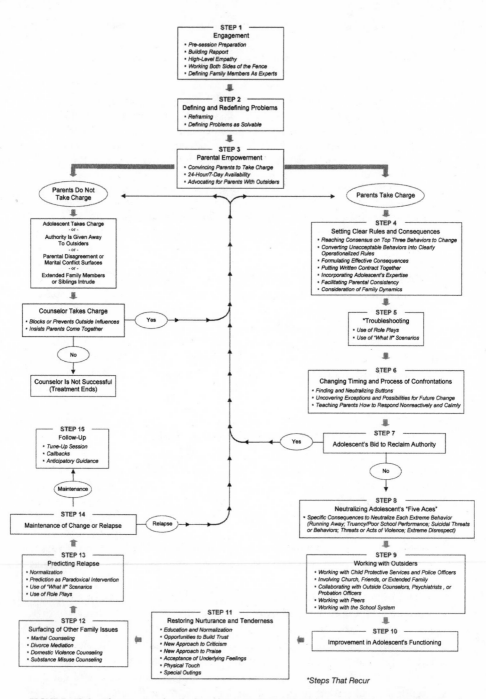

FIGURE 12.8. The 15-step family-based treatment model, with strategies or mini-steps for each step.

plex communications among counselor, parents, teenager, and outside systems. This bridged the gap between research and theory on the one hand, and direct practice on the other.

The key discoveries that reshaped my thought processes during this study centered around four areas: (1) relapse; (2) the "five aces"; (3) the hard and soft sides of hierarchy; and (4) rules, consequences, and troubleshooting. There were other discoveries, but these were the ones that stood out as facilitating substantial amounts of positive client change.

Relapse

From the focus group interviews and analyses of videotaped treatment sessions, exciting discoveries were made in the area of relapse. Each time an adolescent appeared to be doing better and the parents were hopeful, the adolescent would relapse the next week or soon thereafter. When this happened, the parents felt betrayed, angry, and even more hopeless than before. This often caused the teenager to shut down and become recalcitrant. At this point, the family would sometimes leave treatment or commit a series of no-shows.

The treatment model was clearly not working at this point, so I went back to the drawing board to determine what factors accounted for this anomaly. The second idealized model (Model 2/Stage 2) revealed that a teenager relapses following a period of normal functioning. The solution appeared to be to return to the techniques that worked earlier, and to reformulate clear rules and consequences to prevent a second relapse. However, this strategy often proved unsuccessful with the difficult families we worked with. They were too burned out, hopeless, and/or bitter to entertain the idea of refining their rules and consequences. New solutions had to be found.

An intensive analysis of the videotaped sessions in Phase III provided the clues needed to find these solutions. The examinations revealed a common pattern of intervention among the three counselors. In each case, the counselor failed to predict the relapse or prepare the parents for the possibility by discussing what they should do if it occurred. Every time an adolescent relapsed, the counselor appeared just as surprised and frustrated as the family did.

These common patterns led to the creation of Step 13 (predicting relapse) and the development of its mini-steps (normalizing, prediction, and the use of role plays and "what if" scenarios). First, the counselors were trained to normalize the behavior by explaining to the parents that relapse is common and often expected. Most parents understood this rationale, and this helped to decrease the bitterness and hopelessness they felt with a future relapse occurred. In addition, counselors were trained to predict relapse each time the adolescent began to function normally, as a paradoxical intervention to prevent the relapse from actually happening. When a relapse was predicted, the motivation of the teenager and the family to rally together to prove the counselor wrong frequently increased. Finally, counselors were taught to use troubleshooting strategies (role plays and "what if" scenarios) to anticipate all possible occurrences in the event of a relapse.

After the counselors learned these new strategies, more sessions were videotaped and more focus group interviews were conducted. Analysis revealed that the clients' reactions to future relapses were much less negative and destructive. The parents seemed to take the relapses in stride and to work with the counselor to get back on track as quickly as possible. In addition, the parents reported in the focus group interviews that the troubleshooting strategies allowed them to feel prepared so that they were not caught off guard when relapse occurred.

Future research in this area will need to test these mini-steps with a broader population before these findings can be generalized. An outcome measure will have to be developed or located that is sensitive enough to pick up changes in the results of these relapse prevention steps. One specific hypothesis to be tested will be to determine whether relapse prediction immediately following normal adolescent functioning prevents future relapse and allows parents to feel less hopeless and more willing to prevent future relapses. This is a good example of how specific theories about the smaller scale steps involved in change can be generated from process research and tested through outcome research.

The "Five Aces"

The findings regarding the "five aces" were among the most exciting theoretical yields of the study. As the study broadened in Phase III to include other counselors and clients, I began to notice a very interesting pattern: Whenever the parents tried to restore their authority, the difficult adolescent would use an extreme behavior to induce the return of his or her authority from the parents. This use of extreme behaviors initially defeated the counselors in this study, because it was very difficult to come up with effective consequences. The entire process reminded me of a savvy poker player who always has a hidden ace up a sleeve to defeat an opponent at the precise moment the opponent thinks he or she has won. In the same way, adolescents seem to use their own "aces" to defeat parents and counselors any time the adults seem to be winning.

A developmental timeline illustrates how the concept of the "five aces" evolved and how both observational and self-report methods led to this theory.

1. The videotaped treatment sessions revealed a pattern of extreme behaviors by difficult adolescents that neutralized parents' and counselors' effectiveness.

2. The following four extreme behaviors seemed to produce the neutralizing effect on the parents' and counselors' authority: running away, suicidal threats or behavior, truancy/poor school performance, and threats or acts of violence.

3. A closer analysis of the videotaped treatment sessions demonstrated that the adolescents initiated one or more of these extreme behaviors following the parents' attempts to implement predetermined consequences or change their confrontational style. When the rules and consequences were effective and the teenagers were unsuccessful in controlling the mood and direction of arguments, the authority shifted to the parents.

4. As the parents became stronger, the teenagers' typical methods of regaining their authority (yelling, refusing to comply, nagging, inducing guilt, etc.) were no longer effective. The teenagers would then pull out one of their "aces" to counter earlier defeats and regain authority. Parents and counselors appeared not to know what to do to stop these behaviors.

5. If the adolescents were successful, they kept using the "aces" until the parent and the counselor gave up and things went back to the status quo. The parents would then hand their authority over to an outside source (institution, police, extended family), and treatment would often end unsuccessfully.

6. The family-based model was revised to include Step 7 (adolescent's bid to reclaim authority) and arrows to illustrate what happened if the parents and counselor failed to stop a teenager's "ace(s)." The word "aces" was chosen to describe these extreme behaviors because of the similarity to a poker player's actions (see above).

7. Focus group interviews with parents revealed a fifth "ace," disrespect. Some parents report that disrespect often pushed their buttons to a greater degree than all the other aces combined. In turn, this caused the parents to lose control of their tempers and of their rational thought processes. Parents then reacted out of emotion and were unable to maintain consistency or follow through on predetermined rules and consequences.

8. The family-based model was revised again to include this fifth "ace" of disrespect.

9. The literature was revisited to discover methods and techniques that were effective in neutralizing extreme behaviors. The writings of Haley (1980), Schiff and Belson (1988), Price (1996), and Keim (1996) provided helpful suggestions.

10. A menu of strategies or consequences was developed for effectively neutralizing each "ace."

11. The team of counselors was given this menu and trained in the use of these strategies. Counselors then implemented these strategies with parents and teenagers during Step 8.

12. Videotapes of and focus group interviews about these interventions were then analyzed and compared to the final revised performance model.

13. Anomalies were discovered (i.e., times when these interventions failed or were not effective).

In sum, this timeline demonstrates the iterative process involved in operationalizing theory within actual practice. As new discoveries were made, I (as the researcher) had to take the patience and time necessary to explain anomalies at any point during the treatment process. The answers to these questions led to more questions. For example, a discovery of how the parents were defeated through extreme behaviors led to questions on how to stop these behaviors. In turn, these questions led me back to the literature in search of answers. These answers led to the implementation of mini-steps designed to neutralize a specific extreme behavior. A videotape analysis of these mini-steps led to more questions and changes. In addition, collaboration with clients through self-report interviews led to new information and the creation of the fifth "ace," disrespect. Each of these discoveries led to a further refinement of essential concepts and gave counselors a better road map to follow.

The Hard Side versus the Soft Side of Hierarchy

An intensive analysis of Haley's and Schiff's work during Phase II did not result in the discovery of the soft side of hierarchy. Jim Keim's (1996) writing appeared to be the only place in the literature where the concept was described, but details were not provided about its implementation. For example, Keim (1996) wrote about initiating soothing sequences of communication, physical touch, and special outings; however, it was not made clear how or when to implement these interventions in the overall treatment process. Despite this lack of specification, it appeared that these principles were essential contributors to the probability of treatment success. Constant negative communication patterns between parents and difficult teenagers created a dearth of softness, and softness was needed for permanent change to take place. As a result, I decided that it was important to try to implement these procedures somewhere in the overall treatment process. For this to occur, three main questions had to be answered:

1. Where and when should the concept of restoring nurturance and tenderness be implemented within the overall treatment process? In other words, what is the optimal timing of this intervention, and what are the parental characteristics that influence this timing?
2. What are all the mini-steps or strategies that can be used to successfully implement the step of restoring nurturance and tenderness?
3. Once these strategies are discovered, how can they be operationalized in such a way that they can be implemented in a step-by-step fashion?

some of
nce was
and how

ps were
oach to
feelings.
o refine
e third
opera-
by-step

imple-
tinized.
imple-
evealed
l to get
coun-
. After
to in-
of suc-

f com-
ed the
id not
r, but
gs, ac-
physi-
sful, a
t then
operly
uable.
er se,
s.

oreti-
ss re-
nten-
tions
ven-
ients
ation

he developmental process through which these
d. The specific points within this developmental
stions were answered are highlighted.

(1996) work, I decided to implement this con-
project.
ors was trained on how to restore tenderness and
discussed the mini-steps of physical touch, initi-
er outings, and creating soothing sequences or
patterns between parent and child. However, since
developmental stage, the supervisor asked the
ativity and intuition in implementing each step
they should be introduced. The team was told to
which this intervention was used.
us group interviews were analyzed and compared
dels and the final revised performance model.
ons were carefully scrutinized for patterns and

nalysis revealed the answer to the first question
ld restoring nurturance and tenderness be imple-
aracteristics influence this decision? It was discov-
exhibited one or more extreme behaviors (one of
blem was chronic, the counselor had to stop these
ng to introduce the concept of nurturance. Video-
stility whenever nurturance was introduced before
oblems were solved. In addition, parent self-reports
rents ($n = 9$) stated that they and the counselors
leeding" by stopping the problem behavior before
or energy to consider the issue of softness. Parents
t they first had to establish trust and confidence in
help them. Such confidence was in part established
design a consequence to stop an extreme behavior
l failed. When they were armed with this confidence
ere more willing to take the risk of opening their
soft.
ormation, the step of restoring nurturance and ten-
p 11 of the 15-step model. That is, it should general-
es" have been neutralized and the teenager is func-
problems.
erviews partially answered the second question (i.e.,
egies can be used to successfully implement nurtu-
nagers interviewed ($n = 37$) reported that they need-
gain lost trust. Without trust, resentment and bitter-

ness set in, and there was little hope for nurturance. In addition
these teenagers ($n = 17$) reported that the potential for nurtu
blocked when parents constantly criticizes them or failed to under
they felt.

7. Based on this information, the following new mini-s
adopted and implemented: opportunities to build trust; a new ap
criticism; a new approach to praise; and acceptance of underlyin
An analysis of videotapes employing these interventions helped
and operationalize these mini-steps. These results helped answer
question (i.e., once these strategies are discovered, how can they
tionalized in such a way that they can be implemented in a st
fashion?).

8. The strategies of special outings and physical touch we
mented, and the videotapes of these interventions were closely se
Sessions that did not work provided the necessary clues needed
ment these strategies successfully. For example, videotape analysi
that special outing sessions were unsuccessful when a counselor fa
a parent and teenager to set a specific date and time, and when
selor also failed to troubleshoot all the things that could go wr
these problem variables were identified, counselors were shown I
corporate specifics and troubleshooting to increase the probabili
cess.

9. An analysis of videotapes revealed that soothing sequence
munication were conversations where a parent, *not* the child, con
mood, topic, and direction of the discussion. These discussions al
contain elements of criticism or attacks on the teenager's cha
rather elements of praise, acceptance, positive rewards, special o
ceptance of feelings, opportunities to build trust, and/or signs of ge
cal touch. Failed sessions that revealed for this intervention to be su
counselor must first engage in careful preparation. The counselor
show the parent how to deliver soothing communication sequence
through the use of "dry runs" or role plays. These discoveries were i
Finally, it was decided not to describe this intervention as a "strate
but as a means of implementing and pulling together the other stra

In sum, this process is a good example of how a relatively new
cal concept can be field-tested and operationalized by means of p
search. Using task analysis methodology, I studied counseling sessi
sively for clues on how and when to implement the particular inte
involved in restoring nurturance and tenderness. In addition, the
tions were operationally defined. This example also demonstrates h
can collaborate with researchers to direct them to new areas of inv
and strategies that are custom-designed for their needs.

Rules, Consequences, and Troubleshooting

Another important discovery was the correlation between the successful implementation of rules and consequences and the use or nonuse of troubleshooting. In cases where troubleshooting was employed, the parents had a greater degree of success in implementing rules and consequences. In the cases where troubleshooting was not used, the adolescents did something unexpected that often rendered the rule or consequence ineffective. After these patterns were observed, I looked for potential variables within the videotapes to explain these occurrences. Throughout this analysis, I asked myself the following question: "What factors could account for this pattern?"

The answer to this question was revealed when tapes of sessions that employed troubleshooting were compared with tapes of sessions that did not employ it. The following developmental timeline describes how the answers to this question were revealed:

1. The comparison of videotapes with and without troubleshooting revealed the following important discrepancies. The tapes without troubleshooting showed the implementation of rules and consequences without the preparation of role plays or "what if" scenarios. When this happened, rules and consequences were often ineffective, as the teenagers were able either to push their parents' "buttons" so as to make them lose control of their emotions, or to outmaneuver them by thinking two steps ahead. For example, if a consequence was grounding on the weekend for missing school, a teenager would get up early and be out the door before the parent woke up to enforce this consequence. Unexpected behaviors like this were preplanned by teenagers to throw their parents off track and render the consequences ineffective.

2. Tapes using the troubleshooting techniques of role play and "what if" scenarios were analyzed. The tapes showed that parents who used these strategies were able to deliver rules and consequences more effectively than those who had not used these interventions. Parents who had practiced their delivery through role plays did not allow their teenagers to control the mood of the discussion or to throw them off track. In addition, the teenagers would still try to outmaneuver the patients as before, but this time there was a Plan B in place if a particular rule was violated.

As stated earlier, difficult adolescents have both enhanced social perception abilities and the ability to push their parents' buttons. As a result, a comparative videotape analysis revealed the importance of troubleshooting in countering these special skills. The impact of troubleshooting and the timing of its use would have gone undetected without an intensive analysis and comparison of both successful and unsuccessful change episodes. As a result of this analysis, it was decided to make troubleshooting Step 5 of the 15-step model, to stress its importance at this juncture. In addition, an analysis of successful change episodes led to the operationalization of the mini-steps of role plays and "what if" scenarios.

Phase V: Combining Process with Outcome Research

Once it was determined how the model worked, the final phase was to use outcome research to determine whether the model did work. In this section, I report the results of a 2-year pretest–posttest outcome study with 83 difficult adolescents and their families. The ways in which these results supported or disconfirmed the theoretical concepts that emerged from the process study are highlighted. Specifically, standardized outcome measures were used to obtain answers to the following five research questions:

1. At the end of treatment, did the parents show a significant change in negative attitudes toward their difficult teenagers?
2. At the end of treatment, did the results show a significant change in the parents' role, particularly in their ability to be in charge and maintain control over their teenager's problem behavior?
3. At the end of treatment, did both parents and teenagers show a significant change in the areas of affective responsiveness and affective involvement, or nurturance and tenderness?
4. At the end of treatment, did both parents and teenagers show a significant change in negative communication patterns?
5. At the end of treatment, did both parents and teenagers indicate satisfaction with the overall treatment process, even in cases where clients were involuntarily committed to treatment?

In sum, the standardized measures used were sensitive enough to test the effectiveness of four theoretical constructs from the 15-step model: (1) parents' ability to take charge; (2) changing the timing and process of confrontations; (3) parents' ability to neutralize behavior problems (the "five aces"); and (4) restoration of nurturance and tenderness. Other concepts, such as the changes in relapse and in rules, consequences, and troubleshooting still need to be tested. These were not tested here because I was unable to locate standardized measures that were theoretically congruent and sensitive enough to measure changes in these areas. It is important to note that most "measures are chosen because they are widely used and have become standard instruments, not because they provide the best test of the impact of a particular family treatment" (Anderson, 1988, p. 83). As a result, the outcome results in this study could only go as far as the sensitivity of the standardized measures used and the extent to which these were theoretically congruent with the concepts being evaluated.

Target Population Characteristics

Of the 83 families that participated in this study, 68.4% were European American, 18.4% were African American, 7.9% were Asian American, and 5.3% were Hispanic. Almost half the parents participating in the study were married (42.1%); 28.9% were divorced, 18.4% were single, and the remainder (10.6%) were either separated or divorced.

The families had an average of 2.9 children ($SD = 1.3$). Over two-thirds of the parents were employed (69.4%), with 19.4% being unemployed and 11.1% homemakers. Income levels were as follows: 20.8% of the families made less than $10,000; 29.2% earned between $10,000 and $20,000; 25% earned between $20,000 and $35,000; and 15.6% earned between $35,000 and $50,000. The remainder of the families (9.4%) earned more than $50,000.

As stated earlier, most of the adolescents treated were males (78.9%), with an average age of 15 years ($SD = 1.5$). The statistics on these adolescents' behavior problems and arrest records (see the description of clients in Phase III, above) indicate that they were indeed difficult and defiant.

Design and Measures

A nonexperimental pretest–posttest design was implemented. Parents and teenagers completed the Family Assessment Device (FAD) and the Client Satisfaction Inventory (CSI) separately and independently before treatment began and again after counseling ended. Some families completed treatment in 5 sessions and others within 10 sessions, with an average session length of 6.7 sessions. Only the parents completed the Index of Parental Attitudes (IPA). Responses from the pre and post program measures were evaluated to determine the level of change that occurred after the 15-step family-based treatment model was implemented. Descriptions of the scales used are presented below.

The FAD (Epstein, Baldwin, & Bishop, 1983) is a 60-item questionnaire designed to evaluate the overall health and pathology of a family, as well as changes in the family's organizational properties and in communication patterns that have been found to distinguish between healthy and unhealthy families. Family members are given a series of statements (e.g., "We are too self-centered," "Anything goes in our family") and asked whether or not they strongly agree, agree, disagree, or strongly disagree with each statement. The subscales of the FAD identify and distinguish among seven kay areas of family functioning: (1) Problem solving, (2) Communication, (3) Roles, (4) Affective Responsiveness, (5) Affective Involvement, (6) Behavior Control, and (7) General Functioning.

The IPA (Hudson, 1992) is a 25-item questionnaire designed to measure the extent, severity, or magnitude of a parent's overall positive or negative attitude toward a teenager. If the overall pretest or average mean score is above 30, it suggests a clinically significant problem and indicates that the parent has an extremely negative attitude toward the teenager. In addition, there is an increased risk that the parent is experiencing extreme stress, with a clear possibility that some type of violence may be considered or used by the parent to deal with the problem. On this scale, a parent is given statements about his or her child or teenager (e.g., "I really enjoy my child," "I resent my child"), and is asked to respond whether each statement is true none of the time, very rarely, a little of the time, some of the time, a good part of the time, most of the time, or all of the time.

The CSI (McMurty, 1994) is a 25-item questionnaire designed to measure a client's overall satisfaction with treatment and his or her perception of how good or bad the services were in general. If the average mean score is below 30, it suggests a clinically significant problem in the client's perception of the quality of treatment; it indicates that the client is extremely unhappy with treatment or with the counselor's style and "bedside manner." Scores above 30 indicate the opposite. On this scale, a client is given statements about counseling or the counselor (e.g., "I feel much better now than when I first came here," "People here are only concerned about getting paid") and is asked to respond whether each statement is true none of the time, very rarely, a little of the time, some of the time, a good part of the time, most of the time, or all of the time.

Research Questions and Relevant Results

1. *At the end of treatment, did the parents show a significant change in negative attitudes toward their difficult teenagers?* The IPA results showed that parents reported a statistically significant change from pretest ($M = 33.01$) to posttest ($M = 23.17$) in negative attitudes toward their difficult teenagers ($t = 2.69$, $p \leq .05$). The pretest mean score of 33.01 indicated that before treatment the parents had extremely negative attitudes toward the teenagers. Following treatment, however, the mean score dropped below the cutoff of 30, suggesting a decreased risk that the parents were experiencing extreme stress or that violence would be used to deal with the teenagers' problem behavior. This indicates that the family-based model was effective in changing two key areas influencing overall parental attitudes: the timing and process of confrontations, and the restoration of nurturance and tenderness between parent and teenager. During the process study, it was discovered that parental attitudes were affected by these two areas. If the communication was mostly

negative, the attitudes of the parents would also be negative. In turn, these negative attitudes would severely limit the possibility of bringing nurturance back into the relationship. Parents often reported in focus groups that they loved their sons or daughters and that they did not like them any more. In sum, the significant change in posttest parental attitudes supports the hypothesis that changes in confrontational patterns and nurturance can have a positive effect on negative parent–teenager relationships.

2. *At the end of treatment, did the results show a significant change in the parents' role, particularly in their ability to be in charge and maintain control over their teenagers' problem behavior?* Table 12.1 and Figures 12.9 and 12.10 show that both parents and teenagers indeed reported significant changes in the parents' role, especially in their ability to resume authority and keep control over the teens' behavior. This was indicated by changes in scores on the FAD subscales of Roles, Behavior Control, and General Functioning.

The FAD Roles subscale focuses on whether a family has a clear set of rules and consequences, and whether parents clearly assign roles and tasks to the children. Examples of items on this subscale include "We discuss who is to do household chores," and "We make sure members meet their family responsibilities." The posttest mean scores of 1.96 for parents and 1.91 for teenagers indicated that the family-based model was effective in clarifying roles and hierarchy between parents and teenagers. This supports the notion that the parents were able to maintain and accept a position of authority following treatment. In turn, this supports the hypothesis that the family-based model was effective in putting the parents in charge and helping them to maintain this position of authority.

The FAD Behavior Control subscale measures how effective parents are in controlling problem behaviors and setting up rules and consequences. Ex-

TABLE 12.1. Results on the Family Assessment Device (FAD) Roles, Behavior Control, and General Functioning Subscales for Parents and Teenagers

FAD subscale	Pretest	Posttest	t
	Parents		
Roles	2.43	1.96	−3.06**
Behavior Control	1.86	1.56	−2.63*
General Functioning	2.36	1.85	−3.29**
	Teenagers		
Roles	2.64	1.91	−4.16**
Behavior Control	2.08	1.65	−2.76*
General Functioning	2.60	1.81	−4.68**

*$p \leq .05$; **$p \leq .01$.

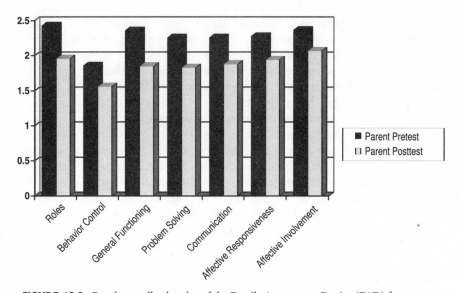

FIGURE 12.9. Results on all subscales of the Family Assessment Device (FAD) for parents at pretest and posttest.

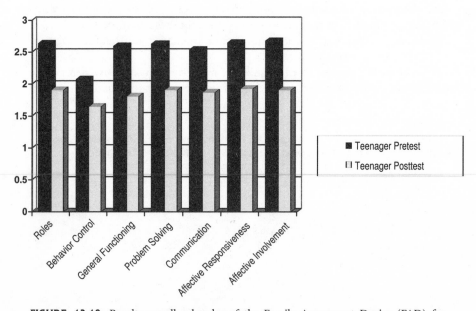

FIGURE 12.10. Results on all subscales of the Family Assessment Device (FAD) for teenagers at pretest and posttest.

amples of items on this subscale include "We have rules about hitting people," and "We have parents who control behavior problems." The posttest mean scores of 1.56 for parents and 1.65 for teenagers indicated that the parents were able to stop or control the problem behavior. In turn, this finding supported the hypothesis that the family-based model was effective in helping the parents to neutralize their teenagers' "aces" by controlling the particular behavior problems. This therefore supported the inclusion of Step 8 (neutralizing the adolescent's "five aces") in the model.

The FAD General Functioning subscale measures the overall health or pathology of a family. Examples of items on this subscale include "We don't get along well together," and "We cannot talk to each other about the sadness we feel." The posttest mean scores of 1.85 for parents and 1.81 for teenagers indicated that the overall health and general functioning of these families improved. A basic premise of the family-based model is that if the hierarchy is congruent and the parents are back in charge, the overall health of the family will improve. These results therefore supported the inclusion in the model of the general principle of putting the parents in charge of the adolescent's behavior.

3. *At the end of treatment, did both parents and teenagers show a significant change in the areas of affective responsiveness and affective involvement, or nurturance and tenderness?* Table 12.2 and Figures 12.9 and 12.10 show that both parents and teenagers reported significant changes in these areas, as indicated by changes in scores on the FAD subscales of Affective Responsiveness and Affective Involvement.

The FAD subscales of Affective Responsiveness and Affective Involvement measure whether or not family members show tenderness, concern, and affection for one another. Examples of items on these subscales include "We express tenderness," and "We cry openly." The posttest mean scores for parents and teenagers on both subscales indicated that both parents and

TABLE 12.2. Results on the Family Assessment Device (FAD) Affective Responsiveness and Affective Involvement Subscales for Parents and Teenagers

FAD subscale	Pretest	Posttest	t
	Parents		
Affective Responsiveness	2.28	1.94	−2.04*
Affective Involvement	2.37	2.07	−1.53*
	Teenagers		
Affective Responsiveness	2.65	1.98	−4.27**
Affective Involvement	2.68	1.91	−4.59**

*$p \leq .05$; **$p \leq .01$.

teenagers were able to show tenderness and nurturance, and to be more concerned for one another's welfare. In turn, this finding supported the hypothesis that the family-based model was effective in helping parents bring nurturance back into the relationship with their teens. It thereby supported the inclusion of Step 11 (restoring nurturance and tenderness) in the 15-step model.

4. *At the end of treatment, did both parents and teenagers report a significant change in negative communication patterns?* Table 12.3 and Figures 12.9 and 12.10 show that both parents and teenagers reported a significant change in this area, as indicated by changes in scores on the FAD subscale of Communication.

The FAD Communication subscale defines the quality of the exchange of information among family members. The focus is on whether or not verbal messages are clear in content and direct, in the sense that the person spoken to is the person for whom the message is intended. Examples of items on this subscale include "We are frank with each other," and "People come right out and say things instead of hinting at them." The posttest mean scores for both parents and teenagers indicated that after treatment there was improved communication in general, as well as a decrease in bitter and negative confrontations. This finding supported the hypothesis that the family-based model was effective in changing communication patterns; it thereby supported the inclusion of Step 6 (changing the timing and process of confrontations) in the model.

5. *At the end of treatment, did both parents and teenagers indicate satisfaction with the overall treatment process, even in cases where clients were involuntarily committed to treatment?* Within a 10-session framework, 88% of the parents and 83% of the teenagers reported on the CSI that they were satisfied with treatment. What makes these percentages *particularly significant* is the fact that a majority of clients came involuntarily to treatment (i.e., they did so only because they were required to do so by probation officers). This was a particularly surprising result, and it suggests that this model has a great deal of promise for the future. Counselors often ask parents to make a great deal of sacrifices to regain control of their households and take charge of their teens' problem behavior. Therefore, unless the clients are satisfied with treat-

TABLE 12.3. Results on the Family Assessment Device (FAD) Communication Subscale for Parents and Teenagers

	Pretest	Posttest	t
Parents	2.26	1.88	−2.89**
Teenagers	2.54	1.87	−4.22**

**$p \leq .01$.

ment, there is no reason why they will make any sacrifices or listen to their counselors. In addition, if the clients are required to come to treatment, they will often enter the first session with a negative attitude and will resist any suggestions for change. This is especially true with difficult teenagers.

Some of the focus group interviews provided clues as to why client satisfaction was so high. Several parents ($n = 7$) reported that this treatment was different and better because it "got down to the business of giving [them] specific tools to solve the problems [they] came in to counseling for." Parents ($n = 5$) also said that "this kind of counseling was not just office work." The counselors were available 24 hours a day and came to where the problems were, whether this required home visits, school visits, or church visits. Teenagers ($n = 14$) reported that the counseling showed their parents how to talk to them differently and without yelling. They also liked the facts that clearly defined rules let them know what to expect, and that the rules had both negative *and* positive consequences. Finally, teenagers ($n = 37$) reported that they liked the fact that they had chances to earn back trust, and that their opinions and ideas were heard and even integrated into the contract.

In sum, these preliminary findings indicated that parents were satisfied with treatment because the model was clear-cut; because it provided specific tools and strategies; and because counselors were available on call 24 hours a day, not just for an hour a week in office sessions. Teenagers reported that they were satisfied because the model provided them with better methods of communication, clear rules and consequences, a voice, and opportunities to earn back trust. Further research is needed to tap into additional reasons why clients were satisfied with treatment. Answers to this question will provide valuable insight into the model's strengths and weaknesses.

BEYOND THE 21ST CENTURY: CONCLUSIONS AND FUTURE IMPLICATIONS

This chapter has demonstrated how process and outcome research can be used within a single study to operationalize key theoretical concepts and build a treatment model directly from clinical practice. Rather than beginning with hypothesis testing, this study moved toward hypothesis testing as the final step of a rigorous program of discovery process research. In this study, outcome measures supported the effectiveness of four theoretical constructs from the 15-step model: (1) parents' ability to take charge; (2) changing the timing and process of confrontations; (3) parents' ability to neutralize behavior problems (the "five aces"); and (4) restoration of nurturance and tenderness. In turn, these findings can lead to future task analysis investigations to find out why clients are so satisfied with this treatment model and which specific parts of these four theoretical constructs produce positive change. In this way, theory-building process research and verification outcome research are interdependent and complementary: Process research has directed outcome research, and now these results are directing researchers toward further process or task analysis research. The use of these two methods can lead to better research questions and a better and more refined definition of theoretical concepts within the 15-step family-based model.

Directions for Future Research

As stated earlier, it is my hope that readers will see this model as a work in progress and will use the research process described in this chapter to refine and develop the model further. The next logical step is to custom-fit the model to an even larger set of variables and possible scenarios. For example, suppose a counselor is presented with these variables and this particular scenario in practice:

> A 15-year-old male comes from a single-parent home. He belongs to a gang, uses drugs, and relapses before Step 13 in the model and before other family issues surface in Step 12. Given this scenario and these variables, what are the best treatment steps and options?

These types of exceptions to the overall model are common. Counselors will want custom-designed road maps for their particular cases and problems. One day in the future, a clinician may be able to sit down in front of a computer and type in a set of variables. After these variables are analyzed, an interactive computer disk will present the counselor with a customized set of procedures that fit the particular scenario and the set of variables presented. This kind of fine-tuning is needed in the future; indeed, it is expected in a society that wants positive change quickly and a health care system that demands it.

As we enter the 21st century, it seems timely for the field to reconsider and reassess its conceptual base by defining its treatment models through process and outcome research. We must struggle to conduct research that moves us closer to answering Frank's (1991) central question in his classic work *Persuasion and Healing*: "The question is not whether psychotherapy works; that goes without saying. Rather, the central question is, what are the central ingredients within a particular treatment method that account for its effectiveness with a particular population and clinical problem" (p. 6). To accomplish this goal, we must return to our roots of discovery-oriented research and to a collaboration between counselors and researchers.

A Return to Our Roots

In the 1950s, family therapy was born of discovery-oriented observations from behind a one-way mirror of family members sitting around a circle in the next room. Initially, the therapeutic goals and procedures, if any, were only vaguely specified. These observations, however, yielded rich theoretical concepts (e.g., metacommunication, family homeostasis, the double bind) and generated new research hypotheses and clinical enthusiasm. In the 1960s, these concepts were incorporated into a diversity of family counseling models (e.g., structural, Bowenian, Mental Research Institute, brief therapy). Family therapy teaching and theorizing flourished and were both conceptually interesting and provocative. From the 1970s to the present, however, family therapy has become disconnected from its discovery-oriented research base and has lost its original zest and focus. The field now either resembles a "flavor of the month club" by moving from one fad to the next, or relies on "who won" outcome studies that fail to move the field to the next step: finding out how a particular treatment works and why, with a particular population and presenting problem. Direct-practice counselors and students are hungry for answers to this question and want mini-steps to find their way within the complexity and multiple layers of a problem.

In addition, a split occurred during the 1970s between those who did research and those who did clinical work. This split is described by Haley (1978):

> In the 1950's it was taken for granted that a counselor and researcher were of the same species (although the counselor had a more second class status). . . . Today it seems more apparent that the research stance and the counselor stance are quite different. The researcher must explore and explain all the complex variables of every issue since he is an explorer of truth. The counselor stance is much different. He must use simple ideas that will accomplish his goals and not be distracted by the explorations into interesting aspects of life and the human mind. It seems evident that the creation of the researcher and the creation of the counselor are different enterprises. (pp. 73–74)

This split continues today. It must end if the gap between research and theory on the one hand, and practice on the other, is ever to be bridged.

In sum, we must ask ourselves this central question: "Is our field's current effort in model building working?" If the answer is no, then we must look for a time in the past when it was working, and must do more of what was done then. I believe that this time was in the 1950s and 1960s, with discovery-oriented research that employed a here-and-now process–outcome template. I hope that this chapter and this book represent a first step toward this future.

The Future of Counseling

At the Evolution of Psychotherapy Conference in 1995, Salvador Minuchin and Donald Meichenbaum gave a joint presentation to answer this question: "What is the future of counseling as we approach the 21st century?" They gave very different answers to this question, but their answers represent both the fears and hopes of many counselors about the future. I present these two different viewpoints here and show how this research chapter and model building may offer one possible solution to the dilemmas presented by each speaker.

Meichenbaum was the first to speak. He stated that the field of counseling will need to move to manualized treatment models whose effectiveness with specific populations (children, adolescents, adults) and treatment issues (anxiety disorders, depression, conduct problems, etc.) can be evaluated. These manualized treatments will have to be able to show documented strengths in order for counselors using them to be reimbursed by third-party payers. Meichenbaum envisioned a time in the 21st century when there will be computerized manuals or interactive disks in which counselors or actors will perform and demonstrate each essential strategy and technique. Family members can then take these disks home between sessions and practice each strategy between sessions. He called these disks "catalytic supplements." In addition, there may be a time when a counselor or client can go on the Internet or tune to a cable TV station and receive interactive supplements through a push of the button.

Minuchin then spoke and presented a different viewpoint. He stated that these manualized treatments will be unable to mirror or reflect all that transpires within a particular session. Manualization will also limit the intimacy of treatment and the therapeutic relationship between counselor and client. Finally, it will lead the counselor toward a rigid application of treatment—one that does not allow for the individual needs of the client or for novel situations and circumstances.

Meichenbaum and Minuchin thus presented different viewpoints, but both posed this central dilemma: How can we produce manualized treatments that do not sacrifice the intimacy of the therapeutic relationship, but are flexible enough to respond to a client's particular needs without stifling the innovation and creativity of the counselor? The 15-step family-based model attempts to accomplish this task in the following manner. First, the model offers treatment guidelines or a generalized template, rather than a rigid application of treatment steps. Even though the steps are numbered, they are done so only to give the counselor a sense of direction. Each chapter of this book provides numerous case examples and "what if" scenarios, to give the counselor as many options as possible within a particular procedural step or situation. For example, Chapter 7 provides the reader with three possible ways to introduce the topic of nurturance, depending on a particular family's characteristics. These different options emerged from the research study and are outlined to give the counselor flexibility.

Second, the intimacy and importance of the therapeutic relationship are never undermined, but are expanded and written about in almost every context. It is described as a separate step (Step 1, engagement), but it is also talked about within many other steps. For example, in chapter 8, I specifically talk about the importance of rapport and trust between counselors and clients and between counselors and outside systems. In this way, engagement is not presented as a one-time step, but as recurring throughout the treatment process.

Third, the model was not developed in a laboratory setting, but emerged from actual practice sessions and from collaboration with expert clinicians (Jay Haley and Neil Schiff), counselors, parents, and teenagers. Each time a new discovery was made, the concept was field-tested with a variety of counselors and clients. These sessions were then analyzed for anomalies. Moreover, clients were asked about their perceptions and feelings about a particular intervention or series of interventions; in turn, this feedback was used to refine the model further. In this way, the model was grounded in direct practice, and the principles reflected all the complexity and "curve balls" a difficult family could present. This gives the counselor information on how to respond to such a family's special needs, without stifling his or her innovation and creativity.

In sum, the 15-step family-based model represents an attempt to address the central dilemmas posed by Minuchin and the needs of the 21st century posed by Meichenbaum. I have already begun the process of experimenting with "catalytic supplements." For example, I have allowed parents to take home and read a draft version of Chapter 6, or have had them view videotapes of actors demonstrating ways to change the timing and direction of confrontations. Preliminary focus group interviews with parents indicate that these additions to treatment have been very helpful in clarifying specific strategies. It will always remain a challenge to juxtapose manualization and the complexity of the counselor–client relationship. However, as we enter the 21st century, we cannot afford to evade this challenge. Theory construction can no longer remain a back-room activity; it must be moved front and center, so that we can improve our methods for constructing testable theories.

References

Alexander, J. F., Pugh, C., & Newell, R. M. (1995, November). *Conduct disorders in adolescents: Clinical update.* Paper presented at the annual convention of the American Association for Marriage and Family Therapy, Baltimore.

American Psychiatric Association. (1994). *Diagnostic and statistical manual of mental disorders* (4th ed.). Washington, DC: Author.

Anderson, C. M. (1988). The selection of measures in family therapy research. In L. C. Wynne (Ed.), *The state of the art in family therapy research: Controversies and recommendations* (pp. 81–88). New York: Family Process Press.

Becvar, D. S., & Becvar, R. J. (1988). *Family therapy: A systemic integration* (2nd ed.). Boston: Allyn & Bacon.

Bednar, R. L., Burlingame, G. M., & Master, K. S. (1988). System of family treatment: Substance or semantics? *Annual Review of Psychology, 39,* 401–434.

Bodenhamer, G. (1988). *Back in control: How to get your children to behave.* Englewood Cliffs, NJ: Prentice-Hall.

Brown, B. B., Mounts, N., Lamborn, S. D., & Steinberg, L. (1993). Parenting practices and peer group affiliation in adolescence. *Child Development, 64,* 467–482.

Campbell, L., & Johnston, J. R. (1986). Impasse-directed mediation with high conflict families in custody disputes. *Behavioral Sciences and the Law, 4*(2), 217–241.

Chamberlain, P., & Rosicky, J. G. (1995). The effectiveness of family therapy in the treatment of adolescents with conduct disorders and delinquency. *Journal of Marital and Family Therapy, 21*(4), 441–459.

Crits-Cristoph, P., & Mintz, J. (1991). Implications of therapist effects for the design and analysis of comparative studies of psychotherapies. *Journal of Consulting and Clinical Psychology, 59,* 20–26.

Crosbie-Burnett, M., & Ahrons, C. R. (1985). From divorce to remarriage: Implications for therapy with families in transition. *Journal of Psychotherapy and the Family, 1,* 121–137.

Epstein, N. B., Baldwin, L. M., & Bishop, D. S. (1983). The McMaster Family Assessment Device. *Journal of Marital and Family Therapy, 9*(2), 171–180.

Estrada, A. U., & Pinsof, W. M. (1995). The effectiveness of family therapies for selected behavioral disorders of childhood. *Journal of Marital and Family Therapy, 21*(4), 403–440.

Faber, A., & Mazlish, E. (1980). *How to talk so kids will listen and listen so kids will talk.* New York: Avon Books.

Fishman, H. C. (1988). *Treating troubled adolescents.* New York: Basic Books.

Frank, J. D. (1991). *Persuasion and healing: A comparative study of psychotherapy* (3rd ed.). Baltimore: Johns Hopkins University Press.

Ginott, H. G. (1969). *Between parent and teenager.* New York: Avon Books.

Goetz, J. P., & LeCompte, M. D. (1984). *Ethnography and qualitative designs in educational research.* New York: Academic Press.

Goldenberg, I., & Goldenberg, H. (1991). *Family therapy: An overview* (3rd ed.). Pacific Grove, CA: Brooks/Cole.

Gould, M. S., Shaffer, D., & Kaplan, D. (1985). The characteristics of dropouts from a child psychiatric clinic. *Journal of the American Academy of Child Psychiatry, 24,* 316–328.

Gurman, A. S., Kniskern, D. P., & Pinsof, W. M. (1986). Research on the process and outcome of marital and family therapy. In S. Garfield & A. Bergin (Eds.), *Handbook of psychotherapy and behavior change* (3rd ed., pp. 595–630). New York: Wiley.

Haley, J. (1976). *Problem solving therapy.* San Francisco: Jossey-Bass.

Haley, J. (1978). Ideas which handicap therapists. In M. M. Berger (Ed.), *Beyond the double bind: Communication and family systems, theories, and techniques with schizophrenics* (pp. 32–43). New York: Brunner/Mazel.

Haley, J. (1980). *Leaving home.* New York: McGraw-Hill.

Haley, J. (1984). *Ordeal therapy.* San Francisco: Jossey-Bass.

Harlow, H. F. (1971). *Learning to love.* San Francisco: Albion.

Hartman, A. (1978). Diagrammatic assessment of family relationships. *Social Casework, 29*(7), 465–476.

Henggeler, S. W., Melton, G. B., & Smith, L. A. (1992). Family preservation using multisystemic therapy: An effective alternative to incarcerating serious juvenile offenders. *Journal of Consulting and Clinical Psychology, 60*(6), 953–961.

Hepworth, D. H., & Larsen, J. (1995). *Direct social work practice: Theory and skills* (4th ed.). Belmont, CA: Wadsworth.

Horvath, A. O., & Greenberg, L. S. (1994). *The working alliance: Theory, research, and practice.* New York: Wiley.

Hudson, W. W. (1992). *The WALMYR Assessment Scales scoring manual.* Tempe, AZ: WALMYR.

Isaacs, M. B., Montalvo, B., & Abelson, D. (1986). *The difficult divorce.* New York: Basic Books.

Kazdin, A. E. (1987). *Conduct disorders in childhood and adolescence.* Beverly Hills, CA: Sage.

Kazdin, A. E. (1993). Psychotherapy for children and adolescents: Current progress and future research directions. *American Psychologist, 48*(8), 644–657.

Kazdin, A. E. (1994). Psychotherapy for children and adolescents. In A. E. Bergin & S. L. Garfield (Eds.), *Handbook of psychotherapy and behavior change* (4th ed., pp. 543–594). New York: Wiley.

Kazdin, A. E., Siegel, T. C., & Bass, D. (1992). Cognitive problem-solving skills training and parent management training in the treatment of antisocial behavior in children. *Journal of Consulting and Clinical Psychology, 60,* 733–747.

Keim, J. P. (1996, October). *Strategic coaching of parents of oppositional kids.* Paper presented at the annual convention of the American Association of Marital and Family Therapy. Toronto.

Kleinman, J., & Whiteside, M. (1979). Common developmental tasks in forming reconstituted families. *Journal of Marital and Family Therapy, 5*(2), 79–86.

Lamberg, M. J., & Bergin, A. E. (1994). The effectiveness of psychotherapy. In A. E. Bergin & S. L. Garfield (Eds.), *Handbook of psychotherapy and behavior change* (4thed., pp. 543–594). New York: Wiley.

Liddle, H. A. (1994). The anatomy of emotions in family therapy with adolescents. *Journal of Adolescent Research, 9*, 120–157.

Liddle, H. A. (1995). Conceptual and clinical dimensions of a multidimensional, multisystems engagement strategy in family-based adolescent treatment. *Psychotherapy, 32*(1), 39–58.

Liddle, H. A., & Dakof, A. G. (1995). Family-based treatment for adolescent drug use: State of the Science. In E. Rahdert (Ed.), *Adolescent drug abuse: Assessment and treatment* (NIDA Research Monograph No. 3, pp. 5–7). Rockville, MD: U.S. Department of Health and Human Services.

Lindblad-Goldberg, M. (1989). Successful minority single-parent families. In L. Combrinck-Graham (Ed.), *Children in family contexts* (pp. 116–134). New York: Guilford Press.

Loeber, R., & Schmalling, K. B. (1985). Empirical Evidence for overt and covert patterns of antisocial conduct problems: A meta-analysis. *Journal of Abnormal Child Psychology, 13*, 337–352.

Luborsky, L., Crits-Christoph, P., Mintz, J., & Auerbach, A. (1988). *Who will benefit from psychotherapy: Predicting therapeutic outcomes.* New York: Basic Books.

Madanes, C. (1991). *Strategic family therapy.* San Francisco: Jossey-Bass.

Mahrer, A. (1988). Discovery-oriented psychotherapy research: Rationale, aims, and methods. *American Psychologist, 43*(9), 694–702.

McMurty, S. (1994). *The WALMYR Assessment Scales scoring manual* (2nd ed.). Tempe, AZ: WALMYR.

Meichenbaum, D., & Minuchin, S. (1995, October). *The future of therapy.* Joint presentation at the Evolution of Psychotherapy Conference, Las Vegas, NV.

Metcalf, L. (1997). *Parenting toward solutions.* New York: Prentice-Hall Press.

Miller, W. R. (1992). The effectiveness of treatment for substance abuse. *Journal of Substance Abuse Treatment, 9*, 93–102.

Minuchin, S. (1974). *Families and family therapy.* Cambridge, MA: Harvard University Press.

Minuchin, S., Montalvo, B., Guerney, B. G., Rosman, B. L., & Schumer, F. (1967). *Families of the slums: An exploration of their structure and treatment.* New York: Basic Books.

Nagel, E. J. (1996). My son the sweet person. *Family Therapy Networker, 20*(4), 28–36.

Neff, P. (1996). *Tough love: How parents deal with drug abuse.* Nashville, TN: Abingdon Press.

Patterson, G. R., & Chamberlain, P. (1994). A functional analysis of resistance during parent training therapy. *Clinical Psychology, 1*, 53–70.

Pinsof, W. M. (1988). Strategies for the study of family therapy process. In L. C. Wynne (Ed.), *The state of the art in family therapy research: Controversies and recommendations* (pp. 159–174). New York: Family Process Press.

Pinsof, W. M., & Wynne, L. C. (1995). The efficacy of marital and family therapy: An empirical overview, conclusions and recommendations. *Journal of Marital and Family Therapy, 21*(4), 585–610.

Price, J. A. (1990). The atom-bomb strategy. *Family Therapy Networker, 14*(4), 46–47.

Price, J. A. (1996). *Power and compassion: Working with difficult adolescents and abused parents.* New York: Guilford Press.

Prinz, R. J., & Miller, G. E. (1994). Family based treatment for childhood antisocial behavior: Experimental influences on drop out and engagement. *Journal of Consulting and Clinical Psychology, 62,* 645–650.

Quay, H. C. (1986). Conduct disorders. In H. C. Quay & J. S. Werry (Eds.), *Psychopathological disorders of childhood* (3rd ed., pp. 35–72). New York: Wiley.

Reid, W., & Epstein, L. (1972). *Task centered casework.* New York: Columbia University Press.

Rice, L. N., & Greenberg, L. S. (Eds.). (1984). *Patterns of change: Intensive analysis of psychotherapy process* (pp. 29–66). New York: Guilford Press.

Satir, V. M. (1988). *The new peoplemaking.* Palo Alto, CA: Science & Behavior Books.

Sandmaier, M. (1996). More than love. *Family Therapy Networker, 20*(4), 20–28.

Scherer, D. G., Brondino, M. J., Henggeler, S. W., & Melton, G. B. (1994). Multisystemic family preservation therapy: Preliminary findings from a study of rural and minority serious adolescent offenders. *Journal of Emotional and Behavioral Disorders, 2*(4), 198–206.

Schiff, N. P., & Belson, R. (1988). The Gandhi technique: A new procedure for intractable problems. *Journal of Marital and Family Therapy, 14*(3), 261–266.

Schmidt, S., Liddle, H. A., & Dakof, G. (1996). Changes in parenting practices and adolescent drug abuse during multidimensional family therapy. *Journal of Family Psychotherapy, 10*(1), 1–15.

Selekman, M. D. (1993). *Pathways to change: Brief therapy solutions with difficult adolescents.* New York: Guilford Press.

Selekman, M. D., & Todd, T. C. (1991). Crucial issues in the treatment of adolescent substance abusers and their families. In T. C. Todd & M. D. Selekman (Eds.), *Family therapy approaches with adolescent substance abusers* (pp. 1–20). Needham Heights, MA: Allyn & Bacon.

Sells, S. P., Smith, T. E., & Moon, S. (1996). An ethnographic study of client and therapist perceptions of therapy effectiveness in a university-based training clinic. *Journal of Marital and Family Therapy, 22*(3), 321–343.

Sells, S. P., Smith, T. E., & Sprenkle, D. (1995). Integrating quantitative and qualitative methods: A research model. *Family Process, 34,* 199–218.

Shadish, W. R., Montgomery, L. M., Wilson, P., Wilson, M. R., & Okwumabua, T. (1993). Effects of family and marital psychotherapies: A meta-analysis. *Journal of Consulting and Clinical Psychology, 61,* 992–1002.

Skeels, H. M. (1966). Adult status of children with contrasting early life experiences: A follow-up study. *Monographs of the Society for Reserach in Child Development, 31* (15, Serial No. 105).

Speck, R. V., & Attneave, C. L. (1973). *Family networks.* New York: Pantheon Books.

Steinglass, P. (1987). Family therapy approaches to alcoholism. In P. Steinglass (Ed.), *The alcoholic family* (pp. 329–364). New York: Basic Books.

Swadi, H. (1992). Relative risk factors in detecting adolescent drug abuse. *Drug and Alcohol Dependence, 29*(3), 253–254.

Turecki, S. (1989). *The difficult child.* New York: Bantam Books.

Webster-Stratton, C., & Dahl, R. W. (1995). Conduct disorder. In M. Hersen & R. T. Ammerman (Eds.), *Advanced abnormal child psychology* (pp. 333–352). Hillsdale, NJ: Erlbaum.

Wynne, L. C. (1988). What should be expected in current family therapy research. In L. C. Wynne (Ed.), *The state of the art in family therapy research: Controversies and recommendations* (pp. 249–280). New York: Family Process Press.

Zastrow, C. (1996). *Introduction to social work and social welfare* (6th ed.). Pacific Grove, CA: Brooks/Cole.

Index